Praise for A Child in Pain

"Applauds to Leora Kuttner! This book should become a "must-have" for all professionals in the field. This informative and entertaining book achieves two goals. First, it provides health professionals from all disciplines with a profound and entertaining overview on the basics of and treatment strategies for relieving pediatric pain. Second, by integrating vivid case examples and easy instructions it enables professionals to integrate these strategies into their clinical practice. This book will help to make the world a bit better for children in pain."

Dr. Boris Zernikow, Professor of Children's Pain Therapy and Paediatric Palliative Care, Witten/Herdecke University, Children's Hospital Datteln, Germany

"In her latest contribution to the well-being of children, Dr. Leora Kuttner has created a gem which is a must read for all child health clinicians. She has masterfully blended her savvy as a scientist, educator, researcher, artist, wife and Mom to create this state of the art *and* state of the science guide to the understanding and comprehensive management of pain in the lives of young people and their families. From the very first page, Dr. Kuttner's well-known skill as a masterful communicator comes alive as Part I illustrates with real-life examples, 'How to Understand, Assess, and Communicate with a Child in Pain." Through vivid vignettes we are painlessly (!) guided to a variety of 'right' ways and best practices in communication around issues of discomfort. In Part II 's elucidation of the most up-to-date understanding of treatment of pain, we read not only the current state of the research, but also how it is best implemented and integrated in the comprehensive plan for the patient which is then detailed for us in Part III. Vignettes of actual patient encounters illustrate what really works, and offers not only suggestions, but also hope for greater comfort for both the clinicians and the families they serve."

Daniel P. Kohen, MD, Director, Developmental-Behavioral Pediatrics Program, Professor, Departments of Pediatrics & Family Medicine and Community Health, and Past-President, American Board of Medical Hypnosis, University of Minnesota

"Dr. Kuttner and her contributors have distilled their rich experience providing integrative care for young people in pain to create an exceptional book that is comprehensive, practical and compassionate. Written with integrity, it speaks to us in the clear voice it would have us use to help children find comfort. This book is profound."

Laurence I. Sugarman, MD, Clinical Associate Professor in Pediatrics, University of Rochester School of Medicine and Dentistry, President, American Board of Medical Hypnosis

"This is a unique and marvelous book. It addresses all the disciplines that work with children, and is very well organized. Dr. Kuttner not only explains the neurophysiology of pain, the assessment, the pharmacological and psychological management of pain, and the anxiety issues, but she also shows the enormous importance of the words spoken by all professionals, and the simple yet effective ways of 'making the pain better.' Throughout the book are numerous case studies, that go a long way in helping the reader understand and put into practice the principles discussed. She also shows how all medical disciplines can collaborate with the child and the family. By reading this book, we can better understand the complexity of pain, and can find numerous ways to improve the pain of a child. This book is a must read for all professionals who work with children, and should be translated into many languages in order to help the children in whatever country they live."

Chantal Wood, MD, Paediatrician and Pain Care Specialist, Unité d'Evaluation et de Traitement de la Douleur, University Hospital Robert Debré, Paris, France.

"This is a wonderful book full of evidence and practical tips. It is a "must read" for any health professional who works with children."

Linda Franck, Professor and Chair, Family Health Care Nursing, UCSF School of Nursing

A Child in Pain
What Health Professionals Can Do to Help

Leora Kuttner, PhD

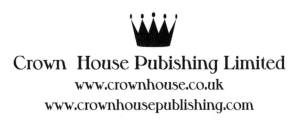

Crown House Pubishing Limited
www.crownhouse.co.uk
www.crownhousepublishing.com

First published by

Crown House Publishing Ltd
Crown Buildings, Bancyfelin, Carmarthen, Wales, SA33 5ND, UK
www.crownhouse.co.uk

and

Crown House Publishing Company LLC
6 Trowbridge Drive, Suite 5, Bethel, CT 06801, USA
www.crownhousepublishing.com

British Library of Cataloguing-in-Publication Data
A catalogue entry for this book is available
from the British Library.

10-digit ISBN 1845904362
13-digit ISBN 978-184590436-4

LCCN 2010920343

Printed and bound in the USA

To my beautiful family, both biological and of the heart,
who are spread all over the world
and remain as close as ever.

Table of Contents

List of Figures and Tables

Chapter 5

Chapter 6

Chapter 7

Chapter 8

Chapter 9

Chapter 10

List of Contributors

Stefan J. Friedrichsdorf, MD
Medical Director, Pain Medicine & Palliative Care, Children's
Hospitals and Clinics of Minnesota, Minneapolis, MN, USA

Helen W. Karl MD
Associate Professor of Anesthesiology
University of Washington, School of Medicine
Former Director of Pain Medicine
Seattle Children's Hospital, WA, USA

Jonathan Kuttner, MBBCh, Dip. Sports Med. FACMM
Musculoskeletal & Pain Specialist
Auckland, New Zealand

Carl L. von Baeyer, PhD
Professor Emeritus of Psychology &
Associate Member in Pediatrics
University of Saskatchewan, Saskatoon, Canada

Acknowledgements

My thanks to Mark Tracten at Crown House Publishing for providing me with a legitimate opportunity to take time and immerse myself in the fascinating pain literature—and for his good humour and reliable guidance from inception to completion. This book outgrew the original invitation to "simply update my book *A Child in Pain; How to help, what to do (1996),* but this time solely for health professionals." With the astounding advances in the intervening period in pain research and technologically, the process of writing became a rich immersion in this material, and the book matured.

I particularly want to thank Dr. Carl von Baeyer. His resourcefulness, knowledge and decency helped immeasurably with many aspects of this manuscript. I am indebted to my four talented contributors for their enriching collaboration: my brother Jonathan Kuttner, my friends and colleagues Carl von Baeyer, Stefan Friedrichsdorf and Helen Karl for contributing their expertise.

Case studies, which are a significant part of the character of this book, were thoughtfully offered by Acupuncturist, Ruth McCarthy; Dentist, Jane Ronen; and Pain Specialist, Jonathan Kuttner. Material contributed by Dan Kohen, Joanne Eland and Penny Leggott from the first book was incorporated into this one. My thanks once again go to them.

One of the great joys was working with our daughter, Tamar O'Shea as she applied her artistic talents to the physiology drawings and charts, and with our son, Daniel O'Shea who gave freely of his computer prowess. My continuing thanks to Kelly Hayton for her manuscript talents and my editor, Susan Liddicoat for her fine attention to detail and professional guidance along the marathon.

Colleagues and friends read sections of the manuscript and generously provided constructive feedback. For this, I am grateful to: Christine Chambers, Andrea Chapman, Ken Craig, Gill Lauder, Julie Linden, Lori Roth and Bonnie Stevens. Additionally, Susan

Tupper read the physical therapy chapter and elucidated the biomechanics of breathing; Joan Fisher and Jonathan Kuttner read the Pharmacological chapter; Jeff Dubin, Bruce Marshall, Jane Ronen & Judith Versloot read and contributed to the Dental Chapter.

My warm appreciation to Lonnie Zeltzer for writing the Foreword and to Neil Schechter for writing the Afterword to this book.

And my ongoing love and gratitude to Tom my husband, partner and companion in all, who thoughout this process was his divinely humoured supportive self – and to the children, parents and siblings who contributed their experiences, their poignant drawings and their guidance on how to help them manage their pain, fear and worries.

Preface

A Child in Pain: What Health Professionals Can Do to Help is designed to help pediatric health professionals of all disciplines gain understanding and skill in how to approach and treat children's pain, and how to help children make sense of and deal with their own pain. Pain is the most common reason for children to seek a medical consultation—and sometimes a common reason for avoiding it. Unaddressed fears and anxiety complicate pain management and recovery. A central theme in this book is the examination of children's fears and anxieties that accompany their need for pain relief, and the communication skills and words that will allay these fears.

Pain is now recognized as a major health problem in its own right. Pain, however, has a history of being one of the least understood and one of the most neglected domains of health care, particularly for children. In this book I have placed a strong emphasis on children's experience of pain and pain treatment, and on their self-expression of their concerns. Wherever possible, children are quoted in the book so that we gain a more nuanced appreciation of their needs. The quotes are from children in my practice or in my documentaries. If the former, their names and identifying factors have been changed to protect their identity. Throughout the book the term *children* includes teenagers, and covers ages three to nineteen. As well, in pediatric medicine today, parents have gained their rightful place as an integral part of their child's care (the term *parent* includes *carer*). This book also demonstrates how health professionals can guide parents to help their child through acute pain, procedures, or chronic pain.

As a clinical psychologist with more than 30 years experience in pediatric pain management, I want to sharpen the focus on behavioral, emotional, and relational aspects of pain management, while simultaneously working with the essential and traditional contributions of physical and pharmacological treatments in our health care system. Affectionately termed the "3Ps," the integration of all three aspects of treatment forms a fundamental principle in this book. The integration of psychological, physical, and pharmaco-logical methods goes hand in hand with our prevailing a biopsycho-social model of care. Today a child's pain (particularly the more complex and chronic pains of childhood) cannot be properly appreciated or treated without applying a biopsychosocial model that incorporates all aspects of the child's world. Dealing with only one aspect of pain and neglecting the other contributing stressors would now be regarded as providing sub-standard care. Explaining why pain may be occurring, how the brain is "the mas-termind" of the pain system, what the child can do to manage or resolve the pain, and how medication and the child's efforts can provide comfort, is now part of state of the art care. With this as a central tenet, I provide examples of, and discussion on, how to navigate this biopsychosocial spectrum of care with greater facil-ity. As fourteen-year-old Jeremy says in the book, "A mind is a terrible thing to waste!"

Today, in the first part of the 21st century, there is still a great deal that we need to do to address and relieve children's pain and suf-fering. To meet this I've drawn from evidence-based literature to provide direction. Our challenge is to bridge the gap between knowing and doing. This book is another in a series of efforts that our international pediatric community has made to close the gap between what we know and what we do.

Our knowledge in pain medicine has mushroomed over the last three decades. On many fronts remarkable progress has been achieved in understanding and developing capacities to assess, treat and relieve children's pain and suffering. This includes basic science research on nerve and brain functioning, technological advances in imaging, and new delivery systems for medications. We have developed new analgesics and anesthetics, and there has been a burgeoning of research into determining the efficacy of psychological, physical, and pharmacological approaches to treat-ing pain. Studies and meta-reviews have examined efficacy with recommendations on how best to apply treatments to relieve dif-ferent types of pain. Pain services in children's hospital are pro-liferating, and there is growing collaboration between the many disciplines within the hospitals to develop standards of care and protocols to manage acute, procedural, and chronic pain. Pain

management has become a collective pursuit across disciplines—
and this is welcomed.

A Child in Pain: What Health Professionals Can Do to Help is addressed
to all disciplines, in its valuing of the professional-patient relationship and in the language used to allay anxiety, address fears and
promote relief and well-being. The book is organized into three
parts: Part I explores our scientific understanding of pain as a part
of children's development. It addresses the physiological processing of pain, how to assess it, and how to explain it to children
who are fearful, anxious, and in pain. Part II explores pain treatments themselves, their efficacies and how to combine them for
therapeutic impact. Part III uses this understanding to help translate knowledge into clinical practice in three domains of pediatric
medicine: the physicians' practice, the dental practice, and in the
hospital. Within the extensive References at the back of the book,
key resources are identified with an asterisk.

I have found it a rewarding and extraordinary privilege to belong
to a vigorous, dynamic, resourceful, and generous international
pediatric pain community. We've shared, learned from each other,
collaborated, and inspired each other. We have worked together,
critiqued each other's endeavors, and matured as practitioners
and researchers. My hope is that this book supports and benefits
those of you entering and participating in this deeply meaningful
and worthwhile field.

Foreword

For all of you who are about to read this book, you are in for a real treat! Dr Leora Kuttner is an experienced pain clinician extraordinaire and her clinical knowledge and sensitivity emanate from each page of this book. Even as an experienced children's pain clinician myself, I found reading this book not only informative but joyful to read as well. I will explain what sets this book apart from many others and makes it a "must read" for any primary care clinician and, in fact, for clinicians across many disciplines who treat children.

First the book is well written, devoid of much medical jargon, and tells an interesting story. I think that Leora's experiences and background as a film maker is apparent throughout the book. She not only explains a phenomenon but shows the reader exactly what she means, as if the reader were viewing the story on the screen. This way of writing is evident in each chapter. She provides a "how to" that makes the book ecologically sound and clinically useful. Further, she then gives clinical examples to demonstrate what she has just described.

There are many unique aspects of this book that have been touched on by other authors of children's pain books but not in the depth that is presented here. For example, two themes intertwine throughout the book that help connect the chapters together—the importance of observation and language. Leora shows how close observation of a child's non-verbal behavior, including body movement and position, facial expression, eye contact, tone of voice, cry, muscle tension, and even what is not said provides important information about a child's pain experience and perceptions of ability to cope with the pain. Observation of the environment is noted to be equally important. For example, she describes the importance of noting context (e.g. are parents present in the treatment room but do not know what to do to help their child, or is a child not crying because peers are present?), as well as parental interactions with their child in pain or in anticipation of pain (e.g. the example provided of parents whose toddler daughter developed diabetes, a condition that required parents to perform multiple finger pricks during the day).

Language is also a powerful tool as noted through the many clinical examples that Leora has provided. The salience of language is especially noted in the chapter on psychological interventions for children's pain (Chapter 5), one component of what Leora calls the "3Ps" (psychological, physical, and pharmacological) of children's pain treatment. In this chapter, she describes in more detail and clarity the concepts of hypnosis and the use of imagery with children than I have read anywhere else. She provides many lovely elucidating clinical case examples to illustrate what she means. Throughout this section, she highlights the importance of language. That is, how what is said to a child and when, can have a profound impact on that child's experience of pain and pain-related distress as well as having the ability to enhance or subvert a child's ability to cope with the pain. As a simplistic example, think of giving morphine to a child who has just had surgery. There might be three ways to administer the morphine. One is to simply give it and not say anything. Another is to give it and say "we can try to lower your pain with this medicine." Yet another way is to say, "I am going to give you some really powerful magic medicine that will likely not only make the hurt better but may even make you feel silly and laugh!" How would you rather receive your analgesia? Leora provides beautiful examples of the power of words and language.

In the chapter on psychological interventions (Chapter 5), Leora also includes biofeedback and presents newer theories related to cognitive behavioral therapies called ACT (acceptance and commitment therapy). Within her description of ACT she also discusses the importance of mindful awareness. That is, the importance of being present, noticing thoughts, sensations, and emotions but not becoming absorbed in or attached to them. In this chapter, she also discusses other creative sensory pathways to help children cope with pain, including music, art, and play.

The chapter on physical strategies (Chapter 6) for pain management in children is just as stellar. Leora provides detailed explanations about self-directed strategies such as breathing with the creative use of bubbles, pranayama breathing and other breathing techniques. She discusses massage, and even provides descriptions of how parents can massage their stressed child. She covers the value of touching, including body to body contact as in kangaroo carrying for newborns and infants and talks about swaddling, rocking, and sucrose for infants. In addition she covers yoga, acupuncture and acupressure in addition to the usually described physical therapy, TENS, heat and cold. However, for each physical strategy, Leora provides specific "how to" details and gives clinical examples to illustrate what she means.

The book also has sections on how to examine a child in pain and how to help a child receive dental care without pain and stress. It describes how to manage children's pain in the hospital setting and how to manage the hospital setting to reduce the likelihood of hospitalized children experiencing pain and distress. It also provides a practical guide to minimize painful experiences in childhood and to reduce the likelihood that early pain experiences will create painful memories that can lay a template for the development of adult chronic pain.

Leora has also brought in some key contributors with added expertise in the neuroanatomy and neurophysiology of pain (her brother, Dr. Jonathan Kuttner, a musculoskeletal and pain specialist), in pain assessment (Dr. Carl von Baeyer) and in the pharmacological management of pain (physicians Drs. Stefan Freidrichsdorf and Helen Karl). She has even solicited a patient, a young girl, to bring together in narrative form a summary of what the book imparts. I applaud Leora in this outstanding book and encourage readers to enjoy.

Lonnie Zeltzer, MD
Director, UCLA Pediatric Pain Program
Professor of Pediatrics, Anesthesiology, Psychiatry and
Biobehavioral Sciences, David Geffen School of Medicine at UCLA

Part I

How to Understand, Assess, and Communicate with a Child in Pain

"Pain is the only condition in which
the patient is the diagnostician."

Unknown

Pain is now regarded not merely as a symptom of a disease, as previously thought, but as a human rights issue (International Association for the Study of Pain, 2004). The relief of pain therefore demands the highest priority. Pain is as important as any disease or illness, deserving of clinical attention and treatment. By definition, pain is a noxious sensation which always has an emotional impact. In assessing and communicating with children and adolescents on their pain, they are the authority on their experience. This is a fundamental principle of pain management in children. Children are to be believed when they say they are in pain.

Pain has its own physiological system. Chapter 1 explores how pain, although unpleasant, can also have a positive function as an intelligent warning system. In its acute form, pain is frequently protective, preventing or stopping further injury. However, in its chronic form, it ceases to protect in any way, and it becomes a problem. Chronic pain is a result of a malfunctioning pain system. Treatment requires a biopsychosocial approach that incorporates appropriate biological, psychological, and social treatments. In the twenty-first century, we need to ensure that misguided messages and myths about pain no longer persist when caring for children in pain.

Carrying out effective pain treatment with children in pain requires a thorough understanding of how the biological, psychological, and social systems interact for pain to be experienced. Chapter 2 takes up the subject of this relationship: how in the pain experience the nerves communicate with one another, the nerve pathways to the brain, the modulation sites, and the brain's neural networks. We draw on the scientific research and theory, such as the gate control theory, that led to a radical change in the understanding and treatment of pain. We explore the more recent neuromatrix concept in pain medicine (Melzack, 1999) to help understand the complexity of brain function in persistent distressing pain, and explain how persistent pain alters its own neural system.

The most common procedure in a hospital is communication. All professionals need to know how to communicate effectively with children and their parents. There are optimal ways of responding to children in pain, children fearful of anticipated pain, or children wanting to understand why they are in pain. It is fundamental to good practice, and to the child's short and long-term outcome, that this process be done well. Chapter 3 discusses this and explores the parents' central role in modeling pain behavior and in helping their child to cope.

Since the 1980s we have seen a burgeoning of well-designed and standardized tools of pain measurement to help assess children's acute and chronic pain. There are tools for infants and for children with developmental challenges, tools for post-operative pain assessment, and questionnaires for children in chronic pain and their parents. There is a simple measure for young children and pain scales and maps with more sensitivity for older children. Designing reliable and valid measures to assess pain across cultures, countries, and languages has been an emerging strength in the pediatric pain field. The most common and key measures are covered in Chapter 4, including a developmental exploration of how children of different ages understand and express their pain – important facets for a full and adequate assessment.

These chapters provide you with the foundation for understanding the role of pain in children's growth and development; the basic physiology of how pain works in the human body, and how to share this knowledge with children – communicating with them when they hurt and are suffering so that they feel heard and helped; and then how to further assess and measure their pain.

Chapter 1

Pain in Children's Lives

"Pain is when it hurts."

5-year-old boy

As children and teens grow and explore the world, they experience many falls, illnesses, and hurts of one kind or another. They turn to their parents to find relief from pain. Too often parents feel anxiety and fear, not knowing what to do in the face of their children's pain, and turn to pediatric professionals for the expertise and guidance to provide their child with sufficient relief. Pediatric health professionals at all levels of care need to know how to provide this necessary help.

Fortunately today many breakthroughs in scientific research have increased our understanding and treatment of childhood pain. The goal of this book is to make this information easily accessible to those working directly with children. With a knowledge of the most effective therapies and treatment combinations in conventional and complementary medicine, professionals can help children and their parents to better manage minor and major pain from injuries and illness. Instead of minimizing, misunderstanding, or dismissing a child's pain, a skilled professional can provide prompt pain relief and empower the child to cope. This requires a combination of helping the child to understand and interpret the pain sensations and to develop coping skills, as well as being aware of the treatment options to ease the pain.

Pain is part of growing up. Young children frequently fall and scrape themselves as they learn to walk, run, climb, and ride a bicycle. This is a time of developing co-ordination and skill and, as a consequence, learning about pain and suffering. Research has shown that preschool children during play, experience an average of one 'owie' or 'boo-boo' every three hours (Fearon, McGrath, & Achat, 1996). Children encounter accidents at home, in parks, in cars, and on the playground at school. They may experience pain when they get a tooth filled at the dentist's office or when they have an injection at the doctor's office. Some children and adolescents struggle for years with painful diseases and hospital treatments.

This chapter discusses the role that pain plays in the human body, the relationship between pain and the brain, and types of pain. A few widely held attitudes or misconceptions about pain have prevented parents and health care providers from dealing promptly and appropriately with children's pain. At the end of this chapter I review and debunk misconceptions about pain.

The Protective Value of Pain

Pain is protective. It provides vital information to guide us in the use of our body, informs us about its condition, and helps us survive and remain intact. As health care professionals, part of our responsibility towards children is teaching them to respect pain signals and to learn how to interpret and cope with them. We know from interview studies on children's concepts of pain that they seldom mention any beneficial aspects of pain, such as pain's diagnostic value, its warning function, or its role in determining whether treatment is effective (Abu-Saad, 1984*a,b,c*; Ross & Ross, 1984*a,b*; Savedra, Gibbons, Tesler, Ward, & Wegner 1982). Children need to know that pain is their personal safety-alarm system, interpreted by the brain in a highly rapid and sophisticated way. Pain messages quickly tell us if there is something wrong with our organs, muscles, bones, ligaments, and tissues, all of which are interwoven with nerve fibers and pain mediators that rapidly carry pain messages to, from, and within our brain. Children need to be informed that part of the sophistication of pain is that memory, emotions, previous learning, beliefs, stress, endocrine and immunological processes, as well as the current meaning of pain, all factor into how the pain message is experienced.

In its healthiest form, short-term acute pain is protective, alerting and preventing damage to one's body. As David, aged four and a half, discovered: "You've got to listen to your stomach when it's hurting, 'cause if you don't, your stomach will get upset!" David knew this firsthand; for five days he had had stomach pains and gastric spasms and had been throwing up. The pain signals had taught him that if he continued eating the tuna sandwich his well-intentioned mother had given him, his stomach might send it back again. Recovering from a gastrointestinal virus, David had come to respect the signals he was receiving from his stomach: to eat only what his stomach could handle and when to stop. Because his actions helped settle his pain and nausea, and because he was being listened to – although he was only four and a half – he learned to manage his own recovery, and set the stage for dealing effectively with the experience of pain in the future.

Children learn about their bodies when we encourage and teach them to pay attention to their body's messages and sensations. They learn to interpret the different pain signals and determine what gives the best form of relief. This learning is refined over a lifetime. Even very young children can be taught to share their pain sensations so that we can determine what is going on, their severity, and what will be most effective in helping the pain to go and stay away.

The value of pain is poignantly evident when we encounter children born with one of the rare conditions of insensitivity or indifference to pain (Nagasako, Oaklander, & Dworkin, 2003). Throughout their lives, these children are at great risk of damaging their bodies, particularly their eyes, hands, fingers, joints, and feet. Pain is disabled by their genetic condition and does not protect them. It does not alert them to stop an action that will cause injury, or prompt them to call for help when they experience the early pain signals of a medical crisis such as appendicitis. These children continue to walk on sprained ankles and damage the tips of their fingers and their legs; frequently they require artificial protection such as braces and guards. By school age, these children have already sustained significant and often irreparable damage to their limbs.

Pain in the Body and the Brain

David Morris (1991), a Professor of Bioethics, writes about the outdated belief that pain can be divided into physical and mental pain. He calls this 'the Myth of Two Pains.' According to this myth, there are two entirely separate types of pain: physical and mental. Morris elaborates: "You feel physical pain if your arm breaks, and you feel mental pain if your heart breaks. Between these two different events we seem to imagine a gulf so wide and deep that it might as well be filled by a sea that is impossible to navigate." (p. 9)

This concept, that pain is either in the body or the mind, goes back to the 17th-century philosophy of René Descartes, who argued that the body and mind were separate. He also maintained that there was a one-to-one relationship between the injury and the amount of pain felt – a theory now debunked. Today's scientific evidence is that there is continual interaction in the nervous system between our physical and mental functions such that any division between them is an artificial construct.

One of the earliest medical practitioners to publicly question this mind-body split was Dr. H. Beecher, a Boston surgeon who traveled to Europe with U.S. troops during World War II. In 1956 he published a paper which described how soldiers who had very similar wounds to the civilians he had treated at home, required significantly less pain medication (Beecher, 1956). In talking with these men, he realized that the meaning of their pain was very different from that for civilians. Pain to these soldiers meant they were alive and were out of active warfare. War wounds were a ticket home. Beecher's reports challenged the thinking of the day and importantly showed that the amount of tissue damage often bore little correspondence to the level of felt pain, and there was no validity in a mind-body dichotomy These conclusions are now widely accepted in clinical practice. We now know that the meaning of a person's pain is subjective, highly personal, and variable from one situation to another, and that this meaning will influence how the pain is experienced. Mental pain can be physically experienced and physical pain mentally experienced. Mind and body are integrated systems.

Definition of Pain

That pain is subjective in no way detracts from the validity of the physical origins of the pain. Pain signals travel through the limbic system, the part of the brain most involved in emotion and motivation (see Chapter 2). When in pain, we are affected emotionally and our feelings can range from distressed, anxious, vulnerable, weepy, to depressed. These emotional or affective correlates are well documented in the literature. The official definition of pain by the International Association for the Study of Pain (IASP) acknowledges this: "Pain is an unpleasant sensory and emotional experience associated with actual or potential tissue damage, or described in terms of such damage. Pain is always subjective. Each individual learns the application of the word through experiences related to injury in early life." (1979, p. 249)

Pain is experienced as emotional and mental suffering, as well as a distressing physical sensation. Above all it is subjectively experienced and so is private and entirely personal. Consider the instructive words of sixteen-year-old Jodi, who coped for five years with severe pain from Guillain-Barré, a neuromuscular syndrome:

> Pain is something that no one can analyze. How can you feel someone else's pain? You can't look at someone and say they are at an eight or a ten out of ten level of pain! How can you do that? It is internal. It's within that person. Only that person can say what level of pain they are in!

She speaks the truth! The primary way of knowing what is going on is to ask each child about his or her experience of pain and its impact on daily life, feelings, and friendships.

How Thought and Imagination Influence Pain

As pointed out previously, in every pain situation, there is an interplay of thoughts, beliefs, emotions, and attitudes with bodily sensations that creates the experience of pain. It is this interaction that enables us to change – increase or decrease – the pain experience. When a child appreciates the impact of these different and personal aspects, it becomes a vital part of success in the treatment process.

Eight-year-old Seana tells what she does to reduce her painful intravenous needles during cancer treatment:

> I learned to use my imagination and go to a place I love, Candyland. I concentrate on what's happening there so I don't even know there's a needle in my arm! It's funny how it happens.
>
> (Kuttner, 1986)

Not all children can attain the level of concentration to turn off pain entirely, but many can find some relief, and with regular practice can improve their outcome. Seana found relying on her imagination so helpful that even when out of hospital, she reported practicing.

In contrast, 12-year-old Josh, a dramatic, highly imaginative young man, who detested coming into hospital for cardiac check-ups, focused his thoughts on all the awful things that could happen. As a result, when Josh experienced a small pain, it quickly escalated into an overwhelming one. He concluded that if he imagined the worst scenario for himself, he would be prepared for any eventuality in hospital. So he imagined that he might die and worked himself up into such a heightened state of anxiety that his routine blood collection became a horrendous and painful experience for him, his family, and the staff. Josh's dramatic reaction is an example of 'catastrophizing,' a cognitive reaction to pain to be discussed in Chapter 3. The instructions his mind gave his body were not, "Shut down on the pain; it is an OK pain," but "MAYDAY! This is the end!"

Our mind and body also interact through the production and release of endorphins – one of the body's own painkillers, an opioid (morphine-like) chemical produced by the body that serves to suppress pain. Endorphins, first discovered in 1975, are manufactured not as first thought only in the brain and spinal cord, but throughout the entire body. We now know that every major internal organ has its own opioid receptors. This means that every organ, including the gut lining, is designed to receive information in the form of neuro-chemical transmitters from the brain, including the naturally occurring opioids for pain relief. These internal pain relievers can be released through physical exercise, and possibly through relaxation, deep breathing, and meditation. Seana probably released enough endorphins to block the sensation of the needle in her arm, whereas Josh released large amounts of adrenaline to boost his panic and terror that heightened his experience of pain. This is the power of our thoughts and beliefs. Pain is after all, a function of a conscious brain.

Types of Pain

As an 'intelligent' signal, pain comes in many different forms. Pain has been divided into acute (protective) pain, recurrent pain, or chronic (often non-protective) pain. Protective pain sensations are referred to as 'nociceptive' or normal, sensory pain. Non-protective pain sensations are referred to as 'neuropathic' or abnormal pain. While the length of time of the pain and its normality or abnormality are aspects used to categorize these types of pain, it is now postulated that acute, recurrent, and chronic pain may be part of a continuum (Cervero & Laird, 1991). Acute severe pain may have some abnormal nerve patterns characteristic of chronic pain, and chronic pain may begin as and have some acute pain episodes (for a full explanation, see Chapter 2). With this potential continuum of protective to non-protective pain in mind, here is an overview of the characteristics of pain in the acute, recurrent, and chronic states.

Acute Pain

Acute pain indicates an episode of tissue injury, potential tissue damage, or inflammation. Examples are pain caused by surgery, a burn, a fracture, or a cut. Acute pain provides continuous, second-by-second sensory information. The pain begins suddenly and follows a predictable trajectory: first warning that tissue has been damaged and over time lessening as the tissue heals and inflammation subsides. Acute pain can be mild to severe. Most of these conditions are readily diagnosed and the source of the pain is fairly easy to determine. The American Pain Society's position statement of children's acute pain (2001) explains:

> Acute pain is one of the most common adverse stimuli experienced by children, occurring as a result of injury, illness, and necessary medical procedures. It is associated with increased anxiety, avoidance, somatic symptoms, and increased parent distress. Despite the magnitude of effects that acute pain can have on a child, it is often inadequately assessed and treated.

With acute pain a host of physiological and psychological responses are mobilized, as different chemical substances, neurotransmitters, are released. The brain immediately receives these pain signals from the injury site, then releases substances such as adrenaline and noradrenaline. Prompt action to relieve the pain, such as removing a body part from danger or stopping an action to minimize further harm, enables the body to return to some equilibrium. These actions occur reflexively and almost without thought. Pain shocks us into being protective. It's a marvelously sophisticated internal survival system that is highly effective – most of the time.

If children with acute pain are provided with adequate treatment and taught to address their pain and distress promptly, relief will be more rapid. Describing the pain can lead to faster relief. "Is that a sting or a tingling feeling, an ache or a sharp pain? Is it a big owie or a pinch?" With guidance, children can describe their pain, clarifying what causes the pain, and learn which treatment might be helpful. Children learn that an ache such as muscle fatigue can be relieved with heat, a rub, rest, or analgesic. A burning or sting-ing pain may indicate inflammation as well as nerve injury, and often feels better when an ice pack or a cool pack is applied and analgesic medication taken. A sharp pain is a signal of more acute tissue damage, or it may indicate muscle spasm, such as the clas-sic 'stitch' in one's side while running. Relaxing the muscles by bending over from the waist and taking deep breaths will ease this pain. A dull, gnawing pain may indicate a more persistent pain, associated with visceral pain, ligament, or tendon injury. Rehabili-tation therapy or wearing a splint to restrain movement will ease ligament or tendon type of pain, giving the tissue time to stabilize and heal.

Acute pain commands attention, causes anxiety, and drains energy. Blood pressure can increase with acute pain, and after an initial drop, the heart rate also can increase. Discomfort and distress continue until this pain is adequately and effectively addressed. When the pain eases, the intervention has been suc-cessful. Generally, acute pain will diminish over a period of days or weeks, becoming less intense as time progresses. It is short-term and unlikely to return. Even though acute pain disappears, it does produce changes that linger in the body's nervous system. The brain remembers this pain. If not properly treated, the injury continues to signal and pain will persist, becoming intermittently recurrent or chronic. It is incumbent on health care professionals to provide this necessary relief promptly, to prevent further harm (Walco, Cassidy, & Schechter, 1994).

Recurrent Pain

Recurrent pain is pain that alternates with pain-free periods, dur-ing which there is commonly complete recovery with no residual pain or disability. Recurrent pains are far more common in chil-dren than are chronic pains. Prevalence estimates of recurrent pain can range from one out of three young school children once a week (Petersen, Brulin, & Bergström, 2006) to 45% of adolescents (Fichtel & Larsson, 2002).

Common types of recurrent pain include headaches (tension, migraine, and mixed types), abdominal pain, irritable bowel syndrome, back pain, and limb pains. While most children cope well with recurrent pain, for some children it accounts for many missed days of school, and if a comprehensive treatment program is not quickly implemented, it can result in disruptions in the school and social life of these otherwise healthy children. Like the treatment for chronic pain, recurrent pain treatment requires the child's active participation in developing coping methods for their pain assessment and management. The school nurse or counselor is often helpful with the child's re-entry by supporting the use of pain management at school. Treatment combines Psychological, Physical, and Pharmacological methods – which I refer to as *the 3Ps* – with each component synergistically empowering the others to improve the overall treatment.

Chronic Pain

Chronic pain has no apparent protective purpose. It is pain that persists long beyond its initial useful, protective, and informative function. It often is a consequence of damaged, abnormally functioning nerves (neuropathic pain). Pain is considered chronic when it lasts longer than three to six months. Examples of such pain are rheumatoid arthritic pain, complex regional pain syndrome, hypersensitivity in a limb following trauma, and diseases causing pain, like Crohn's disease. Children with physical disability from a disease or trauma will often have accompanying chronic pain which affects and limits all aspects of their lives. The American Pain Society's position statement on chronic pain (2005), which includes recurrent pain, further elaborates:

> Chronic pain is a significant problem in the pediatric population, conservatively estimated to affect 15% to 20% of children (Goodman & McGrath, 1991). Children and their families experience significant emotional and social consequences as a result of pain and disability. The financial costs of childhood pain also may be significant in terms of healthcare utilization as well as other indirect costs, such as lost wages due to time off work to care for the

child (Li & Balint, 2000). In addition, the physical and psychological sequelae associated with chronic pain may have an impact on overall health and may predispose for the development of adult chronic pain (Campo et al., 1999; Walker, Garber, Van Slyke, & Greene, 1995).

Chronic pain persists often due to physiological and chemical changes to nerve fibers, which alter the way pain works. In conditions that have not had adequate pain relief, the involved nerves become highly sensitive to touch and pressure. These nerve pathways often do not respond in a predictable way to conventional medication or treatment. Because chronic, persisting pain changes the way the pain system works, it unfortunately often leads to more pain, and may impede the healing and repair process. Our understanding for this comes from animal pain studies that found long-lasting increases in the excitability of the pain-integrating neurons, known as central sensitization (Schwartzman, Grothusen, Kiefer, & Rohr, 2001). Evidence now suggests that long-term plastic changes in the peripheral nervous system and the brain-spinal cord network may represent the mechanisms underlying the persistence of chronic pain. Chronic pain may be a consequence of long-term physiological changes which, in turn, may further generate abnormal nerve impulses (Schwartzman et al., 2001).

These detrimental long-term neurological effects provide a compelling reason why children's pain in the acute stage must be promptly and adequately treated and controlled to prevent the development of chronic and more complex pain. Experiencing chronic pain is wearing and draining for children (see Figure 1.1). The nature of the pain can be constant, with some variation and few pain-free periods. Consequently, chronic pain becomes part of the child's life, changing how the child moves or participates in activities, school, and friendships (Bursch, Walco, & Zeltzer, 1998).The child is likely to lose hope that it will ever go away. Without comprehensive treatment and therapy, children living with chronic pain often feel that there is nothing that will provide relief. This hopelessness compounds with the pain and can lead to depression, isolation, and despair. Reviving and sustaining children's hope, while pursuing multi-pronged 3P treatment (psychological, physical, and pharmacological) is central to successful chronic pain treatment.

Figure 1.1. The Broad Impact of Children's Chronic Pain.

Living with persisting pain impacts the social, psychological as well as physical areas of a child's life, and all need to be understood and addressed in treatment.

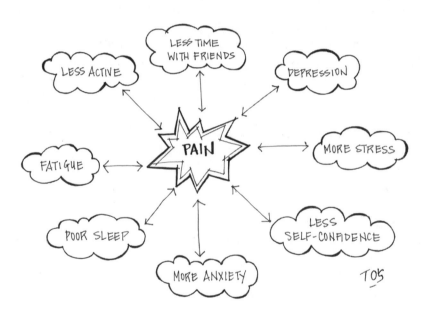

We learn so much from children with chronic pain. Earlier I introduced sixteen-year-old Jodi, who has struggled for five years with the debilitating Guillain-Barré syndrome. She experienced many kinds of pain in the course of her very slow recovery and became an authority on her condition. Cued to these different body sensations, she paid close attention to the pain signals' distinctive characteristics as they indicated important changes in her condition and could guide her treatment. Over the years she became a skilled and patient teacher of the doctors who would come onto the ward. When asked, "Do you have any pain?" Jodi explained that in fact she had three types of pain:

> I have nerve pain, which is a shooting, sharp kind of sensation that comes sporadically and is not there all the time. Then I have muscle pain – I can't call it an ache, because an ache is something that you can put up with. It's more like someone has beaten you internally – it's a severe ache. My joint pain is like an arthritic pain, an osteoporosis kind of pain. (Kuttner, 1990)

After Jodi had described in impressive detail the quality, intensity, frequency, and the subtle differences of pain from different origins in the body, she added, "The hard part was people not believing me!"

We need to let children know that we hear them when they are in pain and that we know they are suffering – whether or not the child's behavior accords with what we conceive of as pain. Remember that when children have had persisting pain, they may no longer 'wear the pain on their sleeve' and may have adjusted to it so that they have a life. In other words, the overt behavioral signs of chronic pain tend to habituate or dissipate as time passes, despite continued self-reported pain (von Baeyer & Spagrud, 2007).

When a child suffers from chronic pain, the entire family must accommodate to the child's increased needs, and this exacts an enormous toll in suffering and disruption for the child, parents, and siblings. For all these reasons, children with chronic pain require a specialized long-term and intensive pain management program that involves changes in lifestyle, psychological treatment, physical therapy, and medication (Krane & Mitchell, 2005; Zeltzer & Schlank, 2005).

Misguided Messages about Pain

There are mixed messages in our world about how to deal with pain, such as, *pain requires a battle,* or *pain is good for you as it builds character!* These conflicting messages often confuse while influencing our attitudes toward pain.

Pain Requires a Battle!

Advertisements on TV or in magazines advocate that to find relief, pain needs to be battled down! "Is this pain killing you?" Often the weapon of choice is a certain medication, which is promoted with happy music behind the softly announced stream of side-effects. Such injunctions promote an adversarial relationship with the pain inside our bodies. The unhelpful, underlying rationale is:

> Pain is our enemy and must be beaten. Guard and fight against pain, against this invader that doesn't intrinsically belong in the body. Tighten and tense up against these inner sensations.

With pain defined as the enemy, fear comes out and panic can reign. In the battle to kill the pain within our own bodies, brain is pitted against body. Acceptance and commitment therapy (discussed in chapter 5) is a recent development to effectively counter this misinformed attitude.

Using the language of war, we lose the concept of pain as an intelligent guide and messenger helping us live more harmoniously within our body. Believing that pain is an invader and an enemy, relief against pain comes in the form of 'shots'. Shots come from guns. They wound and hurt. No wonder children don't want anything to do with them! In our hospital we teach the use of the word 'injection' or 'needle' instead.

In a hospital clinic parents have been heard to use the threat of a needle to force obedience from a child, "If you don't behave yourself, the doctor will give you a shot!" Health care professionals can promptly counter, "No! We're here to help you to feel better and to manage!" Unfortunately, the child has already had fear instilled and will remain distrustful until the health professional's hard work of building trust breaks through. This is part of our cultural legacy of war, fear, and threats.

There is a further insidious message found on television and in magazines and newspapers. In the battle against pain, the only means to arm yourself is to rely on something outside of your body – a bottle of pills. Faces smiling with relief in advertisements try to convince us that reaching for a pill is the only option. Rarely are other options revealed. Pharmaceutical companies do not make a profit by teaching pain sufferers that actively using their inner resources, such as imagery or relaxation, together with a pain medication, will control pain and reduce discomfort. However, in pain clinics throughout the world, these brain-body techniques are now a key part of pain programs – one of the three Ps of pain treatment: psychological, the 'top-down' treatment approach.

Pain Builds Character

Another common misconception is that being stoic when in pain is admirable, as if pain is good for you. Pain builds strength and character. "Pain will make a man out of you!" "No pain, no gain" reflects this stiff upper-lip attitude toward pain. The truth is very different. Suppressing one's pain adds considerably to the strain of experiencing pain and depletes energy, joy, and vitality. When pain is present, efforts need to be made to relieve it. Pain especially has no place in the lives of growing children. It is not needed for character, growth, or achievement.

This stoic position further suggests that pain medication should not be used, or that we should feel shame or defeat when we 'give in' and use it. Taking medication means weakness, as if it weakens character. This attitude obstructs successful pain management.

Medications appropriately given to a child in acute or persistent pain by a knowledgeable health professional will go promptly to the source of the pain and provide relief. Analgesics are, without question, the method to use when pain overwhelms and drains, as when a fractured bone is being set in a cast. Pain medication will help break a continuous cycle of pain, as when a child has a migraine headache. Medication provides relief and a chance to sleep and heal. When pain is reduced, the analgesic can be gradually withdrawn and other pain-reduction methods such as physiotherapy, heat pads, or hypnosis can come into play to further the child's recovery. Controlling pain promptly and keeping it well controlled until it abates is the fundamental principle of effective pain management.

Neither the belief that pain is a battleground in which fear reigns and medication is the only help, nor that pain builds character and taking medication is a weakness, is true. Like life, the truth is more complex, and a lot more interesting! When pain is kept under control with adequate, regular doses of pain medication, the child can develop inner resources using imagery and self-regulation to better manage the pain so that less medication is then required.

Debunking Myths About Children and Pain

The belief that children don't experience pain pervaded medical and nursing teaching and practice until the 1980s. If children expressed pain, it was ignored or underestimated and undertreated. "It's not really that bad. It can't be hurting that much!" These attitudes harmed children in pain. The following case study shows the long-term consequences of practices that neglected babies and children in pain:

Rod is highly respected 46-year-old police officer. He is decisive, physically tough, and capable on the job. Few people knew that vigorous Rod was born prematurely. He spent the first four months of his life in an incubator in a neonatal intensive care unit (NICU). He had many painful medical procedures to aerate his lungs, feed him, draw blood, and check blood oxygen levels. After leaving the NICU and over the next five years, he had regular check-ups, which included many blood tests. He has no clear memory of these early experiences, just his parents' stories. But Rod has one serious problem: he cannot stay in a room where there is a needle. Since the age of 12, he has never allowed blood to be taken. He can't tolerate any invasive medical procedure. Try holding down a 230-pound man, let alone a man trained to fight! No blood technician, physician, or nurse had taken on the challenge.

Health difficulties forced Rod to consult a doctor, who required a series of tests for a diagnosis. Suddenly faced with a serious health issue and medical tests, he needed help. Rod's terror was visceral and overwhelming: "I feel like such a wimp. I can face and wrestle an armed man to the ground. But when a pint-sized nurse comes toward me with a needle, I clear out of the room! It's irrational. It's crazy!" No, it's not crazy at all. At a very early age Rod had become sensitized to pain. In those early years he probably had not been given analgesics to control the pain before invasive medical treatments, since it was believed then that newborn infants did not feel pain. As an infant he experienced that there was nothing he or others could do to stop the pain. Now any medical procedure caused terror to overwhelm his six foot three inch frame, and without knowing why, he would flee to safety.

Rod came for a consultation to conquer his deep, reflexive fear. He was ashamed, and he wanted to learn how to desensitize himself to needles, manage that pain, and overcome this Achilles heel. Highly motivated, he became skilled in using deep-breathing methods and self-hypnosis. After six weeks of cognitive-behavior therapy and coping techniques with graduated experiences with needles, Rod learned to regulate and lessen his own anxiety and to exercise his coping skills. He then calmly had his blood drawn – a triumph!

If Rod's pain in infancy had been recognized and better controlled, he might not have developed this understandable, so-called 'irrational' terror. (See chapter 8 for further discussion about the amygdala in the limbic system and our built-in survival responses.) If over the next five years, during regular check-ups, his fear had been noted and discussed, giving him more control, he would not have felt ashamed or powerless. There was much that his parents and the various health care professionals could have done during those early years to alleviate his pain by supporting him to learn coping skills and to develop confidence, and thus prevent his 45-year-old phobic response to medical interventions.

There are a number of myths about children and pain that scientific evidence has now proven wrong. These myths and their refutations are summarized in Table 1.1 and discussed individually in the following sections

Table 1.1   Common Myths and the Refuting Scientific Evidence

Myth	Scientific Evidence
1. Newborns don't have the mature nervous system needed to experience pain	By 26 weeks, a fetus in utero is capable of experiencing pain. Infants premature or at term are highly sensitive to pain. Even though a newborn's nerve fibers are not fully myelinated, this does not alter the generation of the pain messages which are still transmitted, and newborn infants feel pain exquisitely.
2. Children do not feel as much pain as adults do	Children on average report higher levels of pain than adults for similar pain-producing events
3. Children will get used to pain	Untreated ongoing pain has deleterious effects, causing long-term changes in the child's nervous system

4. Children cannot reliably explain their pain	If asked, and listened to, toddlers and children at a very young age are capable of indicating where it hurts, how much it hurts, and what helps the hurt to feel better
5. If a child complains of pain but does not appear to be in pain, the child does not need relief	The child is the authority on whether or not he or she is in pain. If the child says, "I have a hurt," the pain usually needs attention
6. If a child can be distracted, the child is not in pain	Momentary distraction does not exclude the existence of pain. For example, children commonly play in hospital play rooms despite high levels of pain
7. Opioid analgesics are dangerous for children and cause addiction	Opioid analgesics are powerful pain-relieving medications that are invaluable for children in pain

Myth 1. Newborn infants don't have the mature nervous system needed to experience pain

Until the 1980s newborn babies were considered physiologically incapable of processing pain and insensitive to pain (Anand & Hickey, 1987). The rationale at that time was that pain medication for painful invasive procedures was unnecessary due to newborns' physiological immaturity and, specifically, their lack of nerve myelination (the protein sheath that surrounds the nerves, enabling the nerve impulse to rapidly travel).

What We Now Know

It is true that newborns do not experience pain in the same way as an older child since their nervous systems are still developing. However, research with newborns, and particularly premature newborns, indicate that from 26 weeks of gestation or earlier, these infants have developed the central nervous systems necessary to feel pain (Anand & The International Evidence-based Group for neonatal Pain, 2001). The belief that the nerve fibers necessary to transmit pain messages lack myelination, thereby reduce the newborn's pain experience is now known to be invalid. Pain is transmitted over poorly myelinated and unmyelinated fibers, even in adults. Although pain messages are conducted more slowly in newborn babies, these messages have a shorter distance to travel. Moreover, because the nervous systems of newborn infants are developing, they do not have the ability to modulate the transmission of pain signals and exert control from the brain to the spinal cord. Pain signals therefore persist in the infants' systems, and painful procedures produce a much stronger physiological response in an infant than in an adolescent or adult.

Certainly, the behavioral reactions of newborns and infants to painful events, including crying, facial reactions, and limb and body movements, demonstrate clearly to observant adults the presence and severity of painful distress. The newborn's exquisite sensitivity to pain combined with immaturity in the ability to modulate or shut down the pain signals, as found in older children and adults, makes the pro-active pain management of newborns and babies imperative – especially for the more vulnerable premature infants in hospital care.

Circumcision provides an important example of the underestimation of newborn's pain: the myth that circumcising an infant is not painful has been discredited. It is surprising that otherwise caring, compassionate human beings are convinced that since circumcision has been practiced without anesthesia for centuries and the baby cries for only 5 to 15 minutes, it can't be painful. Evidence from controlled studies of the infant's immediate reaction to the surgery found increased irritability and wakefulness during the first hour following the circumcision, signs which were decreased if analgesia was used (Malnory, Johnson, & Kirby, 2003). Furthermore, ninety percent of circumcised newborns showed changes in behavior and greater difficulty in quieting themselves for up to 22 hours after the operation. These behavior changes are absent when babies are given local anesthesia for their circumcision. Research has also found long-term behavioral changes in circumcised boys, indicating that circumcision performed without analgesia or anesthesia has persistent effects (Taddio, Katz, Ilersich, & Koren, 1997).

Not very long ago, analgesia and anesthesia for the newborn undergoing surgery were considered too risky. Witness these words from a surgery textbook written in 1938: "Often no anesthesia is required. A sucker consisting of a sponge dipped in some sugar water will often suffice to calm a baby" (Thorek, 1938, p. 2021). Today sucrose analgesia is now widely recommended and strongly supported by evidence, though only for minor painful procedures and certainly not for surgery. We now know that doing major or minor painful procedures without proper pain management is putting the newborn at even greater risk, increasing the baby's post-surgical complications and mortality risk, and delaying healing and recovery – as well as being inhumane.

Newborns do metabolize opioids, the strongest analgesics used in surgery, very differently than do children and adults, thereby requiring careful clinical attention. Their systems do not break the opioids down as quickly as children's systems. The analgesic therefore remains in their blood longer, and the side effects can be greater and less predictable. Nevertheless, with careful monitoring, it is now recommended practice that preventing and controlling pain is less harmful to the infant than allowing uncontrolled pain. Pain management of newborn infants up to six or nine months of age requires special nursing and medical expertise (Fitzgerald & Walker, 2009; Yamada, Stinson, Lamba, Dickson, McGrath, & Stevens, 2008).

Myth 2. Children do not feel as much pain as adults do

Children's pain is often underestimated in places where painful procedures most frequently occur, such as in blood collection laboratories. "Oh, this won't hurt!" says the person giving, not getting, the needle. Insensitive remarks like these – "You don't have to be scared," "Oh, let's be brave," "Don't cry; be a big boy!" "It'll be over in a minute," – reveal a lack of empathy for the child and/or appreciation that the child's fear of pain will amplify the pain experience. Furthermore, if you're five years old, isn't a minute of pain something to object to? A minute is an eternity for most children, particularly if the experience is sharp pain and the needle breaks your skin. Children have their own ideas about procedures, and we only discover them by asking. For example, six-year-old Marcos was upset about having blood drawn. When his mother asked him what was especially upsetting him, he answered, "When they take my blood, will they give it back to me?"

What We Now Know

Children feel as much pain as adults do and perhaps even more. Infants, toddlers, children, and teens are at risk of developing anticipatory fears of painful procedures.

When health care professionals understand the multi-factorial nature of pain and have compassion, they can help children prepare for the procedure with remarks such as the following:

> Do you know how to help yourself during this procedure? ... Let me show you how to blow away your scary feelings in these bubbles. [Child and professional blow together.] See – that blows it out of your body and so you're not bothered by the procedure. That's it! ...You can help yourself! You have got an important job to do to help your body feel better!

Faced with performing painful medical procedures, health care professionals have a choice: either provide a supportive and understanding climate in which to do procedures, or emotionally cut themselves off from the experience and act merely as technicians. The latter group of individuals appear to have numbed themselves, building protective walls so that they don't need to address the emotional demands inherent in these painful situations. Frequently, their attitude appears to be: "Let's just get it over as quickly as possible." Faced with this insensitivity, parents and other pediatric staff must speak up and advocate for the child, creating a more child-centered, resourceful, and manageable situation.

Myth 3. Children will get used to pain

Children's pain is often undertreated. Some children in pain may become very quiet and withdraw, not playing as they used to. Often they may feel exhausted by the pain, unable to articulate the degree or intensity of the pain, so they suffer in silence or become restless or agitated. It's incumbent upon us as health care professionals to inquire and assess whether pain may be a factor in a child's change in behavior.

Seven-year-old Mark jumped off a wharf into shallow water and gave a yelp. His parents saw that he had sustained a small cut on his foot. From that moment his behavior gradually changed. He had been a rough-and-tumble, sociable child, brought up on a farm. He became a listless pale boy who wouldn't play with his friends. Over the next 6 weeks he didn't get any better. The parents consulted his family physician and then an emergency physician. They both reassured the parents that he was "OK." The concerned parents sought out a third consultation with a pain specialist, who listened carefully to their concerns and observed Mark's guarded movements. He dropped his pen and asked Mark to pick it up. Mark kept his back rigid and only bent his knees to retrieve the pen. An MRI revealed a discitis, a rare infection. The initial bacteria entered through the cut in his foot, traveled in the blood stream and settled in his disc. By this stage, this low-grade infection had completely destroyed the disc. Mark had been in pain the entire 6 weeks, but he could not articulate this fact to his parents. He was a stoic child who had managed his pain by not moving. The fact that there was something significantly wrong had been missed by the earlier two physicians, because they had not attended to his change in typical behaviours. (J. Kuttner, Personal Communication, September 2009)

What We Now Know

With good care, children with chronic or recurrent diseases or syndromes do learn about the nature of their pain. Over time they become sophisticated in their diagnostic ability to determine what the pain may indicate – but they don't 'get used to it,' accept it as normal, like it, or dismiss it. Pain is a fact of their lives, and they have to deal with it and manage it, otherwise it disrupts their attempts to live a normal life (See Helen in Chapter 10).

Experiencing pain over time drains and debilitates children – as well as adults. Prolonged pain also causes changes in the nervous system, along with increased sensitivity and irritability. As pain persists, achieving relief becomes more difficult. Nor do children get used to acute or recurrent pain, such as recurring migraines, Crohn's disease, flares of juvenile idiopathic arthritis, or frequent blood-draws.

Children also do not become used to needles with increased frequency of injections. In fact, the opposite is the case. Children build up greater fears and quickly learn to resist subsequent procedures unless a therapeutic plan to prevent this fear has been developed. Anticipating a needle can disrupt a child's sleep, destroy the child's appetite, and make an otherwise normal child preoccupied, anxious, and clingy (Kennedy, Luhmann, & Zempsky, 2008; Walco, 2008).

Never underestimate the fear of pain. For children, the fear of a painful procedure can be worse than a disease itself (Zeltzer & LeBaron, 1982). Children will go to great lengths to avoid pain. Sensitive nurses can identify children who are in pain because they're not playing or moving about in their usual way. When asked if they're in pain, some children have denied their pain because they suspect they'll be given a needle to make the pain go away! A child who has had a bad experience with injections and has developed a fear of needles may show great ingenuity and desperation in bartering and negotiating to get out of an injection. In extremes, a child has even hidden away on the ward or physically battled with medical staff to avoid the upcoming 'shot' (replace the word 'shot' with the more apt term 'injection' to remove the notion of wounding). These extreme situations result from not empowering the child with better ways of coping.

Myth 4. Children cannot reliably explain their pain

All children feel their pain, but whilst some children are spontaneously able to explain their pain, others need help to do so. The case of Mark above shows how difficult this process can be – especially with a stoic child. With careful coaching and good assessment skills, the vast majority of children should be able to talk about their pain; once this dialogue is established, children will engage and provide reliable reports. Exceptions to this are children who are developmentally delayed, where the parents, or caregivers' observations are paramount and where clinicians need to be attuned to gauge whether the child is in pain. The myth that children are not reliable in their pain assessment comes from not working closely with children of all ages and knowing their capacities.

What We Now Know

Clinically we know that children as young as 12–15 months can let you know very clearly if it hurts or not. Even very young children are capable of expressing in their own words, what they are experiencing or what is occurring. I recall a toddler of twenty months, recently diagnosed with diabetes. Little Mackenzie and her family were having a difficult time establishing a smooth routine of assessing blood sugar levels and giving insulin injections. During a consultation with me, her father said that since her diagnosis all her favorite stuffed animals had developed diabetes, and he started naming them. Turning to his toddler, he said, "And who else?" Without missing a beat, Mackenzie replied, "And me!"

Children are capable of reliably reporting about their pain and disease. If children are asked with non-leading questions where they hurt and how much they hurt, young children (even at twenty months) will answer by pointing to the site of their pain. With experience, even young children can become reliable interpreters of their pain signals. For example, six-year-old Jeffrey was chasing his older sister around the house, and he slammed into the side of the dining room table. His father winced, "Oh, boy, that must have been a big hurt!" With a look that implied, "Well, really, Dad, you should know better," Jeffrey replied, "Dad, that wasn't a hurt; that was a whack!" "What's the difference?" asked his puzzled Dad. "Well, don't you know that a whack isn't serious? It's like a bump," said Jeffrey with authority. "But a hurt is serious, like when I cut my leg or when you bleed."

First, to explain their pain, children need to be asked where they are hurting. Second, the questions need to be in age-appropriate language, using familiar words or preferably, the child's own words (refer to Table 3.2 for child appropriate language for medical terms). The word 'pain' is rarely used by children younger than 6 years of age; the word 'hurt' is better understood. (Stanford, Chambers, & Craig, 2005). Third, the child must not feel intimidated by the person asking the questions. If all three conditions are met, the child can become a helpful ally in the process of diagnosing pain and monitoring changes.

If children feel the need to please the questioner, they may say what they sense the person wants to hear. When children feel intimidated by an authority figure, they will again not convey a reliable picture. Younger children are more at risk for this than school-age children. Feeling intimidated or overwhelmed, however, indicates a problem in the clinician-child relationship and can be avoided if the child develops a sense of comfort and trust with the clinician.

32

Myth 5. If a child complains of pain but does not appear to be in pain, the child does not need relief

Some children who report ongoing pain still wish to play, either by themselves or with others. Playing is the normal 'work' of childhood. Central to this myth is the notion of disability that assumes when one is in pain one should not be able to function adequately. This is far from the truth. Pain does not equal disability.

Allie, a ten-year-old patient with juvenile rheumatoid arthritis, had set her heart on joining her brothers and sister water-skiing during their summer holiday. Even though she reported experiencing significant pain in her right wrist and ankle, she chose to go ahead and water-ski. If someone had based a decision on the evidence of her water-skiing, her pain would have been inadequately treated.

You only know if you ask the child directly. These children's desire to maintain involvement in their normal daily life, doing the things that give them meaning and pleasure, despite the pain, is a sign of their psychological resilience and health. This myth persists if pain is regarded as an objective measurable phenomenon, which it is not.

What We Now Know

Pain is a subjective, private, and highly personal experience. It is therefore difficult to assess the presence or absence of another's pain merely by looking. Some children will openly exhibit their pain, some will hint at it, and others will cope by acting as if the pain were not there. If a child says he or she is in pain, the child's pain needs to be attended to and in the process, better assessed. The child is asking for help, and as professionals, we must respond promptly and with compassion. The child does not need to convince us through certain behaviors of the existence of the pain; the child is the authority on whether or not he or she is in pain. Our job is to help.

Myth 6. If a child can be distracted, the child is not in pain

Some nursing or medical professionals have used the method of distracting children from their pain as a diagnostic tool. If the child can be distracted, the myth goes, the pain isn't real. This is based on the assumption that if a child is able to be successfully distracted by a conversation or question, such that the child no longer winces, cries or complains, this indicates that the child's pain isn't that severe.

What We Now Know

Distraction does not exclude the existence of pain, and it cannot be used in that manner as a diagnostic tool. Distracting a child from pain – that is, shifting the child's attention away from the pain – does not indicate that pain is no longer being experienced. It merely indicates that the child is capable at that moment of using cognitive capacities to move his or her focus away from the pain, and so minimize the perception of it at that moment – a useful coping method. It could also indicate that, for the moment that the child chose to focus on something more engaging, like play or a game-boy, the pain was not all-consuming. The gold standard, when assessment is needed, is to ask the child if the hurt is still there. The child's attention will then return to those physical sensations, and the child will accurately assess what is happening in his or her body.

Myth 7. Opioid analgesics are dangerous for children and cause addiction

Until recently, a child in pain post-surgery did not routinely get adequate analgesia. The undertreatment by professionals of children in pain was first exposed in a study in Iowa in 1974, and it took some time for this finding to have the full impact on surgical practice (Eland, 1974). Dr. Joanne Eland compared the medical charts of 25 children with those of 18 adults who had undergone similar surgeries. She found a startling and significant undertreatment of the children's pain, and a wide discrepancy in medication given to children compared to that given to adults. The common finding by other researchers in the 1980s was that because of an ill-founded fear of addiction to opioids and the effects of opioids, medical and nursing staff gave young children and infants significantly less opioid medication than adults for similar pain conditions.

In a landmark case in 1985 in Washington, D.C., Jeffrey Lawson was born prematurely and required heart surgery, common for premature infants (Lee, 2000). His parents were told that he would receive proper anesthetic analgesia. Baby Lawson later died following cardiac surgery. Upon reviewing the chart, his mother discovered he had received anesthesia and a paralyzing agent, but he had received nothing for pain. She pursued legal action, and this case heightened public and professional awareness that infants feel pain and require and deserve effective analgesia during surgery.

Twenty years after Eland's first study, a study re-examined the pain treatment practices for children and adults in the same hospital (Asprey, 1994). This time, children in pain received 968 doses of medication, compared with 24 in the earlier study. Clearly there has been an increased willingness to give children opioids, although attitudes and practices had neither changed overnight, nor everywhere.

What We Now Know

This fear of using strong pain medications, such as opioids (the most common opioid is morphine), especially with children, has had a long history and still persists in some countries. It has hindered the provision of adequate pain relief all over the world. Even in countries where morphine is readily available, there has been the misplaced concern that giving a child morphine will cause respiratory distress. We know that this will not occur when opioids are appropriately administered and monitored carefully .

It is important to dispel immediately the concern about opioid addiction. When a child is in severe pain, the use of opioids will not create an addiction. Unlike people who become addicts when they take drugs for recreation or pleasure, children (or adults) in pain do not become addicted when they take strong analgesics for pain relief.

Over time the child may become more tolerant of the medication and higher levels may be required to relieve pain. This is a physiological dependence, not drug addiction which is a psychological and physiological dependency (see Berde, 2008 p. viii, for a clear and succinct summary). Unlike substance abusers, children on opioids for pain relief are not psychologically dependent on their medication. They use the medication until their pain no longer interferes with their lives. Treatment of a physiological dependence requires a gradual reduction in the medication to control withdrawal symptoms. Using available pain reduction methods and medications with a child before or during a pain episode encourages the child's active participation in reducing the pain and fear and thus prevents feelings of victimization. Children will learn to become 'boss of their own bodies,' even when they are in pain. This goal, a central focus of this book, is valued in child-rearing and pediatric practices, as it promotes a healthy sense of self-efficacy and self-empowerment for children.

Conclusion

In 1986, the International Association for the Study of Pain formed the Special Interest Group on Pain in Childhood (www.child-pain.org) to promote the study of children's pain and to educate the public and practitioners. As pointed out earlier, pain is now regarded as not merely a symptom of a disease, as had previously been thought, but as a human rights issue. It deserves clinical attention and treatment, and is as important as any disease. Today in many pediatric hospital charts, pain is now charted as the fifth vital sign. If present, pain requires ongoing assessment, monitoring, and adequate and comprehensive treatment.

The IASP position is to acknowledge what the child is experiencing, and clinical practices should be based on the conviction that children require being listened to and their pain is to be believed and acknowledged. Pain is real, and children and adolescents are the ultimate authority on their pain. This is the fundamental principle of pain management in children.

Treating children in pain requires a thorough understanding of how the biological, psychological, and social systems interact for pain to be experienced. Chapter 2 takes up the subject of this relationship and draws on the scientific research that led to a radical change in our understanding and treatment of pain.

Chapter 2

How Pain Works

With Jonathan Kuttner, MBBCh, Dip. Sports Med. FACCM

"If there is one experience where the human condition's
universality and the species' biological unity is manifest,
pain is certainly it."

Roselyne Rey, 1995, p. 5

Pain is a function of a conscious brain. The brain is a highly active system that first filters, then selects, modulates, and finally integrates input from various sensory, emotional, and thought processes. The sensory signal is only one of many inputs which will ultimately influence a child's response to pain. Historically we have a great deal of research and information available on sensory input, particularly how acute pain is processed in the periphery of the body and how the nerve impulses move up the spinal cord to the thalamus in the brain (spinothalamic processes). This scientific endeavor, prominent in the nineteenth century, is what the pain pioneer Dr. Ronald Melzack (2008) calls the 'bottom-up approach': how sensory input ascends through neuronal pathways to the brain. For centuries it was believed that a message – like a searing burn in a singed foot – would go up a pain pathway and reach the brain unchanged from when it started in the foot (see Figure 2.1). The notion that the pain system was 'hard-wired' persisted through to the 1960s.

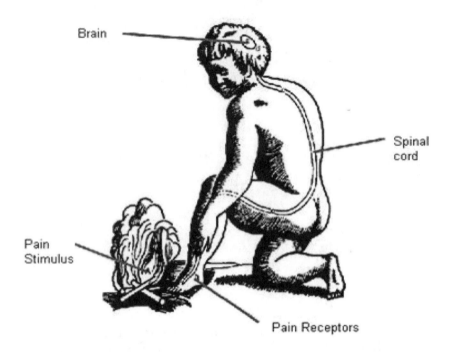

Figure 2.1. The Historic Model of Pain by Descartes. 'The Bottom-up Approach'

It was believed for centuries that pain from an injury would travel through the pain pathways and reach the brain unchanged. The system was thought to be 'hard-wired' such that there was an exact one-to-one correspondence between injury and the perception of the pain.

Our future progress in pain management lies in a 'top-down' approach. Twenty-first century pain research is focused on understanding how the descending pathways of the brain and spinal cord modulate pain. With functional Magnetic Resonance Imaging (fMRI), we now know that there are extensive brain areas involved in pain processes, and these connect to a widely distributed neural network. The major challenge in future work is to better understand the complexity of how the brain functions, and the role it plays in all types of pain – particularly chronic pain – as well as in recovery.

This chapter provides some of the current understanding on how pain works. We'll examine how the pain message is transmitted from an injury occuring in the body to the brain and becomes the experience of pain. We'll discuss how pain can be controlled at different sites and some of the puzzles of pain. We'll look at Melzack and Wall's gate control theory and Melzack's current concept of the 'neuromatrix', proposed to better understand how stress, emotions, cognitive functions, and heredity interweave in the experience of chronic pain. Children are empowered to handle their pain once they understand how pain works in the brain-body system and how interventions could potentially reduce their pain. This chapter will conclude with providing this information in a conversation with a child in pain.

A definition of pain, first used in nursing in 1968 by Margo McCaffery, is still widely accepted today: "Pain is whatever the experiencing person says it is, existing whenever he says it does" (1972, p. 8). Pain is an 'inside' experience, and there is no reliable external measure for it. The scientific evidence described in this chapter further endorses the simple wisdom and accuracy of this definition. Pain is highly individual and governed by the brain.

The Processing of Pain

A favourite ditty of mine is, "The strain of pain lies solely in the brain." As Dr. Melzack says the central nervous system, consisting of the spinal cord and brain, is highly dynamic. Sensations arising from the body, perceptions, emotions, memories, and behavioral responses constantly interact within this neural circuitry. When pain is experienced it is a unified stream of these experiences generated by the brain (Melzack & Wall, 2008).

We begin the story of pain at the periphery, when pain has just occurred.

A child trips in the playground, falls, and skins his shin. He feels an immediate sharp stinging pain and yells out "Ow!" A few seconds later a deep aching pain arises which makes him moan and hold onto his leg. We will now explore how this happens. This everyday accident sets off a cascade of events in his body and nervous system ending up in his brain.

Nociception

The beginning of this cascade is called *nociception*. This refers to the unconscious detection of tissue damage in the sense receptors, peripheral nerves, spinal column, and brain. This is different from the perception of pain, which is a conscious experience.

The initial process of nociception is *transduction*. Noxious stimuli are detected by the free nerve endings in the viscera (organs) or somatic tissue (joints, ligaments, tendons, muscles, and fascia). Transduction involves either a mechanical or a chemical process or both.

Mechanical nociception occurs when tissue is stretched. These tissues contain nerve endings that weave between collagen fibers. When stretched, the fibers twist and squeeze the stretch receptors in the nerve endings, thus stimulating them. This process occurs in ligaments, tendons, joint capsules, and the capsules around organs such as the liver and kidneys.

Chemical nociception occurs when the nerve endings are exposed to pain-inducing substances. These are part of the so-called 'inflammatory soup' which is released in the body after injury. Hydrogen ions, potassium ions, serotonin, histamine, prostaglandins, and Substance P are all liberated into the damaged tissue. These stimulate the chemoreceptors at the terminal of the peripheral nerves.

Nerve-Fiber Transmission

The next step in the child's pain process is *nerve-fiber transmission*, which occurs initially within the peripheral nervous system. The child's nociceptive signal is very rapidly transmitted via nerve fibers to the spinal cord and brain.

Two kinds of nerve fibers transmit messages about injury or tissue changes: C fibers, which are small and transmit sensation slowly, and A delta fibers, which are larger and transmit sensation more rapidly. Both have smaller diameters than the A beta fibers which rapidly transmit sensations of touch, vibration, and position sense. C fibers transmit messages very slowly because they are unmyelinated. Yet C fibers are polymodal: they respond to mechanical, thermal, and chemical stimuli. Although both A delta and C fibers relay messages from heat, chemical, or mechanical stimulation, they produce different qualities of pain.

So, revisiting the child hugging his sore, bleeding shin ... The immediate sharp, stinging pain of the injured tissue on the child's shin was produced by the more rapidly activated A delta fibers. A second or two later, the smaller and more slowly conducting C fibers produced a burning, more diffuse pain sensation that outlasted the initial stinging pain, and kept the child guarding and protecting his leg. It is essential that we have both of those types of pain fibers. If we didn't have the A delta fibers, the first sharp pain may not have been felt which warns a child to pull his leg immediately away from danger.

Central Transmission

The following step in the pain process is *central transmission*. The nerve-fiber transmission from the child's shin injury then enters the dorsal root entry zone in the dorsal horn of the spinal cord (see Figure 2.2). Different zones have been mapped out, and these nerve fibers enter and divide mainly in lamina 1 and 2 (in Figure 2.2) in this part of the spinal cord. The peripheral nerves end in the nuclei and then synapse with second order interneurons (see Figure 2.2). There are excitatory and inhibitory interneurons in the spinal cord.

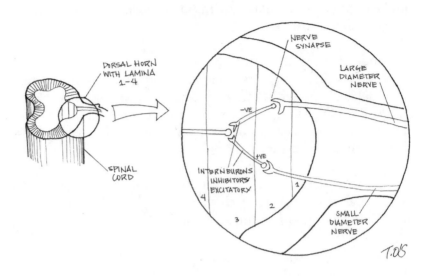

Figure 2.2. Central Transmission

In central transmission, pain signals from the child's leg enter the dorsal horn in the spinal cord at lamina 1 and 2. The synapses that occur with the second order interneurons there can be either excitatory or inhibitory, which leads to pain modulation.

Modulation

This complex interaction sets up the subsequent step in the pain pathway – which is *modulation*. This vital concept of modulation furthers our understanding of how all messages coming from the body can be altered within the pain system. The modification of the pain signal as it travels from one neuron to the next, results in feeling more pain, or beginning to feel some relief. It is also the basis of most chronic pain problems.

When one nerve fiber, such as a C fiber, converses with a neighboring nerve cell in the spinal cord, neurotransmitters are released from the first cell to its neighbor (see Figure 2.3). The transmitter carries the message across the synaptic gap. There are many different functional types of neurotransmitters or neuropeptides.

44

These include glutamate, Substance P, cholecystokinin, neurotensin, somatostatin, and many others. The peptide Substance P is considered to be the main nociceptive transmitter. (P stands not for pain, but for the powder in which it was isolated!) Researchers found that C fibers synthesize substance P, and it is carried into the spinal cord where it is stored to be released when 'pain' messages are activated.

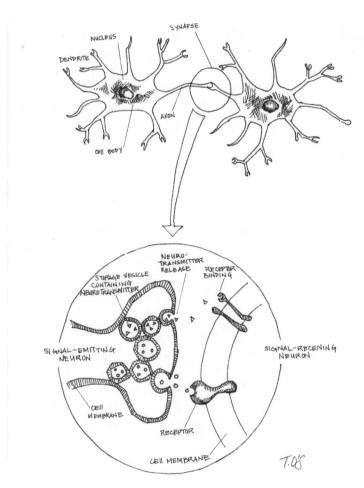

Figure 2.3. Nerves talk to one another.

When one nerve converses with a neighboring nerve cell, neurotransmitters, carrying the signal, are released from one cell to the other across the synaptic gap.

Substance P, released following injury, can spread over large distances in the spinal cord, exciting those cells which transmit the injury message to the brain. It comes closest to being the 'pain' transmitter in the body. This wide release can also explain why some pains are difficult to localize and why some injuries often result in an achy sensation over a large region of the body, persisting longer than expected.

The transmitters attach to receptors in the second-order neurons. The message can be suppressed or facilitated by different transmitters attaching to specific receptors on the second-order neurons. The most important is the NMDA receptor. This is an amplifier that is difficult to turn on. However, once it is turned on, it is very difficult to turn off, and forms the basis of much chronic pain. This is the first level of modulation, and is fundamental to our present understanding of how plastic or changeable the pain system is. The message coming in is not the same as the message going out.

The message then crosses the midline of the spinal cord to ascend the spinothalamic tract to higher levels along the tract. You can follow this pathway in Figure 2.4. Here the level of complexity rapidly increases. When the message reaches the brain stem, there are some structures that inhibit transmission (the peri-ventricular grey matter, nucleus raphe magnus, and the lateral medullary reticular formation).

There is also an extremely important *descending modulatory system* (see Figure 2.4). This is part of the 'top-down' system and arises in the brain from the cortex. The descending modulatory system also acts as a form of filter to increase the clarity of incoming nociceptive stimuli. If this modulation does not work, then biologically important noxious stimuli could be lost in the background noise from the other neural activity in the spinal cord. It acts by inhibiting all spinal segments except the one receiving the noxious stimulus and therefore increases the clarity of the incoming signal.

Once the message of pain reaches the brain stem, it divides into two pathways, which appear to transmit different types of pain information. Sharp or acute pain travels up to the thalamus (a complex central integrating and relay center), whereas achy pain, which is

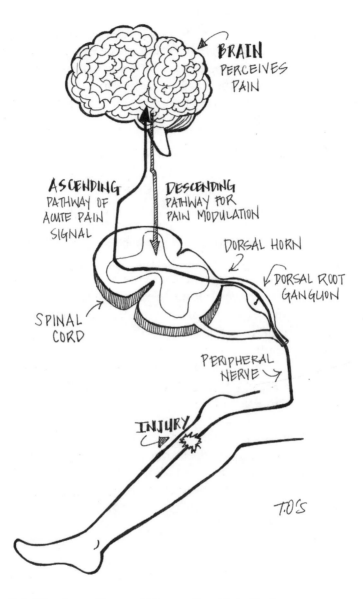

Figure 2.4. The Ascending and Descending Pain Pathways.

When the child skinned his knee the sensory message travels to the brain stem and brain where modulation of the pain signal can occur. The descending modulation arising from the cortex travels down and is part of the 'top-down' system in which brain actively filters, selects, modulates and integrates all of these dimensions in the final pain experience.

more diffuse and difficult to localize is carried to the reticular formation in the brain stem. As the pain message reaches the higher brain centers, it combines with a wide range of other information in the brain, including beliefs, thoughts, emotions, memories, and sensory input, such as smell, sight and sound. The brain actively filters, selects, modulates and integrates all of these dimensions in the final pain experience.

The brain decides if what is being experienced is 'pain' and how to deal with it. If alarmed by the nerve impulses, the system speeds up the transmission and intensity of the pain. If the brain determines that the pain is tolerable and not alarming, a descending inhibitory control system is activated. The child's cortex for example, recalls having experienced a fall before, and remembers that he needs a Band-aid to feel better. This accessed memory triggers a complex set of decisions which activate his descending modulation system. He stops crying and limps his way to the school's nursing station for the Band-aid solution. As mentioned in Chapter 1, natural body-based pain-relieving substances (endorphins – morphine-like substances produced by the body) are released by the brain through the spinal cord, and together with other modulating substances, such as serotonin and norepinephrine, ease the experience of pain.

The nerve impulses alone are not the pain; only after they have reached the brain and have been processed, are they defined: to be or not to be experienced as 'pain'. For convenience, terms such as 'pain message' or 'pain pathways' are used to describe the nerve impulse. Bear in mind, that until this impulse reaches the brain, it is just that – an impulse, devoid of meaning.

Pain Control

Pain can be physiologically controlled within the brain and body in numerous ways. What begins as a potentially strong pain message in one part of the body is not necessarily transmitted to the brain and interpreted as a strong pain message. Let's explore what is known about brain-body pain control systems.

During the twentieth century, the pain network ascending along the spinal cord to the brain, as well as the descending control from the brain to the spinal cord, were extensively researched. One of the most celebrated pain researchers is Canadian psychologist Dr. Ronald Melzack, who with British physiologist Dr. Patrick Wall, wrote the 1964 classic *The Puzzle of Pain*, revised in 1973 and 2008 as *The Challenge of Pain*. They proposed the Gate Control Theory of Pain.

The Gate Control Theory of Pain

A pain signal goes through various physiological 'gates' which either increase or decrease the amount of pain information transmitted along the pain pathways (see Figure 2.5). These gates occur at many sites, from the source of the pain to spinothalamic tract, up to the brain and down again from the brain to the pain – allowing pain to be modulated at any site. Here are some examples of gating along the brain-pain network.

Gating in the Spinal Cord

Nerve fibers converge as they enter the spinal cord. The spinal nerve cells respond to both painful and non-painful stimulation, because they receive input both from large touch- and movement-sensitive A beta fibers and from the smaller pain A delta and C fibers. Rubbing a painful area stimulates the large movement-sensitive A beta fibers that respond to tactile stimulation and muscle movement but not to painful sensation. This inhibits cells in the spinal cord that transmit the pain message from the small C fibers, and so the message in the cord is decreased before it reaches the brain. Children learn quickly that if they gently rub a sore leg, it feels better more rapidly than if they don't rub it. By rubbing the injured site, they activate a pain 'gating' mechanism.

Another way to activate large fibers is to use a device to produce transcutaneous electrical nerve stimulation (TENS). This

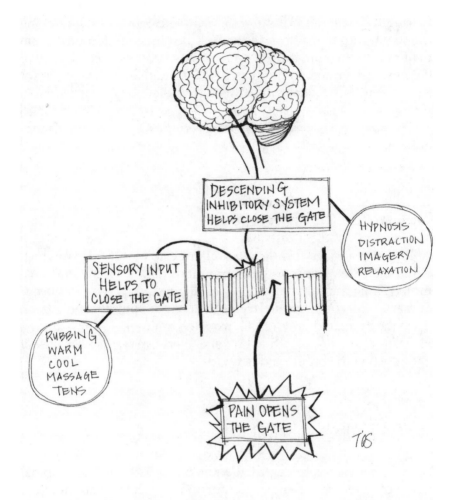

Figure 2.5. Gate Control Theory of Pain

Melzack and Wall proposed that the degree to which the various gates are open or closed determines whether the pain signal is inhibited or moves on. Sensory input that is competitive, such as massage or rubbing helps close the gate. Cognitive-behavioral methods, such as distraction or hypnosis work through the descending inhibitory system to close the gate.

technique, developed by Drs. Melzack and Wall, consists of a small battery-powered unit with electrodes that are placed on the skin at specific sites. The pulse interferes with the pain signal before it reaches the brain. Pain relief can sometimes continue for several hours after using TENS. This is described in more detail in Chapter 6.

Gating in the Brain

Biofeedback clearly illustrates how the brain can 'gate' those physiological functions previously considered outside voluntary control, such as heart rate and body temperature. With biofeedback, a body signal, such as heart rate, muscle tension, or temperature, is electrically monitored and fed back so that child can change the signal. Children can successfully be trained to use biofeedback techniques to alter their biological functions. These include decreasing the tension in the frontalis muscle in the forehead to relieve tension headaches, increasing fingertip temperature to help manage a migraine headache, and increasing rectal sphincter control for bowel problems. Biofeedback demonstrates in a measurable way a child's capability for enhancing well-being by using brain-body interaction (discussed further in Chapter 5).

The Role of Emotions in Gating Pain

Deep in the center of the brain is the limbic system, key to emotion. Stress, mood and emotions interact and are affected by the endocrine system and corticol release (a stress hormone). These influence the experience of pain. In the following examples, three children of the same age have a leg injury, but their different moods and circumstances change their pain experience.

Sara with a sore leg is distressed and getting increasingly wound up. The adults around her are attending to her pain, trying to make her more comfortable. She is watching everything, and this intense attention, in turn, leads to greater responsivity to the pain signals. However, when Sara's attention is directed to a playful pop-up book that she finds quite engrossing, she is able to distract herself from her sore leg for a few minutes and calm down. Her shift of attention temporarily and partially closes the gate on the pain signal in her brain, modulating the pain experience so that she is not bothered as much by the pain during that time. Without this alternative focus, she would feel the pain more intensely. This use of selective attention is the principle behind cognitive-behavioral pain management techniques of imagery and distraction.

Lizzie has a sore leg and is distressed and anxious. She is not absorbed in anything other than her pain. She is wound up and becoming more anxious, which leads to greater behavioral reactions and distress about the pain. Lizzie has become intensely focused on the pain, absorbed in its every aspect. With this anxiety, she releases adrenaline and other substances which lower her pain threshold and heighten her pain sensitivity. The pain gates in her brain are wide open, allowing all of the pain information to flood into her brain. Lizzie feels more pain than Sara.

Meghan, in contrast to the other children, has had leg pain on and off for several months, which has interfered with sports so that she is hardly active anymore. She feels disappointed and frustrated, and is in despair, believing that her leg will never recover. With depression, the brain's pain gates tend to stay wide open, allowing for fuller pain perception and with little downward inhibitory modulation. The pain leads to greater fatigue and feelings of hopelessness. We now know that neurotransmitter substances, such as serotonin, become depleted with depression, which in turn increases the pain. Meghan's pain is not well managed. She is in a depression-pain cycle, deconditioned, and the persistent pain tires her. This increases her feelings of helplessness and maintains her responsiveness to her leg pain. Of the three children, Meghan suffers the most. (Antidepressant medication in low or normal doses can be very helpful in treating persistent pain associated with irritability, anxiety, and interrupted sleep and eating patterns. Even if Meghan appears not overtly depressed, such medication can relieve both pain and its associated problems.)

Endogenous Opioids

Now let us explore the specific pain control systems in our brain. Electrically stimulating the periaqueductal gray (PAG), a key gating area, was found to activate a powerful pain control system, blocking pain messages from the spinal cord to the cortex. It became evident that the PAG electrical stimulation activated the same brain mechanisms as the opioid analgesic morphine. How do morphine and other opioids provide such powerful pain control? The short answer is that they produce pain relief by mimicking the action of the brain's own opioid system, our *endogenous opioids*.

As noted earlier, scientists have discovered that our bodies are capable of producing our own opioids – endorphins – and that we have receptors for these opioids throughout our peripheral and central nervous systems. Dr. Christoph Stein (1995), an anesthesiologist at Johns Hopkins University, demonstrated that many cells of the immune system also synthesize endorphins. In the presence of inflammation, for example, the immune system can mobilize cells that travel to the site of injury, releasing endorphins, which reduce the transmission of pain. We now know that when morphine is injected into the bloodstream it travels to the brain, binding with opioid receptors in the PAG and turning on the same pain control system that was activated by electrical brain stimulation. The brain and other organs, including the stomach and bowel, have opioid receptors, which explains why pain control isn't the only effect that is produced by opioids such as morphine. Adverse effects, including lowered blood pressure, constipation, and depression of the respiratory, cardiovascular, and gastrointestinal systems also occur, and need to be taken into account when using morphine (see Chapter 7).

Hypnosis

Hypnosis is an altered state of consciousness, achieved through a narrowing of attention and focused concentration. During a hypnotic trance, the subject focuses on reducing, altering, or creating distance from the pain – and in this process changes pain perception. Children are highly responsive to hypnosis and can be trained to use self-hypnosis for injuries and many illnesses. For example, it has been found effective in the treatment of burns, cancer, chronic headaches, asthma, wart removal, enuresis, tics, and eczema management (Olness & Kohen, 1996). Naloxone, which is used to reverse the effects of morphine (an antagonist), did not block the effect of hypnotic pain reduction, so it appears that hypnosis acts by a different mechanism (Goldstein & Hilgard,1975; Barber & Mayer, 1977). The neurophysiological mechanism by which hypnosis enables a child or adult alleviate their suffering is not known. We know that the rate and the degree of pain modification achieved by hypnosis can be dramatic. This has been experimentally and clinically well-documented (Hilgard & Hilgard, 1994; Barber & Adrian,1982, Barber, 2004). Hypnotic pain control is a fascinating reminder that our complex pain network does not faithfully transmit the pain signal, and our consciousness appears to be the final arbiter of pain. (For a fuller discussion of hypnosis, see Chapter 5.)

How and Where Medications and Other Common Treatments Work in the Pain System

Pain, particularly severe pain, can be effectively controlled by analgesic medication. The medications available for use in hospitals and home are detailed in Chapter 7. Following is a brief explanation of how these commonly used analgesics work (see also Figure 2.6).

- *Acetaminophen,* one of the most popular analgesics. It is used to lower temperature and to provide pain relief. Although it is widely available and generally safely used, scientists still do not know exactly how it achieves both peripheral and central pain relief. We do know that it acts primarily in the higher centers of the brain.

- *Non-Steroidal Anti-Inflammatory Drugs (NSAIDs)* have a dual action. They work at the site of the pain by counteracting the chemicals, in particular prostaglandins which cause local inflammation, and therefore they reduce pain transduction. They also act in the central nervous system in a similar manner to acetaminophen. The purely analgesic action occurs at lower doses and is actually their major effect in most painful conditions.

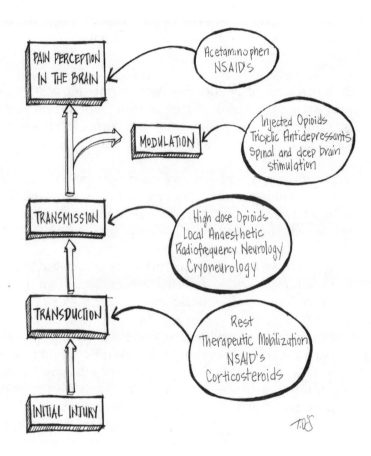

Figure 2.6. How and Where Medications and Other Common Treatments Work in the Pain System [Modified from the original. Used with permission from Dr. Nikolai Bogduk]

- *Corticosteroids* are potent anti-inflammatory agents. Although not primarily analgesics, they can be used to control pain, particularly cancer pain. They work by blocking chemical reactions earlier in the pathway for the synthesis of prostaglandins. If taken over a long time, they have serious side effects, such as interfering with bone growth, elevating blood pressure, and interfering with blood-glucose control.

- *Local anesthetics* block transmission of messages; however their effect is temporary. They can be useful blocking pain during procedures that would otherwise cause pain.

- *Radiofrequency Neurotomy* and *Cryoneurotomy:* coagulating and freezing the nerve can destroy the transmission of impulses. These are used for longer term relief of painful conditions such as neuralgia or pain arising from facet joints in the spine. This treatment is more commonly used in adults.

- *Opioids,* such as morphine, a synthetic compound derived from the opium-producing poppy plant, alter transmission and modulation of the pain message mainly in the brain and spinal cord. They work in two ways:

  1. Opioids decrease the pain messages sent to the brain by inhibiting the nerve cells in the spinal cord that receive C nerve fiber messages, and

  2. Opoids alter the manner in which the brain perceives the pain stimulus. By binding to the brain's opioid receptors, opioids activate the powerful descending inhibitory control systems that shut down the transmission of pain messages in the spinal cord. These receptors are also used by the body through its own endorphins and enkephalins, which are powerful short-acting natural pain relievers.

  Opioids are effective for severe acute pain, post-surgery pain, pain during medical procedures, and pain related to cancer, AIDS, and sickle cell disease. They create a feeling of distance from the pain, and so there is less awareness of the pain. As pointed out earlier, because opioid receptors occur in many organs of the body and brain, they produce some adverse effects, such as lowered blood pressure (usually associated with rapid administration), constipation, and slowing of the respiratory and gastrointestinal systems.

- *Epidurals: spinal injections of morphine* can block pain for up to 24 hours, whereas the same dose given through the bloodstream will control pain for only three or four hours. As a result, spinal injections of morphine are now commonly used for children in the hospital. Although this method produces very good pain relief, especially for certain surgical procedures, it is not a panacea. The opioids infiltrated into the fluid surrounding the spinal cord travel up to the brain, and can produce unpleasant side effects, such as nausea, vomiting, itching, and urinary retention. Spinal opioids can be mixed with local anesthetics, adding to their pain coverage to combat pain from surgical procedures, injuries, or invasive diseases. They are also used pre-emptively to prevent the onset of pain, or the return of pain post-surgery.

- *Spinal cord and deep brain stimulation* involves the insertion of wires either into the epidural space around the spine or into the grey matter of the brain. These create a tingling sensation which interferes with transmission or perception of pain signals. Spinal cord stimulation has been used to treat Complex Regional Pain Syndrome (CRPS) that has been unresponsive to other therapies.

Puzzles in the Pain Process

There are some puzzles in the processing of pain messages. With our growing understanding of pain, some of these puzzles can now be explained, but others remain unsolved, and remind us of the intricacy and complexity of the pain process.

Why don't we experience the same pain every time from the same injury?

One might think that a large injury should always result in a large amount of pain. This is not necessarily true because, as we have discussed, the pain message can be altered via modulation in many areas along the pain pathway. Many variables influence the quality and intensity of the pain experience. The meaning, mood, and context of the pain for a child varies, affecting and interacting with the physiologic release of chemical substances. Our pain systems are not fixed or rigid but are highly plastic. Children may respond differently to the same pain stimulus, depending on a multitude of factors, including genetic patterns, culturally learned attitudes, the social context, and their energy and emotional state.

As an example, this was four year-old Callie's experience. She had a diagnosis of Acute Lymphocytic Leukemia, which required regular blood drawn from her finger. When she went into the lab and Anna was there, she relaxed knowing that Anna would warm her finger in a playful way before directing her to squeeze the scrunchie in her other hand at the same time as her finger was deftly 'poked'. However, when Anna wasn't there Callie immediately tensed up, called for her Mom and clung to her, because she did not feel safe with the new lab technician. These blood draws always took longer and were more distressing and more painful for her.

Why is pain in one area felt in another area?

Pain isn't always what it appears to be. Our complex pain system has a curious manifestation known as *referred pain*. For example, an injury to the upper neck is often referred upwards and you perceive it as a headache. Headaches are a very common symptom in children. The mechanism of referral is by *convergence*.

This is how it works. First the injury occurs in the upper neck segments of the C1, C2, or C3 spinal nerves, and the painful messages are picked up by the nerve endings in those segments. These messages are transmitted to their respective nuclei in the grey matter of the upper spinal cord and lower brain stem. The nucleus is the actual living cell, the nerve is an extension from the cell. The nucleus needs to be stimulated for the message to be transmitted upwards to the brain.

The fifth cranial nerve or the trigeminal nerve in the body transmits its information from the head and face to the trigemino-cervical nucleus. This is a very long structure, and as you can see in Figure 2.7, the lower portion of this nucleus runs parallel and very close to the nuclei of C1/2/3. Any activity in the trigeminal nucleus will result in the perception of a headache.

The information from your neck arrives at the C1/2/3 nuclei. It spreads or converges into the fifth cranial nerve nucleus and stimulates it as well. All this information then moves upwards to the thalamus and cortex. Unable to distinguish the origin of this information, the brain interprets activity in the trigeminal nucleus (actually evoked by the upper cervical spine stimulation) as a headache, which is typically perceived as pain in the forehead, behind the eyes or in the temples. This is one very common cause of the so-called 'tension headache'.

Appendicitis pain is another example of referred pain. An acutely inflamed appendix, located in the lower right quadrant of the belly, can be first experienced as diffuse pain around the belly button and not pain in the location of the appendix. The nerve supply for the appendix is T10. When the appendix is inflamed, the nociceptive impulse is localized by the brain to this segment. The information, as is the case with all visceral pain, is poorly differentiated so that the brain perceives it as a deep, dull, and diffuse pain in the T10 distribution, which is the peri-umbilical region. This is visceral referred pain. Later the actual inflammation irritates the abdominal wall in the right lower quadrant of the abdomen. This is a somatic structure and the information is now localized to the actual area of the appendix. This presentation may be initially confusing and reminds us of the particular complexity of visceral pain.

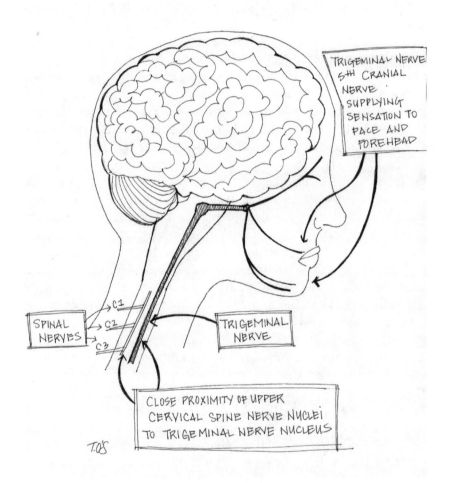

Figure 2.7. Referred Pain: How a headache is experienced from cervical nerve injury.

Because of the close proximity of the C-spine nuclei to the trigeminal nerve nucleus, if there is in any injury to C 1, 2, or 3, this can affect the trigeminal nucleus and will be felt as pain in the head. This is the concept of referred pain. Pain occurs at one point in the C-spine, converges, stimulating the fifth cranial nerve nucleus and spreads along the nerve to be experienced in the head as headache.

Why do some muscles become painful without experiencing direct injury?

Pain also affects muscles and ligaments and is called myofascial pain. This pain arises from the fascia, which are the thin but tough membranes covering muscle. It can manifest in many different ways, such as recurrent tension headaches, back pain, or widespread achy muscles. There are tiny structures within skeletal muscle called *muscle spindles*. These consist of nerves coiled in a spiral pattern which will fire when the spindle reaches a critical length. When it fires, the message synapses in the spinal cord and returns via a motor nerve to stimulate the muscle to shorten. This is the simplest reflex arc, part of a protective reflex used constantly for posture. When this reflex malfunctions, the muscles become tight and painful, developing sensitive trigger-point areas. These points trigger or radiate the pain into another point of the body, especially when the muscle is used or the trigger point of the muscle is pressed (Lavelle, Lavelle, & Smith, 2007).

One kind of pain can cause another kind of pain. For example, arthritis in a joint can turn on myofascial trigger points on muscles around the joint. The contracted muscles themselves become a source of pain. In addition, chronically painful muscles may cause changes in posture and spasms of surrounding muscle groups, spreading the pain. The main cause of pain spreading most probably occurs in the central nervous system where areas in the thalamus and cortex are 'turned on'. We then perceive the pain area as widened. Treatment options such as physical therapy, relaxation techniques, TENS, ultrasound, massage, and medication are necessary to break the persisting cycle.

How does persistent pain develop from acute pain?

Another piece of the pain puzzle is how the various nerve fibers interact with each other and change as a result of an injury. Neuroplasticity is now regarded as a significant contributor to chronic pain. Nerve fibers themselves can be damaged when the body suffers injury and cause various effects. Their moderating influence on the C fibers decreases or is lost. When nerve fibers are injured, they no longer behave normally, as they do in an acute pain situation, but become irritable. Often the fibers spontaneously send impulses and are not able to stop. The pain signals can be insistent and troubling. The brain may interpret the increased C fiber activity as arising from severe injury even though the actual damage is mild or non-existent, and with this, changes occur in the brain and greater pain is felt (see the discussion later in this chapter of the 'neuromatrix').

Pain due to nerve injury (neuropathic pain) usually has a burning quality. This pain is no longer protective or helpful, as it is not representative of actual damage. The nervous system has changed. There is altered or sometimes enhanced transmission of pain-sensory information. Specific nerve fibers have become irritated and more sensitive. Neuropathic pain is a devastating consequence of injury to the peripheral nerves and is difficult to treat. In neuropathic conditions there are two specific phenomena. The first is 'hyperalgesia' in which a pain sensation is perceived as more painful. The second is 'allodynia' where normally innocuous sensation is perceived as pain: for example, just touching the area may provoke significant pain. With neuropathic pain there are both neurochemical and neurophysiological changes that are still poorly understood, but can impede the healing and repair process.

How does injury cause a 'memory' of pain?

When an injury persists and pain is not effectively controlled, long-term changes in the spinal cord and brain occur which creates a 'memory' for pain. A fascinating breakthrough has been the discovery of genes that are 'turned on' by pain. With painful stimulation, the gene activity that synthesizes and regulates neurotransmitters dramatically increases. Instead of thinking of the pain-transmission pathway as a telephone cable that merely sends information from one place to the next (as shown in Figure 2.1), think of it as a voice mail system. As the pain message enters the central nervous system (CNS), molecular changes occur that establish a memory trace of the injury. This is able to be stored for long periods of time. Furthermore this memory trace in the CNS is able to influence the subsequent transmission of information along this pathway. The memory of pain can therefore be more damaging than its initial experience (Song & Carr, 1999). This finding provides a compelling reason for treating children's pain as soon as possible (von Baeyer, Marche, et al., 2004).

Why may surgery not be the best intervention for persistent pain?

The discovery that the body 'remembers' pain throws more light on why surgical interventions to relieve chronic pain have only limited success. It used to be thought that simply cutting the fibers, as one would a telephone wire, that carry the pain message to the brain, would provide pain relief. We now know that cutting the fibers rarely relieves pain, or does so only transiently.

Unlike a telephone wire, the body tries to heal the severed nerve portions of the peripheral nervous system. If the outer sheath of the nerve has been cut, then the actual nerve grows out into a bundle called a *neuroma*. This is exquisitely tender, and even minor pressure causes an electric-shock-like pain. Consequently, surgical interventions for chronic pain where the nerve is actually cut are now infrequently performed. Instead, techniques that do not destroy the outer sheath but only the nerve within it are now preferred. In this case, either a heat probe (most commonly using microwave and called Radiofrequency Neurotomy) or cold probe (cryotherapy) is used. The nerve will regrow in months to years, but by this stage the chronic pain cycle has been broken. Often the original chronic pain does not return. If it does, the process can be repeated. If the ganglion (the actual nerve cell) is destroyed, then the nerve will not grow again. However there is a small risk of setting off a phantom-limb-like pain after such a procedure, and thus it is infrequently used with children or adolescents.

The use of spinal cord stimulators has been increasing. In this, a fine lead is inserted into the epidural space just outside the spinal cord. This is attached to a device which gives a small electrical stimulation to the spinal cord. This 'closes the gate' and effectively reduces pain messages from the painful area, such as for CRPS.

Damage to the central nervous system was previously thought to be irreversible. It was believed that the nerves that have been cut in the brain and the spinal cord never regenerate normal connections. There is growing evidence that nerve cells may regenerate. Recently researchers discovered that we produce substances which inhibit the regeneration of damaged nerves. The search continues for ways to turn this inhibition off so that the nerves will regrow and reconnect. This has extraordinary implications for recovery from spinal cord injury, strokes, and neurological diseases.

How can pain last when the painful site no longer exists?

Sometimes practitioners cannot find a reason for the child's pain and conclude that it is not 'real' pain, despite the child's evident distress and reports to the contrary. Phantom-limb pain exemplifies the fallacy that pain has to be located in the body to be real. Phantom pain is not physically located in the body, but is an experience generated in the brain that feels as if it were in the body. One report indicated that 48.5% of children and adults experience pain in an absent limb after it was amputated as a result of an injury or disease (Wilkins, McGrath, & Finley, 1998). Children will report sharp, throbbing pain or itching in a limb that is no longer there. It is evident that the child is in pain and suffering, yet the source of the pain, the injured limb, had been surgically removed, weeks, months or years before. Some report that over time the sensation of the limb either telescopes or shrinks upwards. This is truly a memory held in the central nervous system.

Phantom-limb pain reveals the powerful role of the brain in pain perception. The brain does more than detect and interpret sensory input – it can generate pain. The child knows the limb is gone, but the child's brain spontaneously generates and interprets signals within its neural networks as pain. While the neurological mechanisms of phantom pain are still not fully understood, we do know that if the child had severe pain before amputation, it is more likely that the child will experience phantom pain after surgery. It seems that the brain and neural pathways had mapped in that input. This can cause a lot of suffering. Sometimes, with appropriate treatment and over time this pain may diminish. Some studies suggest that by blocking this pain with intensive pre-, intra-, and post-operative epidural infusions of local anesthetic and opioids, phantom limb pain may be reduced (Berde, Lebel, & Olson, 2003).

The ingenious use of the mirror box that creates the illusion that the amputated hand has returned, has been an exciting and novel approach to therapy devised by neurologist V. S. Ramachandran (Ramachandran & Blakeslee, 1998; Ramachandran & Hirstein, 1998). The mirror is placed vertically in the centre of a wooden box whose top and front surfaces have been removed. The patient places his normal hand on one side and looks into the mirror, seeing an illusion of the returned amputated hand. This experience can help the somatosensory and motor cortex reorganize and remap. In the first reference the researchers report their findings of mirror box therapy with 10 patients. In four patients the mirror had no effect. However in six patients, when the normal hand moved so that the phantom hand was perceived to be moving in the mirror, kinesthetic sensations were experienced in the phantom hand, which was also felt to move. In one patient with three weeks of practice ten minutes per day, the phantom hand telescoped back into the shoulder stump for the first time in ten years. This led to the permanent disappearance of his phantom arm and the pain. Further studies with adults with upper limb phantom pain have found this approach to have therapeutic merit. They found a higher amount of motor reorganization with amputees whose daily used of their prosthesis was less frequent, which also tended to be related to experiencing more severe phantom limb pain (Karl, Mühlnickel, Kurth & Flor, 2004). Phantom pain exemplifies the primacy and complexity of the brain in maintaining the pain experience and the challenge of providing timely pain management to prevent ongoing traumatic pain.

Understanding Chronic Pain

Pain hurts. Yet understanding this in children with chronic pain isn't straightforward (Figure 1.1). While acute pains, such as the child's shin injury, have been meticulously investigated and their sensory transmission is now well understood, in contrast, much of chronic pain remains a mystery. As previously explained, chronic pain persists long after the healing is complete. It is often out of proportion to the original injury and is usually not successfully treated by conventional methods. In many ways chronic pain is itself the disease – the result of neural mechanisms gone awry.

Pain that persists can lead to anxiety and depression. There is a great deal we need to know about the mechanisms by which persistent or chronic pain causes alterations in pain perception, changes in mood, and impaired decision-making ability. We know that patients suffering from anxiety and depression experience pain more strongly and are more likely to develop chronic pain. Pain also impairs cortical function such as the ability to think clearly and make advantageous decisions. Acute pain appears to activate the prefrontal cortex, while pain that persists deactivates it (Neugebauer, Galhardo, Maione, & Mackey, 2009). Understanding these complex interactions will greatly improve the assessment and management of chronic pain.

Scientists are actively exploring the neural pathways in the brain using neuroimaging. Findings indicate that neither the cortex nor the thalamus can be identified as a single 'pain center' (Neugebauer et al., 2009). The areas of the brain involved in the pain experience and behavior are very extensive, including the limbic system, vestibular and visual mechanisms, cognitive processes, and somatosensory projections. To make sense of these multiple neural inputs and circuitry processing possibilities, the pain pioneer Dr. Ronald Melzack (1999) has proposed a new theory of pain, the Neuromatrix.

From the Gate Control Theory to the Neuromatrix

The gate control theory, discussed earlier, emphasized the central neural mechanisms in pain processing. The neuromatrix theory goes further in an attempt to understand brain function during chronic pain. Research using imaging techniques revealed that pain occurs in widely distributed areas of the brain that are highly interconnected (Melzack,1999). This led Melzack to propose the concept that pain is generated by a 'body-self neuromatrix' – a highly integrated neural network comprising many sources of neural inputs to the body-brain (sense of self) and outputs to brain areas that produce pain perception, action, and stress-regulation (see Figure 2.8). This, Melzack proposed, creates a unified experience of self, and produces the multiple dimensions of the pain experience:

> Pain is not injury; the quality of pain experiences must not be confused with the physical event of breaking skin... the qualities of experience must be generated by structures in the brain... by in-built neuromodules whose neurosignatures innately produce the qualities.... We do not learn to feel qualities of experience: our brains are built to produce them. (p.87)

The output patterns, the 'signature' of the body-self neuromatrix, activates perceptual, homeostatic, and behavioral patterns after an injury, illness, or chronic stress. This proposed matrix is the primary mechanism that generates the neural pattern that produces the pain. It is genetically determined and is modified by sensory experiences – but this sensory input is only one of several contributions. Mood and fearful or anxious thoughts also converge to modify this neuromatrix.

How the Neuromatrix Helps Explain the Puzzle of Complex Pain

Melzack's neuromatrix theory incorporates and recognizes the role of the stress system in pain processes. It proposes that the individual's neurosignature pattern can also be modulated by physical and psychological stresses which act on the body's complex stress-regulation systems. Psychological stress is not the only type of stress that pain causes. As Hans Selye (1956) articulated many years ago, stress is a biological system, triggered by any threat to the body's homeostasis including physical injury or pain. Research into immune and hormonal factors has shown that pain disrupts the brain's homeostatic regulation systems producing both the experience of stress and complex systems to reinstate the body's homeostasis.

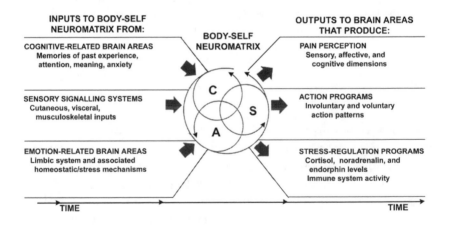

Fiure 2.8. The Body-Self Neuromatrix.

There are cognitive (C), emotion (A) and sensory (S) inputs into a highly integrated brain neural network (the interacting circles), and outputs to brain areas that produce pain perception, action and stress-regulation, and create a unified experience of the 'body-self'.

[Reproduced with permission from Dr. R Melzack]

In Dr. Melzack's (2005) words:

> The stress-regulation system, with its complex delicately balanced interactions, is an integral part of the multiple contributions that give rise to chronic pain... The neuromatrix, as a result of home-ostasis-regulation patterns that have failed, may produce neural 'distress' patterns that contribute to the total neuromatrix pattern, and may also produce destruction of tissues [because of sustained cortisol release with ongoing stress]...

> I propose that some forms of chronic pain may occur as a result of the cumulative destructive effect of cortisol on muscle, bone and neural tissue. ... The cortisol output by itself may not be sufficient... but [it] provides the conditions so that other contributing factors may all together produce these [problems]. (p.90)

The concept of the neuromatrix helps to further unravel some of the complexity of brain function and consciousness in persisting, distressing pain.

Explaining to a Child How Pain Works

Returning to the child who had skinned his shin, this is how you could explain the pain to him. With this knowledge his anxiety should reduce and he should consequently manage the pain better (you could also use the diagram shown in Figure 2.4). We wrote this for a child approximately seven years old, but of course it could be used for a younger child cognitively more mature, or adapted to any age of child or type of pain.

"Here is where you hurt yourself. Do you know how pain works? The nerves in your skin have picked up the pain message, and this message races up the nerves very quickly from your leg to your spine. It then zips amazingly quickly up your spine to your brain to tell you that you have cut your leg. That's why you know that you've hurt yourself. So now your brain can make good decisions. You got help, you are taking care of your leg, and you're now starting to get better again.

"But here's more about this amazingly intelligent pain system. Do you remember how you grabbed your leg to stop the pain? Pressing it like that helped a bit – didn't it? It also stopped the bleeding. Pressing it sent some more messages up to your brain that the situation is now under control. Now, once your brain got the message that you are managing, your brain told your nerves to settle down by closing the gate on the pain message. This is just like when you turn down the dimmer switch when the light is on full so that it goes softer and weaker. Isn't that cool! Your brain is really the boss. When your brain knows that everything is under control, it makes your pain go dimmer and weaker, and calms those nerve messages. Then you start healing."

Conclusion

The brain decides if what is being experienced is 'pain' and how to deal with it. We have learned a great deal about how these signals travel to the brain. However, we know a lot less about how the various brain networks make sense of these signals, or the role of stress and emotional distress in our experience of pain. We do know however, that this processing is widely distributed over the entire brain including sensory, emotional, and thought processes.

The gate control theory of pain modulation has provided us with a very helpful model in clinical practice to explain how body and brain work in an integrated manner for pain to be experienced. Melzack's concept of the neuromatrix proposes how the brain's multiple inputs and outputs maintain chronic pain. This provides health professionals with background knowledge so that they can approach and communicate more effectively with children in pain, anxiety, or distress – the topic we take up in Chapter 3.

Chapter 3

Communicating with a Child in Pain

"If an adult tells you not to worry and you weren't
worried before, you better hurry up and start because
you're already running late!"

C.P. Curtis (1999, p. 42)

Witnessing children's pain is distressing. What can we as pediatric health-care professionals do to relieve such suffering? The first step is to affirm the child's experience and acknowledge the child's pain – no matter what your culture, belief system, or attitude. What about the child's crying – how best to deal with that? In this chapter we explore how to respond to children in pain, what words to use and those to avoid, and what is important in this communication. This is an area that is under-researched, apart from research into optimum responses for parents of children in pain. These findings are useful, for as professionals you will be in a position to guide parents on how best to deal with their child. We'll examine children's and parents' coping responses, as well as the role of attention and pain catastrophizing as a response to the threat of pain.

Effective Responses to a Child in Pain

If you know a child and have a trusting relationship, it is often easy to gain the child's confidence and cooperation. If you have to deal with a child in pain and you do not know the child, there is still a great deal you can do in the first few moments to turn a painful, fearful situation into a more manageable one. The guidelines in Table 3.1 are based on what children, health professionals, and researchers know is helpful to a child in acute or persistent pain. Each guideline will be explained in more detail below.

Table 3.1 Effective Responses to a Child in Pain

- Respond promptly to the child's pain in an empathic, professional, practical manner.

- Explain in child-oriented language what is happening in his or her body.

- Make physical contact with the child in the way that feels best for you both.

- Acknowledge the pain, as you examine, palpate, observe, and/or attempt to gain some measure of the child's pain.

- Encourage the parent to remain with the child or teenager until the pain is under control.

- Tell the child calmly and slowly what positive steps are being taken or will be taken to reduce the pain and provide comfort.

- Provide hope, wherever possible, as it is sustaining.

- Instruct the child on using pain management strategies (see Chapter 5).

- Be an attentive coach and track what would therapeutically support the child's coping.

- Keep yourself calm, as this will help allay the child's anxiety.

- *Respond promptly* to children's pain in a caring professional and practical manner, and direct their attention to the sensations that would be soothing so that they are orienting themselves toward more comforting sensory input.

  - To a child who has sustained a laceration, you might say, "That's a painful cut. We must first cool and clean it up. The coolness of the water will soothe it. Feel the cool and focus on it, because that helps your body find comfort."

  - To a child complaining of a headache, you could say: "Ah, you have a headache. You know the buildup of the pain will stop when you lie down. Lie down now close your eyes. That's it, feel how that position helps the pain to start draining away. I'll close the blinds to keep the light out, and bring your medication. While I'm away, let the darkness sooth your eyes, and do some slow easy belly breaths to bring more comfort back into your body."

- *Tell the child what is happening* in his or her body. For example: "You've had an accident. You're shivering because your body has had a shock and is sore and hurting. It's best not to move at all. Be so still so that you feel your whole body settling. It's good to be still as I carefully check your leg, so lie perfectly still. That's good. I'm going to cover you with a blanket, because your body feels cold even though it's hot outside. Feel how that helps. You'll be OK now that you're here. Focus your attention on feeling the warmth growing. You can squeeze Mom's hand while we have a look." The repetition of what you need the child to do, spoken in a comforting tone of voice while providing concise explanations, is likely to be immediately experienced as beneficial.

The next case from our emergency room shows how important for a young child in pain to understand what is happening to his or her body. This child demonstrates his assessment skills by authoritatively giving the emergency physician his own diagnosis!

> *Four-year-old Clarence was brought to the emergency department of a children's hospital with a dislocated elbow. His mother told the attending nurse the circumstances that led to his elbow being sharply pulled. Clarence was in pain and unable to bend his arm. Tense, he held onto his mother with the other arm. The physician examined his arm carefully and then pronounced, "This looks like a pulled elbow!" "No, it's not!" said Clarence. "It's a swollen hand!" The physician gave a big smile and took a few extra minutes to explain to Clarence about the mechanics of his arm and why it caused his hand to swell and elbow to hurt – important information for this anxious bright child.*

- *Make physical contact* with a child in the way that feels best for you both. Depending on your relationship, the age of the child, and the situation, you can touch the child's shoulder and/or encourage the parents to provide some comfort and protection. Physical touch is part of a physical examination to determine the nature and extent of the child's pain, but it can also give comfort or encouragement. Making physical contact provides physical and psychological relief when words are just the start, or when the child is hurting and too distressed to listen.

- *Acknowledge the pain;* don't minimize or deny it. Children feel discounted and disrespected when their pain is not acknowledged. If a child has stomach or bowel pain, you could say: "These stomach cramps are hurting you a lot. I can see that you're very uncomfortable. Is the pain hurting more or less than when it first started? How has it changed? What made it change? Tell me what it feels like – dull, throbbing, achy, or shooting stabbing pain? Show me now where it is hurting… and where it is not. Has this stopped you doing what you like to do?" This is the principle of *joining with the patient,* wherever the patient is. Then you can begin to gauge the nature of the child's pain in this first encounter before making a more comprehensive assessment later (see Chapter 4 for more detail on assessing and measuring children's pain).

- *Encourage the parent to remain with the child.* Acute pain is an intensely subjective experience. Both the pain and its accompanying sense of separation from the outside world can be frightening. Children feel vulnerable and do not want to be left alone to struggle on their own. Wherever possible, have a parent or family member remain with a child until the pain is under control. Over and over children say that what counted the most when they were in pain was having Mom or Dad present with them (Gonzalez, Routh, Saab, Armstrong, et al.,1989). The presence of a known and trusted adult makes the experience bearable for both children and adolescents in a myriad of obvious and subtle ways, and enables them to cope.

Even with teenagers parental presence is important. Older adolescents may say, "I can handle it on my own." That may be true, but check at the beginning whether the teen needs support until they are coping. Dismissing parents who are no longer needed is then a positive step, indicating growing competence and self-reliance. Adults can then step back and support from an acceptable distance. Teens appreciate the opportunity to feel stronger and more independent. Situations vary, so listen to what the teen wants. Sometimes trusted adults who are not the teen's parents can provide the necessary support, as they are at an acceptable emotional distance, and the teen can hear their message without a dependency battle.

Caution: Ensure that teens who want to handle the pain on their own don't cut themselves off from accepting the essential analgesic or physical treatment that will support their full recovery. For example, taking less than the recommended analgesic dose is not a sign of 'being strong'; rather, it is inviting more suffering.

- *Tell the child what positive steps are being taken* to deal with the pain. Don't lie to the child, withhold essential information, sugar-coat it, or give false reassurance. Give accurate age-appropriate information sensitively so that the child and parents can make sense of what's happening. You might say as you enter a cubicle in the emergency department: "I know it seems a long time since you came into the emergency room. The nurse who first saw you has told us what happened to you on your BMX bike. The accident sounded dramatic. The good news is that I'll get you some pain medication to take the edge off your pain. And while it is starting to work, I'm going to very carefully examine you, and you can help me by telling me how this feels... Thank you... Then we'll do an X-ray to see your bones and find out what may be causing your pain."

- *Provide hope, wherever possible.* Children need to know that the pain will get better because of the steps being taken: "You know, of course, that now that you're doing your physio program regularly your body is going to heal. Young bodies know how to do that well!" Providing hope can spur a child on to face difficult procedures or trying times. It is more than a placebo, it is an active sustaining energy. We don't fully understand it but recognize that its absence is often problematic. Robbing a child of hope that things can get better creates despair and may hamper recovery. Hope can be destroyed in a number of ways – by the words said, an attitude, and any underlying sense of phoniness or cynicism which children are quick to note. Use language that conveys your concern and genuine conviction. Remind children of their body's natural potential for healing and relief from suffering. This helps children to let go of terror, doubt, fear, and pain.

- *Instruct the child in some pain-management strategies.* As you listen attentively to a child's concern, you can suggest or invite the child to begin helping him or herself. These strategies include diaphragmatic breathing, blowing bubbles, using imagery and relaxation techniques, or listening attentively to a favorite story (see Chapter 5). When the child participates in becoming comfortable, pain and distress eases. The active involvement required by these strategies moves the child from helplessness to actively finding more comfort – and more trust in the treatment team. For example, take out the bubble kit. "Here's the bubble wand. I'll blow first, and you count and see how many bubbles. Three? I bet you can do better! Here, blow! See how good that makes you feel. As you blow out, let the scary feelings go? That also helps your pain to go down and down and down."

- *Be an attentive coach and track what would be most therapeutic to support the child's coping.* Distinct from your professional role working with a child, you have a part to play in developing the child's coping. Coping is a learned skill that varies from one situation to another. Encouragement and active guidance help children to cope and set the stage for more confidence and complex coping skills. Here is a child-centered example of how one dad drew on a prior experience of coping to coach his anxious seven-year-old son through the removal of his leg cast:

"I can't do it, Dad!" cried a weary Sam. Uncertainty and fatigue nearly wrecked this child's first coping steps. His dad responded with soothing, consistent support: "I'm right here with you, Sam. You're doing OK, just hold still for a short, short while. The cast is nearly off. You've held wonderfully still, and it's been very awkward. This is almost like the time you were wedged into the canoe with your legs twisted around our gear, remember? Remember how you had to just sit there so still because we didn't want to tip the canoe? No-one risked moving around. It's like that time. The waves were coming, and it was sitting-still time. You're doing so well right now. You'll soon be free."

- *Keep yourself calm,* as it will soothe the child's anxiety. Check your own breathing. If it is shallow and rapid, breathe out and release the tension, allowing yourself to settle and regroup. Maintain this breathing in a regulated fashion, inhaling for three and exhaling for three, until you feel yourself calmer.

I learned this important lesson when I worked with children with cancer during their painful procedures. When the procedure was not going well, the tension in the treatment room would spiral, everyone would tense, and the atmosphere could be cut with a knife. We learned to cue each other with: "Breathe!" Everyone exhaled and grinned, releasing our tension. From then on the procedure would invariably go better. Before that, we would end up with a variety of symptoms, such as neck or back tension, feeling wrung out, or with a headache. The children naturally picked up our tension and inevitably did worse than if we had been relaxed and playful. I learned how crucial it is to help myself if I wish to help others.

Choosing Words That Clarify and Don't Confuse

Young children tend to understand words at their surface and concrete level, and language can be confusing when words are used that have more than one meaning. To add to this, medical terms are like a foreign language for most children who are naïve to hospitals and their procedures. We have an obligation to ensure when children are in a clinic or hospital, that they understand what is said to them and what is happening. We need to use child-oriented terms that are simple, clear, and understandable to the different ages of children. Table 3.2 provides a list of the many ambiguous and confusing hospital terms, as well as the clearer terms we should use when speaking to children. Note particularly the words that could frighten a naïve child.

Table 3.2 Considerations in Choosing Language

Words that have different meanings can be confusing. If it is likely that the child will hear the standard medical expressions used, these words should be explained or defined. Ideally the child should be asked if he/ she knows what nurses and doctors mean when they say these words. Compare, for example, the phrases in the left column with the suggested alternatives in the right column.

Potentially Ambiguous	Clearer
The doctor will give you some "dye". *To make me die?*	The doctor will put some medicine in the tube that will help her be able to see your ____ more clearly.
Dressing; dressing change *Why are they going to undress me?* *Do I have to change my clothes?* *Will I have to be naked?*	Bandages; clean, new bandages

Potentially Ambiguous	Clearer
Stool collection Why do they want to collect little chairs?	Use child's familiar term, such as "poop" or "BM"
Urine *You're in?*	Use child's familiar term, such as "pee"

Shot
    Are they mad at me? When people get shot, they're really badly hurt
 	
    Are they trying to hurt me?
	Medicine through a small, tiny needle

CAT Scan Will there be cats? Or something that scratches?	Describe in simple terms, and explain what the letters of the common name stand for
PICU *Pick you?*	Explain, as above
ICU *I see you?*	Explain, as above
IV *Ivy?*	Explain, as above
Stretcher *Stretch her? Stretch who? Why?*	Bed on wheels
Special; funny (words that are usually positive descriptors) *It doesn't look/feel special to me*	Odd; different; unusual; strange

Potentially Ambiguous	Clearer
Gas; sleeping gas *Is someone going to pour gasoline into the mask?*	Medicine called anesthesia. It is a kind of air you breathe through a mask like this to help you take a nap during your operation so you won't feel anything
Put you to sleep *Like my cat was put to sleep? It never came back*	Give you medicine that will help you take a nap; you won't feel anything until the operation is over
Move you to the floor *Why are they going to put me on the ground?*	Unit; ward. Explain why the child is being transferred and where
OR (or treament room) table *People aren't supposed to get up onto tables*	A narrow bed
Take a picture (X-rays, CT and MRI machines are far larger than a familiar camera, move differently and don't yield a familiar product).	A picture of the inside of you. Describe appearance, sounds, and movement of the equipment
Flush your IV *Flush it down the toilet?*	Explain

Words can be expressed as "hard" or "soft" according to how much they increase the perceived threat of the situation. For example, consider the following word choices.

Harder	Softer
This part will hurt	It (you) may feel (or feel very): sore, achy, scratchy, tight, snug, full, ...
The medicine will burn	Some children say they feel a very warm feeling
The room will be very cold	Some children say they feel very cool
The medicine will taste (or smell) bad	The medicine may taste (or smell) different than anything you have tasted before
Cut, open you up, slice make a hole	The doctor will make a small opening. (Use concrete comparisons, such as "our little finger" or "a paper clip" if the opening will indeed be small
As big as ... (e.g., size of an incision or of a catheter)	Smaller than ...
As long as ... (e.g., duration of a procedure)	For less time than it takes to ...
As much as ...	Less than ...
(These are open-ended and "extending" expressions)	(These expressions help to confine, familiarize and imply "manageability" of an event or of equipment)

The unfamiliar usage or complexity of some common medical words or expressions can be confusing and frightening.

Potentially Unfamiliar	Concrete Explanation
Take your vitals (or your vital signs)	Measure your temperature; see how warm your body is; see how fast your heart is working. (Nothing is "taken" from the child)
Electrodes, leads	Sticky, like a Band-Aid, with a small wet spot in the center and small strings that attach to the snap (monitor electrodes)
Intravenous; IV	Medicine that works best when it goes right "Into a Vein" (IntraVenous). It's the fastest way to help you get better. (First ask the child if he knows what a vein is, and why some medicine is OK to take by mouth and others work best into a vein. Explain the concept of initials if child is old enough)
Hang your (IV) medication	Bring in new medicine in a bag, and attach it to the little tube already in your arm. The needle goes into the tube, not into your arm, so you won't feel it
NPO	Nothing to eat. Your stomach needs to be empty. (Explain why)

Potentially Unfamiliar	Concrete Explanation
Anesthesia	The doctor will give you medicine called 'anesthesia'. It will help you to take a nap during your operation so you don't feel anything at all. The doctors know just the right amount of medicine to help you stay comfortable through the entire operation
Incision	Small opening (Follow with discussion of how cuts and scrapes received while playing have healed in the past)
Tourniquet	Rubber band that squeezes your arm
Veins	Blue lines, tubes that move blood through your body
Sterile	Really clean, no germs
You will have to say "Goodbye" to your parents	That will be the time when you say "See you soon"
Lots of children feel sick to their stomachs and throw up when they wake up	Your stomach has also been sleeping and resting. It may need some time to wake up. As your stomach wakes up you will slowly be able to drink, and eat food again
You will have a sore throat when you wake up	Your throat may feel very dry when you wake up

Gaynard, L., et al. (1990). *Psychosocial Care of Children in Hospitals: A Clinical Practice Manual from the ACCH Child Research Project.* (Used with permission from Child Life Council, Inc.)

Unhelpful Responses to a Child in Pain

Sometimes when witnessing a child in pain, health care professionals feel not only the desire to help but also fatigue, hopelessness, irritation, or helplessness. It is crucially important to acknowledge and understand how our clinical work impacts us. How do the various children and tough situations emotionally affect us? It is natural to feel empathy and emotional pain when a child is in distress, and we need to be aware of our reactions. Yet when events do not go well, how do you deal with it? How does one process or ward off feelings of helplessness that may occur. If this is done by avoiding or verbally minimizing a child's distress, this may be self-protective but is ultimately a blunted and negligent clinical response. Psychologist Dr. Joseph Barber (1989) expands on this:

> Many of us, trained to be 'clinically objective' suppress even our awareness of our natural reactions to a child's suffering. Eventually, of course, such habitual suppression becomes a more automatic repressive response and we become unaware of our actual feelings towards suffering children. If we become deaf and blind to the suffering of children we severely impair ourselves as clinicians. (p. 121)

An essential element of being a professional means finding a balance between being emotionally responsive to a child's distress, yet not being overwhelmed by this situation. The balance between too detached and too involved is a dynamic one. It may vary from one child to another. However, as clinicians dealing with children in pain, "we need to be neither overwhelmed by our feelings of compassion for our patients, nor estranged from them" (Barber, 1989, p. 121). This requires taking the time to be aware of ourselves and heed our own responses to the demanding work we do and to our patients. Unheeded uncomfortable feelings lead to negative reactions that can stand in the way of our providing effective and necessary care. Table 3.3 summarizes what not to do with a child in pain, and a fuller explanation follows:

Table 3.3 Unhelpful Responses to a Child in Pain

- Don't ignore the child's pain.

- Don't rob a child of hope.

- Don't be inconsistent with preparation or follow-through.

- Don't use reassurance and sympathy with the child.

- Don't engage in the myth of two pains.

- *Don't ignore the child's pain.* People who are emotionally distant or out of touch with a child and themselves are more likely to deny the child's pain. For example:

  A clinician known for her cold approach in the procedure room began the procedure by injecting some local anesthetic into a child's back. The child responded with a yelp, "That hurts!" and without missing a beat she retorted "That doesn't hurt!" The others in the procedure room were startled. The staff all could see from his face that he was in pain. The nurse moved to comfort the child, but the damage was already done.

  There is no doubt that most who come to work with children do so because of a love of children and motives of wanting to ameliorate pain and suffering. Yet when professionals are distressed by a child's pain and defend their discomfort by denying or minimizing the pain, this response has long-term negative consequences on their capacity to deliver good care. Over the years they build up a protective wall to keep themselves from experiencing these uncomfortable feelings of having to deliver care, such as collecting blood or doing a lumbar puncture, that initially may cause pain and suffering. In so doing, they shut themselves off from an essential part of their humanity. Working through this challenging process of "How do I do this procedure in the most humane way possible for the child, as well as take care of my own feelings of discomfort?" requires training, discussion, team work, and coming to terms with this difficult aspect of the job. Processing this dynamic balance requires integrating 'learning with the head' with 'learning with the heart' and is aided by modeling those who have achieved this balance.

Downplaying a child's pain tends unfortunately be a gender-biased phenomenon. Researchers in a study of everyday pain among young children found that girls receive physical comfort twice as often as boys (Fearon, McGrath, & Achat, 1996). Girls also receive physical comfort more frequently than boys when the caregiver is nearby and is aware of a pain incident, without being prompted by the child's sobs, cries, or screams. In contrast, boys are more likely to receive physical comfort only when they are in tears. This preference to comfort young girls and expect young boys to 'tough it out' has long-range effects on boys' sense of support and on their right to express distress when in pain. We need to ensure that young boys get their fair share of nurturance, enabling them to develop compassion for others in turn.

- *Don't rob a child of hope.* In the struggle with pain or illness, it is inexcusable to rob a child – or anyone – of hope that their suffering and pain can ease. Communicating when someone is in pain requires thought, sensitivity, and tact. In the human interchange there are often multiple layers of message, meaning, and sometimes miscommunication, such as in this not uncommon scenario:

  A teenager, Taz, had to see his physician for the fourth time for pain in his back, a pain that worried him. His doctor recommended various treatments with little or no change in Taz's pain. Taz, feeling disheartened, talked to his physician who said things that Taz does not want to hear:

  Physician: We've tried everything and there's not much more that I have to offer you. You're just going to have to live with it.

*Inwardly Taz thinks: He's telling me I'm a hopeless case and he's giv-
ing up on me!*

A helpful remark would have been:

*Physician: Even though we haven't managed to pinpoint the cause
of your back pain, it is not uncommon with this kind of pain. We
know for sure that it's not a disease or a tumor. There are still things
we could do, and there's no reason to give up. How do you feel about
starting a progressive physical strengthening program? Even though
your pain is there, when you gain muscle strength, the pain is likely
to decrease. Also as a teen it's good to be in good physical condition.*

- *Don't offer inconsistent responses.* Children in pain need their
  concerns to be consistently heard, believed, and addressed.
  This includes reliably providing adequate preparation for
  procedures, painful or not, so that the child is fully supported
  through the process. It also means that you respond sincerely
  and promptly and stay engaged with the process until the
  child's pain concerns become history. Inconsistent responses
  – sometimes heeding the child's concerns, and at other times
  dismissing them with the put-down, "It's time that you
  learned how to handle it!" – may lead the child to prove to
  you that his or her pain is real. The child may grimace more,
  cry more intensely, becoming over-concerned about having the
  pain acknowledged. Children sometimes develop other symptoms, such as headaches on top of the original pains, because
  of their sense of neglect or their fears. In the following case,
  consider the experience of this girl who was referred to me for
  consultation:

*Ten-year-old Prabjot recently immigrated from India. Her history of
headaches worsened with the challenges of adjusting to a new school,
language, and culture. The pain of her headaches was usually around
3 out of 10 and bothered her although she attended school and did
fairly well. A CT scan was recommended. This occurred on a hot day,
and she was unprepared for the injection of Contrast. She reported
to me that 'this made her headache increase to a 6, and it had never
gone down since then' – 6 months ago. It was hard to know whether
it was the shock of the invasive procedure or her feelings of being out*

of her depth and unprepared that compounded her headaches. It was clear to me that effective treatment would require trust and sensitivity over time to develop a relationship with her. It would also be pivotal in her treatment that I quickly learn the cultural issues and negotiate their nuances.

It is always best to engage with the child and the pain directly. If you feel that the child is becoming caught up with anxiety or embroidering the pain, start by accepting and addressing the child's experience. Say in a kindly, matter-of-fact way: "I can see that you're still bothered by the pain; could you tell me what's happening... And what else?" After hearing the child, enlist the child in determining what needs to happen to help ease the pain. In this way you're establishing a working alliance, essential for any pain therapy to succeed.

- *Don't use reassurance and sympathy.* Research has shown that when parents and professionals use pain promoting language, such as giving reassurance ("It will be OK!" or "It will soon be over!"), being empathic, apologizing to or rebuking the child, this increases the child's pain reports (Blount, Zempsky, Jaaniste, et al., 2009; Chambers et al., 2002). Sympathy and reassurances send a message of alarm to the child about the pain: "Feel those pain signals, they must be bad. No wonder you're so upset!" This weakens the child's ability to learn to cope or draw maximum benefit from analgesics and pain-relieving strategies. Conversely, studies have shown that when pain-reducing language is used by parents – language that uses distraction and humor, and encourages the child's coping – reports of pain decrease (Chambers, et al., 2002).

- *Don't engage in the myth of two pains.* That is, if it isn't easy to diagnose the pain in a child's body, it must be in the child's head! Children experience puzzling kinds of pain, such as recurring headaches, or abdominal or limb pains that don't fit neatly into a recognizable syndrome, disease, or trauma. They can struggle to gain sound professional help and a clear idea of what is happening. Unfortunately at clinics and during hospital visits they encounter remarks that are at best unhelpful and at worst reveal a poor appreciation of the complexity of pain pathways: "Since we can find no organic cause for the pain, it must be just psychological" – as if pain in the body does not involve the brain!

Children and teens are very sensitive to the judgment or diagnoses made about their pain experiences. Fifteen-year-old Crystal had made two emergency room visits to the local children's hospital for acute abdominal pains. When the hospital staff could find no clear organic cause, she said, "I felt a failure and confused. Maybe it was in my head; maybe I was making it all up? But it hurt so much I didn't know what to do! They put me through all these tests, and they all came up negative. Now I really felt awful. Maybe they thought I was making it all up!"

What Crystal needed was validation that, although it was difficult to identify exactly what was causing her pain, it was clear to all that she was in pain, and that she would not be dismissed just because her pain did not fit neatly into an easy diagnostic category. Some children who do not feel heard or supported in their pain and distress become angry, and sadly end up not trusting the very people they have come to for help, as in the following case:

Eleven-year-old Bryan, who had irritable bowel syndrome, said to his mother on the way home from a clinic visit: "I could see that the doctor did not believe me. He thought I was exaggerating my pain... I feel so alone... No one can help me! It's no use." Bryan then told his Mom that he would not return to that clinic, or that doctor. His Mom felt quite desperate. She knew that his trust had been broken, and it would be a struggle to get him to go for the help he needed.

The Role of Crying

Crying is one way we know when a child is in pain, as it is a natural and automatic response to pain. Tears release the physiological tension produced by trauma and pain. From birth, babies cry spontaneously in response to distress, such as when feeling hungry, unsettled, or in pain. When a baby feels distress, the body tenses, the lips or jaw trembles, the eyes squeeze tightly together, the mouth opens wide, the tongue becomes taut and cupped (Grunau & Craig, 1987; Hadjistavropoulos, Craig, Grunau, & Johnston, 1994; see Figure 4.1) . The baby emits sobs of different degrees of intensity, which together with deep inhalation and howling exhalations, release the tension from pain and alert the baby's caregiver.

Hunger cries are higher pitched than pain cries and become more like pain cries if the infant is not fed – being hungry can indeed be painful. Parents over time learn to identify the sound of their infant's pain cry and facial expression of pain. Crying therefore has survival value as a distress signal. It is the most immediate way that parents and caregivers are alerted that the baby is in distress, and they respond by finding out why.

Cultural attitudes toward crying can confuse and complicate this natural emotional and physical release. Children naturally respond to pain by crying, and they in turn are responded to in different ways, depending on age, gender, and the social implications of the situation. Whether we are aware of it or not, we all carry beliefs and attitudes about the display of emotion – particularly crying – and convey these attitudes to our children from early on in life, such as: "Crying is OK in private only," "Crying means you're weak," "It's OK to cry at weddings or funerals," "To cry is humiliating," "Big boys don't cry," "Girls can cry, but boys have to be brave," and "If a boy cries, he's a sissy." All cultures and societies have well-defined attitudes about whether crying is allowed, under what circumstances, and what crying means at those times. In most cultures, girls are given greater freedom to cry than are boys.

As children grow, crying is increasingly inhibited or repressed. Adults do harm when they disapprove of children's tears instead of supporting their efforts to gain control of their distress. If a child is told that it is not acceptable to cry, his or her ability to express distress in a natural and healing way is impaired. Because of the powerful ways in which cultural beliefs and child-rearing practices intertwine, how crying should be handled can be controversial. There are however, a number of things we know about crying:

- *Children generally don't like to cry.* They don't feel good about crying. If there is a choice in a situation, most psychologically healthy children prefer not to cry, whether or not it's physiologically relieving. School-age children and adolescents, in particular, are very concerned about 'losing it'. For them crying represents failure and potential humiliation. Conversely, learning how to manage these difficult situations and to control the distress and pain becomes a worthwhile challenge and growing step. If they successfully manage pain and don't cry, children report experiencing an increase in self-esteem and competence.

- *Children in pain need to express their feelings, which develops a sense of self.* We need to acknowledge children's emotions, not only those of pain but also of anger, fear, joy, envy, jealousy, gratitude, or grief. When adults say disapprovingly, "There is nothing to cry about!" or "That doesn't hurt! Now stop your crying," this effectively shuts the child down, suppressing those feelings. This disturbs the child's sense of self and ability to cope. Central to a child's emotional health is the affirmation of experience. An adult's acceptance of a child's expression of self is formative in developing identity. A young child's emotions and internal sensations form the nucleus of the emerging sense of self.

- *It's unhelpful to tell a child that "it's OK to cry" when the child is facing a painful procedure.* Years ago physicians in training were taught that a suitable response to imminent pain would be to tell the child that "It was OK to cry." Saying this would only be helpful if the child was embarrassed by crying or if parents are trying to quiet the child because they thought he or she is creating a scene. Then the response of "It's OK to cry" is sympathetic and supportive of the crying child, and instructive to the parents that crying is acceptable. However, telling a child who is about to have a painful procedure that it is OK to cry, conveys doom: "What I'm about to do will hurt so much that I expect you to cry, so if you do it's OK!" This is likely to provoke tension and tears because there clearly is no other way out. A child who does not cry is likely to remember the situation as less frightening and distressing than one who does cry.

Crying in a sense proves to the child that it was a big problem. By diminishing the intensity of the experience, such as, "You only cried a little bit", and emphasizing coping "and your concentrating on your iPod made it go quicker" could shift the child's memory of the pain in order to help them next time (von Baeyer, Marche, Rocha, & Salmon, 2004). There are many reasons why encouraging crying isn't a good idea – although discouraging it is also not a good idea. Pay close attention to the subtle messages in the language you use!

Responding to an Angry Child

Some children get frustrated and angry when their pain persists. It is unusual for children to take their anger out on the health care professional; most times the only 'acceptable' target for this anger is a parent. How can you guide a parent to manage this? Remember what the child is really angry about – that the hurt or disruption to their normal life won't stop. The anger is a protective reaction and venting of frustration. Instruct the parent not to take the child's anger as a personal attack. Anger is the child's natural defense. However, if the child physically lashes out, as younger children can do, it's important that you empower the parent to physically protect him or herself and encourage putting that understanding into words, as did the mother in the following example:

> *Seven-year-old Juan lashed out at his mother during a lab test for blood. She dealt with it by saying: "Juan! Stop! Don't hit me! That is not OK! I know you're mad as anything that the needle hurt. I'm so sorry that it did. But hurting me, punching me, isn't going to take the hurt away! Here take these bubbles and start blowing to get rid of the owie! That's much better way to help yourself. That's better! Thank you."*

Children understandably become angry if they're tricked or not told about a procedure that lies ahead, or the pain is downplayed in the mistaken belief that it will decrease the child's anxiety. Research has shown that under-predicting imminent pain negatively affects children's coping: pain that is worse than expected creates extra stress (von Baeyer, Carlson, & Webb, 1997). Some staff think that it's best to not address the upcoming pain, to avoid upsetting the child. This strategy does not work and will back-fire. The child may feel justifiably angry and betrayed, and strug-gle internally to make sense of the being surprised by a painful experience.

Your best insurance is to provide a child with sufficient understand-ing of the upcoming plan, procedure, or treatment. Sensitively provide as much accurate sensory and procedural information as is helpful or tolerated, so that there are no surprises (Jaaniste, Hayes, & von Baeyer, 2007). (The timing of when to provide this information and the legal and moral aspects are covered in Chap-ter 10.) Using child-oriented language (refer to Table 3.2), discuss:

• What is happening with the child's body right now.

• What needs to occur for the pain to reduce and the child to get well.

• What the plan of treatment is.

• If a procedure will occur, what it is called, what will happen, how it could feel.

• What the child can do to help him or herself get through it.

• What or who will be there to support and what they could do too.

When children are invited to become part of the planning team, then the staff as well as parents are experienced as supportive and concerned, rather than as accomplices in causing, or not prevent-ing, the pain from occurring.

Parents' Central Role in Health Care

Parents rated 'taking care of pain' as one of their highest priorities, second only to getting the right diagnosis (Ammentorp, Mainz, & Sabroe, 2005). Historically, pediatric health care professionals did not permit parents to have a central role in the care of their child in pain. Major changes over the last 30 years have occurred in how health care is delivered. One of these is the shift in pediatric hospitals from a service model to a family-centered model. This change has promoted an alliance between health care professionals and parents in how best to provide for a child's care. In this progressive change, parents are regarded as:

• Experts on their child: health, history, temperament, and needs.

• Key resources in caring and managing their child's health.

• Partners in decision making and future planning.

These principles also apply to the management of children's pain. Parents are an invaluable aid in assessing, observing, and interpreting their child's symptoms, behavior, and responses. As mediators between the child and health care professionals – who don't know the child as well, yet have to provide the child with medical attention – parents play a pivotal role in ensuring that the medical intervention is beneficial for the child. Parents encourage the child to follow through with medical recommendations and interventions, such as taking medications, coping with necessary medical procedures such as blood draws, practicing self-hypnosis, and using biofeedback or other self-regulatory methods to ease chronic pain and illness.

Today, as health care dollars are constrained, parents often must provide care in a hospital that used to be provided by hospital staff. This could include bathing, comfort massages, adjusting and positioning their child. Children are now being discharged from hospitals earlier after illness or surgery to be cared for by their parents at home, often without home nursing support. Surgical procedures such as the removal of tonsils and adenoids that used to require a child to remain in hospital for a few days following surgery are now routinely done as day surgery. Parents have to assume more of the responsibility, care, and management of their children in pain.

The days are gone when parents would take their child to a health care professional and the child would be taken away for treatment. Gone also are the days when parents handed over their child for medical treatment and were not permitted to remain in the room – with the exceptions of surgery and emergency and life-threatening interventions. The 21st-century philosophy of 'parents as partners-in-care' requires health care professionals to reassess their current practices for dealing with pain. They need to include how to prepare and educate the parents to support nursing and medical treatments in order to help children in pain. Parents are now regularly included and consulted as members of the diagnostic and pain-treatment team. With such a crucial role, parents will need to learn more about pain and how to help their child to learn and respond in non-fearful and flexible ways of coping with pain. It is the pediatric health professional who has to provide this information (see Chapter 10 for legal issues in providing information) and to do so sometimes in situations of duress and under time pressures!

Key points

Some key points on what we know about parental involvement in their children's health care:

- Children have consistently reported that their parents' presence during medical procedures is the single most important factor to help them cope with fear and pain.

- Parents, as well as children, need to be given adequate information about their child's condition and be adequately prepared for any planned interventions, including where to sit/stand, what their role is, and importantly, what they can do.

- Parents should be invited and prepared to be present at medical examinations or procedures – with the exception of those teens who prefer their independence. However, if parents feel emotionally overwhelmed or unprepared, they should not be made to feel guilty if they are unable to remain. Rather, once the most stressful part of the procedure is over, the parent can be invited back to provide essential comfort for the child. This is a learning opportunity for the parent. Sometimes they feel distressed that they couldn't protect their child or prevent the pain. Some anticipate that the child will be angry and take it out on them. It's important to soften this process by providing flexible access and support for the parent until the process is better tolerated.

- Parents empowered in this way will be an ally for pediatric health professionals. They will help prepare their child, and assist by mediating or explaining to the child or the professional what the other means.

- Parents, however, should never be required to coerce or restrain their child. This is not their role in medical care.

- Parental anxiety in medical situations has been found to predict their children's anxiety (Jay, Ozolins, Elliott, & Caldwell, 1983). An increase in parental heart rate, blood pressure, and anxiety during a child's venipunctures predicted the child's increase in behavioral distress. This gives another meaning to 'family-centered care'! It points to the importance of considering the child and parent as an interdependent whole that requires care. If we want the child to do well, we must ensure that the parent is doing well too – they affect each other. The parent is a key to the child, and a key to the success of the treatment plan and its follow-up.

Parents Teach Children the Meaning of Pain

Learning to make sense of inevitable pain, both trivial and serious, starts early in a child's life. Parents explain and interpret confusing and alarming pain signals. Whatever their temperament, infants, toddlers, preschoolers, and school-age children learn from their caregivers, absorbing information like sponges. The early years are a time of particular rapid learning to establish pain attitudes and potentially develop the brain's neural patterns for pain processing, modulation, and inhibition. When alerted by a child's cries that he or she is hurt, caring adults across most cultures run to the child to relieve the pain. Prompt responses with a hug or words similar to "Let me kiss it better!" help the child in distress. Glad for the attention and comfort, the child learns that the sharp pain is eased with comfort and loving attention.

Trust, reliance, and understanding develop with these experiences over months and years. The parent's accessibility, quick response, and offer to kiss it better sends the message that "with a kiss, the hurt will begin to get better." Just as in fairy stories where a kiss has magic properties, as when a kiss wakes the princess, in real life a kiss takes the pain away. Having experienced this wonder with a parent, the child trusts that it will work again and probably starts learning to turn on the brain's downward inhibitory modulation. By helping the child make sense of pain, giving it a name, and putting it in its place, the parent may influence the formation of the early circuitry of the child's neuromatrix – the patterns of the 'body-self' that regulate, interpret and select actions to re-establish homeostasis and down-modulate pain and stress reactions in the hormonal and immune systems (see Figure 2.8).

Recognizing the Influence of Parental Pain Responses

Children experience and observe how their parents deal with pain, talk about pain, and cope with pain. I learned this years ago after a particularly demanding day of work at the hospital. I returned home complaining about how sore my head was. Later my three-year-old son came into the room holding his head, saying my words complaining of his sore head! I was stunned – the little mimic! I realized I needed to be more thoughtful about how I cared for my sore head and to practice what I teach. I invited my wriggly son to lie down on the bed with me. Together we put our heads on the soft pillows "so that the pain could drain away."

Here is the lesson: All children, particularly pre-schoolers, are masters at learning by observation. They absorb their parents' values, attitudes, and behavior toward pain, with or without their being aware of it. Not only do children demonstrate behavior toward pain similar to that of their parents, but they also have the same fears and attitudes about treatments. Also a parent's belief about a pain treatment effectiveness will influence how the child responds to treatment and the child's expectations of outcome. For example, when parents tell their child that any pain treatment other than medication is hocus pocus, they stand in the way of that treatment's success. But if parents tell their child how they used breathing and imagery during the child's birth to get through painful contractions, then the child knows that Mom and Dad will support his or her efforts to make breathing work.

Two-year old Caitlin was diagnosed with Juvenile Diabetes Type 1, which required insulin injections twice a day to control her blood sugar level. She also needed frequent finger pokes throughout the day to test her sugar levels. All of these were painful, a shock for her to experience. Her parents Kyle and Susan were even more distressed. Their adorable first child was sick with a potentially life-threatening illness. To add to their distress, they had to ensure she stayed well – her health was in their hands. They had to do painful finger pricks a couple of times per day and give insulin injections morning and evening.

The nurse at the hospital had taught them how to give the injections into Caitlin's thigh while she was sitting on their lap. But Caitlin had become sensitized and was becoming more and more worked up, fighting and wriggling with each successive insulin injection. Susan and Kyle felt they were traumatizing their child. As they discussed with me their loathing of doing 'the pokes', they slowly came to terms with what they needed to do to make it better for her. They accepted to do this work as a cool, calm, collected team. I suggested that they buy a Raggedy-Ann Dolly who curiously also had Diabetes, and introduce her to Caitlin – as

Dolly needed Caitlin's help with regular pokes and injections. The simple predictable procedure was set up at home with Caitlin helping Dolly to sit and blow bubbles to keep calm and ease the brief needle pain. Her parents became so good at doing this daily routine with her that within 3 weeks, one parent was able to do it alone without the other's help. Now months later Caitlin is an active part of the blood checks and insulin shots. She no longer even cries. Now these procedures only take a brief minute, and Caitlin helps her parents. Susan and Kyle realized how their fears about pain had unwittingly escalated the procedures. With their distress and fears out of the way, everyone copes well.

Guiding Childhood Attitudes Toward Pain

Toddlers are at particular high risk of developing fears. They are rapidly developing receptive language, but can't yet adequately express themselves. They're making sense of their world – but often pediatric health professionals don't take the time to explain a medical condition or procedure in simple concrete language so that the toddler can integrate this new information. Health professionals often underestimate the comprehension capacity of toddlers, and with that oversight, their essential needs are not adequately addressed. They become at high risk for developing fears and behavioral patterns of self-protection and resistance.

Maturing into a well-adjusted young person or adult requires developing confidence and authority about one's body. Since pain is a protective intelligent system, toddlers of thirteen months or older, gaining some independence as they begin to walk are easily alarmed and sensitive to any threat to their bodies. Toddlers' reactions show that they are aware of other people's pain and that they are sensitive to pain in their own body, even if they don't yet have the expressive language. I saw this clearly while working with eighteen-month-old Narjit, who was diagnosed with systemic juvenile rheumatoid arthritis.

Narjit noticed a small hole in my stocking. She pointed her chubby little finger at the hole and chimed with alarm and distress: "Owie-owie!" She was alarmed by the hole. She seemed to be asking if it was hurting me, a possibility that appeared to worry her. I showed her in a playful way that this owie didn't hurt me. It belonged to my stocking and was painless. She then did what toddlers do to gain mastery over something distressing. She repetitively poked her finger in and out of the hole, with considerable delight as she fully understood that this 'hole' over my leg didn't hurt me. She seemed relieved by this, an early sign of her developing empathy for others and an important aspect of early child development.

Research has shown that children in their toddler and preschool years spontaneously use words such as 'ouch' and 'hurt'. They rarely spontaneously used words such as 'pain' or 'sore' before the age of 6 years (Stanford, Chambers, & Craig, 2005). The expressions that children use to describe pain and discomfort vary as the child matures. With clear and developmentally appropriate language, and active guidance over months and years, children learn to make sense of their body signals. When health care professionals and parents put this learning into words, actions, and play, it helps ease toddlers' distress, and they gain a mental map of these body experiences – perhaps the beginning of the neuromatrix. For instance, when a toddler is rubbing her forehead or pulling her ears, one could say, "Does your head hurt?" Or, "Does pulling your ears make them feel better... are they hurting?" By two-and-a-half or three years of age, a child can say, "I have an owie" or "My ears hurt!" and expect understanding and help.

With recurrent or persisting pain, toddlers and young children need consistent coaching to learn how to deal with their pain. This empowers the child, however young, to work with pain:

Four-year-old Tyler had migraine headaches. He would become irritable, whine, and be clingy. Initially his mother wasn't sure what was happening to her little boy. She knew that he was unhappy and demanded all of her attention. After multiple visits to doctors, a pediatric neurologist diagnosed childhood migraine. (This is not uncommon in children, particularly in families with a strong history of migraine.) With the diagnosis, and information she's been given about how headaches present, his mother, now alert to the early warning signals of eye rubbing and irritability, could intervene promptly. "Remember what the doctor said: you'll take your headache medicine, then I'll tuck you in with your blankey, put a cool cloth on your head and you can sleep so that the pain goes away."

Tyler became accustomed to this pain relieving ritual. This was evident when he began volunteering, "Mommy, my headache is coming back!" Tyler was no longer bewildered or helpless. He heeded his pain and took the action he had learned, which included asking his parent for help.

An interesting post script: I saw Tyler seven years later on an unrelated matter, and enquired about his migraines. Despite his strong family history and perhaps because of his prompt responsiveness and possible repatterning, he now rarely gets migraines.

Children can change fearful responses to pain as they grow. Depending on the nature and degree of exposure to painful experiences, children can develop ways of adjusting to pain signals that regulate their stress responses and re-establish feelings of well-being. The following vignette illustrates that pain does not necessarily lead directly to distress, when a child learns to modulate pain and cope instead of being threatened, fearful, and panicky.

Jason, a rapidly growing five-year-old, who only months before wailed and demanded immediate attention whenever he hurt himself, stunned his mother as he landed flat on his face in the playground, skinning his hands. "Don't worry, Mom, it's only a scrape!" he called out from the gravel. "What was the difference this time?" wondered his mother in amazement, as she stopped herself from her usual 'run to rescue'. Was it modeling of the other children present? Was it his stronger sense of self-confidence now that he had turned five and had begun kindergarten? Or was it the story-books they were reading about how the body works? She was not sure if it was one or all, but she was thrilled that Jason was now coping. He's growing up, she mused.

Differentiating Parental Strategies

As children grow and develop, the ways of assisting them when they are in pain also need to change. Teens tend to cope more independently with their pain and may object to having too much parental attention. Those shifts are not always easy for parents to make, particularly when the teen is ill and in pain, and health care professionals may need to sensitively mediate between the two. Some teens and older children reject or scorn their parent's attempts, however helpful they were in the past. In family-centered care, parents sometimes require guidance, humor, and the opportunity to discuss their own coping options with a health care professional.

Parents often tell staff about their need to use different pain strategies with the various children in the family because of individual or temperamental differences. Parents learn to deal with a 'dramatic' child in pain in one way and a quieter, more introverted child in the family in another. Parents, like health care professionals, also recognize they sometimes need to use different strategies at different times with the same child. This flexibility represents an intelligent adaptive coping response on the part of the child, and warrants further examination, as it is a central process in successfully self-regulating the stress of pain.

The Process of Coping

Within our current biopsychosocial model (See Figure 3.1), coping is a key process to understand how children respond to stressful medical experiences. Coping with a stressful situation depends on its nature and inherent meaning for each child. Furthermore, the same child in the same situation may cope very differently at different times. Since coping is a very personal process that varies with each situation, a child's coping will change when pain or context changes, as will that of the parent. In interacting with children and their parents, health care professionals need to be able to recognize individual coping responses and the efforts that constitute less effective coping.

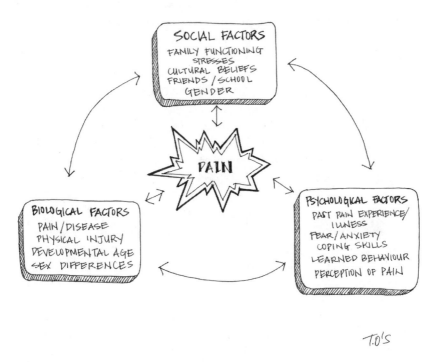

Figure 3.1. Biopsychosocial Model of Pain.

The prevailing biopsychosocial model depicts the stressful event of pain and its interactional effects on the biological, psychological and social equilibrium of the child in pain. Coping is an attempt to re-establish homeostasis and well-being. It plays a central role in the relationship between the stress of pain and biological and psychological outcomes.

Understanding Children's Coping Responses

Coping has been defined as "conscious volitional efforts to reg-ulate emotion, cognition, behavior, physiology and the environ-ment in response to stressful events or circumstances" (Compas & Boyer, 2001, p. 326). Children demonstrate these efforts in order to regulate their stress responses and to re-establish both biological and psychological homeostasis. The best coping is goal-directed, organized, specific to the stressful context, planned, strategic and draws on children's language capacity.

Research to develop further understanding of children's coping has proposed a common structure on the range of coping responses consisting of three dimensions (Compas & Boyer, 2001):

- *Active efforts to regulate* emotion and act on the source of the environmental stress. These include problem solving, decision making, modulating emotion and its expression, as well as obtaining social support that is focused on the problem, or focused on emotion.

- *Accommodating efforts* aimed at achieving some adjustment to the stress. These include distraction, acceptance, cognitive reframing, self-encouragement, minimizing or positive thinking.

- *Disengaging efforts* to orient attention away from the source of the stress as well as any emotional responses. This is considered to be passive or avoidant coping. These efforts include withdrawal or isolating oneself, wishful thinking, denial, and avoiding thoughts or action associated with this stressor.

Coping processes are recruited and activated when children encounter acute stressful events, and chronic stressful conditions of pain, illness, injury, or disease. When a children's coping involves actively engaging with the stressful event or condition, or with their emotional responses, this tends to be associated with better functioning and fewer emotional, behavioral, or physical problems (Compas & Boyer, 2001). In addition, when a child is faced with stressors that are beyond his or her personal control and adjusts by accepting, distracting, or reframing thoughts and beliefs, this too is associated with a better outcome. When children's efforts go into attempting to avoid or to disengage from the stressor, and they experience unwanted thoughts and feelings, this in contrast is associated with a poorer emotional, behavioral and physical outcome (Compas, Conner-Smith, Saltzman, Thomsen, & Wadsworth, 2001).

Coping and Attention Under Stress

There is a natural interdependent relationship between children's coping and their attention when faced with a stressor, such as pain. A child's attention acts as a mental filter. Paying attention orients the child towards a potential stressor to appraise its threat, before any coping is initiated. The child then selects among various competing sources of information to process what may be relevant. The above abilities develop gradually. Younger children require significantly more health care staff and parent support and more concrete, simple language and distraction than older children. When children are under stress and in pain, these abilities may be lost during a regression to earlier modes of functioning. Appreciating this stress response, allows health care professionals to identify those children who demonstrate ineffective coping responses to their illness, pain, or hospitalization. Sometimes this may be due to temporary fatigue, the impact of the illness or disease, the child's temperament, or family intergenerational patterns. It is important to identify these potential vulnerabilities early in care, so that referrals for further interventions that support and promote more adaptive coping patterns are initiated early.

Some children experience being overwhelmed by the potential threat, or may initiate ineffective coping responses to the stressor. For example, some children find themselves unable to re-orient their attention away from the pain and towards activating their coping responses to deal with this stressor, such a child who catastrophizes. These children have become pre-occupied, over-focusing on their pain symptoms, and consequently may experience more pain for longer than children who are able to divert their attention to more helpful coping strategies. This has significant and potential long-term consequences for children's health care.

Catastrophizing

Pain is a nasty experience and a threat to our well-being. Some children develop an anxious anticipation, heightened vigilance, and an exaggerated fear of pain. Catastrophizing is the manifestation of unwanted persisting negative thoughts and distressing feelings, reflecting the high threat of anticipated or experiencing pain. For example, if a child has persistent thoughts like these, it is called catastrophizing: "This stomach-ache will *never* go away. I must have a bad disease that nobody has found. I think I'm going to die." There is a lot of evidence that children (as well as parents) who catastrophize suffer greater distress than those who don't (Bédard, Reid, McGrath, & Chambers, 1997; Crombez, Bijtebier, Eccleston, et al., 2003; Eccleston, Crombez, Scotford, Clinch, & Connell, 2004; Piira, Taplin, Goodenough, & von Baeyer, 2002).

Research to better understand the components of catastrophizing have identified related dimensions of ruminating on the pain event, magnifying it and accompanying feelings of helplessness, all subsumed under this construct of pain catastrophizing (Crombez et al., 2003). It has been found that the more children catastrophize about pain, the greater their pain severity and disability (Crombez et al., 2003). Catastrophizing is also related to a lower pain tolerance (Piira et al., 2002), more anxiety, and greater depression (Eccleston et al., 2004). Children who have developed catastrophic patterns also tend to use more analgesics (Bédard et al., 1997).

The function of pain catastrophizing appears to be an attempt to escape from pain and to communicate this distress to significant others. Despite that, this pattern of anxious thinking and heightened emotion about pain promotes the experience of pain. Children who have developed this 'coping' strategy tend to over-predict the threat of the pain, how bad it will be and their helplessness in adequately dealing with it. In short, pain catastrophizing is a cry for help that requires early, skilled and ongoing intervention to prevent its many known adverse effects. It also has considerable spill-over and negative impact on other children, staff, and the child's parents.

Giving Parents Support to Cope

Parents and grandparents experience distress when their child or grandchild experiences pain. You may hear: "This is not fair. I wish I could have the pain so that my child didn't have to suffer," or "I wish this had happened to me rather than to my child." Sometimes a parent has admitted, after the fact: "I wanted to simply gather her up in my arms and whisk her away – away from the pain, upset, and confusion."

The worst part of seeing their child in pain for some parents is their own sense of helplessness. Being dependent on nursing and medical professionals to provide relief, that may or may not be forthcoming, can be distressing and frustrating. Parents tend to emotionally carry their child's pain and consequently feel overwrought, worried, or desperate unless they see evidence that adequate steps have been taken to address and ease their child's pain. We as health care professionals need to be alert for this: a child in pain has a parent in pain. Parents also need understanding and support to regain perspective and lighten their emotional burden.

To facilitate parents coping more adaptively in the treatment room, the practice has been for the health care professional to discuss and rehearse the strategies that both the parent and child would be able to use at the various states of the procedure, that is, before, during, and after the painful event. Research suggests that in some cases when the staff model coping-promoting behaviors, rather than individually training every parent, this may be sufficient to indicate to untrained parents how to promote their child's coping (Cohen, Blount, & Panopoulos, 1997).

Gathering support and information from health care staff, friends, and other parents is a natural way to cope. The simple act of expressing their distress away from their ill child, conveying it to someone who hears empathically and can appraise the situation, eases parents' feelings of anger or helplessness. Parents in similar situations quickly become allies for each other. They provide support, strength, and the invaluable knowledge from their and their child's suffering and experience. These friendships can provide help in a way that friendships outside the current stressful situation cannot. Pediatric health professionals need to be attuned, involved, and accessible to parents, who sometimes spend a long time on their children's ward and create a subculture. Guiding and promoting healthy exchanges can benefit the ward or clinic climate – well beyond the child's pain.

Many of the methods recommended to relieve children's pain and distress can also be recommended by health care professionals to parents to ease their tension, strain, and distress. These coping techniques include:

- Taking breaks to listen to a relaxation, imagery, or favorite music CD or iPod, to return refreshed with a clearer vision of the situation and its possibilities.

- Breathing deeply to help when energy is fading or strained.

- Exercising regularly, such as walking, practicing yoga, swimming, or cycling, to rebalance emotional and physical energies.

- Having a massage or a refreshing warm bath or shower.

- Using meditation or prayer as natural ways to draw on extra strength.

- Reading books or materials on pain management (such as Krane & Mitchell, 2005; Zeltzer & Schlank, 2005) or the child's particular condition or disease.

- Writing to family and friends by email, blogging, or keeping a journal.

Parents have commented that blogging or keeping a journal to track their child's episodes of pain is a valuable coping and assessment aid. This narrative process focuses, contains, and increases the parents' understanding of their own and their child's experience. It helps to identify the pain patterns and lessen uncertainty. A journal can help in assessing more complex pain or the patterns of factors that worsen the child's pain and in parents' advocacy for better pain relief. Encourage parents who wish to journal to address these questions:

- What time of day or night does the pain occur?

- What else coincides with the pain or has preceded the onset of the pain within the last hour?

- How long does the pain last?

- What worsens it?

- What helps the pain to settle?

- How long is your child pain-free?

The value of a parent's journal is shown in this incident with fifteen-year-old Tamiko:

During hospitalization and routine medication administration, an antibiotic capsule became stuck in Tamiko's throat. It dissolved and burned her esophagus, and was acutely painful. Her pain treatment in the hospital consisted of an opioid IV infusion. Her mother was puzzled about why Tamiko had increased pain episodes during the day yet seemed much more comfortable at night. The house staff maintained that she had been given enough pain-relieving medication during the day to keep her comfortable but, according to Tamiko and her mother, during these acute pain episodes she was far from comfortable.

Her mother decided to keep a journal of Tamiko's pain episodes, and asked her daughter to rate her pain using a 0–10 pain scale and recorded it. Through her careful documentation over two days, a pattern emerged. Tamiko's mother could see from her journal that within half an hour after a meal, which consisted of a smoothie or liquid food, Tamiko's pain would increase, getting progressively worse at each subsequent meal. Thus, her pain after her dinner smoothie was the worst. She requested that the staff observe Tamiko half an hour after her lunch and half an hour after dinner. It became clear to the physician that the food was irritating her esophageal burn and causing a spasm. She was immediately taken off food by mouth so that the tissue could heal uninterrupted by irritants. Her pain medication was changed to include a muscle relaxant to reduce the muscle spasm after drinking.

As an observational tool, the parent's journal helped clarify the nature of Tamiko's pain giving staff information that led to changing the treatment plan and improved pain control.

In this case, a father used a blog to cope with his pain, grief, and sorrow during his baby girl's prolonged illness:

The father of desperately ill Hannah was encourage by her bedside nurse to create his own blog during the long days and nights of his little daughter's treatment for a congenitally malformed heart. The nurse noted his quiet despair and thought it may be therapeutic for him to write and make some sense of this experience – and inform his extended family. Processing his grief in this way, he stayed connected to his support system. At night and in the early morning hours he blogged. It became his means of making some sense of the pain and suffering his five-month-old girl was undergoing in her fight to live. He wrote as he sat at her crib after holding her hand for long quiet stretches. This private man found energy to relate how fragile human life is, how elemental he found parenthood, how deeply bonded he felt to his frail daughter with her wide dark eyes. He blogged of the physical aching in his chest – pain that felt both emotional and physical. This process enabled him to deal with the anticipatory grief knowing he could lose her during her struggle to hold onto life.

Which Parent?

Some children do not have the luxury of choosing a parent for an imminent stressful medical procedure. However, if both parents are available when a child is in pain, which one would do a better job of supporting or coaching the child through a painful episode or procedure? In most parenting relationships, jobs are distributed in such a way that each adult deals with what she or he does best. This distribution evolves over time. Children in the family intuitively know about this distribution of labor. For example, a child will know that Mom is the real disciplinarian or that Dad hates the sight of blood, even though he is great as the decision-maker about plans when someone is sick. A child will approach one parent rather than another about certain problems or coping with pain. If both parents have experience and feel competent, ask the child whom he or she would like to have present when dealing with pain, as having both there is not advisable.

Eight-year-old Leanne required frequent blood work and IVs. She knew that her mom was the better of the two parents to accompany her into the clinic. Her dad, a lawyer, could relate to the staff, but when his daughter became distressed, he would fume at the nurse. In the confusion of not having control, he had on one occasion ended up yelling at his daughter, who was already in tears. His response to her pain was deep rage that he couldn't stop his daughter from hurting. In contrast, Leanne's mom had a sensitive stomach and although she easily became queasy, she was able to talk quietly and encouragingly to her daughter through her fear while the nurse found a vein. When Leanne's mother became light-headed, she would fix her eyes on her daughter, take deep breaths to steady herself and say to herself, "If this little kid can go through this, I can too!" Over successive treatments, Leanne's mom's concentration and focus on her daughter strengthened, becoming quite intense. "It was like I was sending strength to her and our bond became much stronger. I got as much strength from her as I gave to her – it's funny how this works!"

Conclusion

Responding to a child in pain requires prompt, sensitive, and practical skills. How we respond in words, tone, action, and attitude to children in distress has a significant impact on how they deal with their anxiety and pain. Children require explanations in developmentally appropriate language that is clear and provides sensory and procedural information. Differing developmental needs require health professionals to be versatile in their communication skills. Light humor (never at the child's expense!) distractions, and invitations to cope help to mitigate against the threat of pain.

Considering parents and child as a system or interdependent unit requiring treatment brings all players onto the same field to work together. Sometimes parents are themselves distressed and need direction in order to cope. Children, particularly in their early years, absorb, model and learn their parents' behavior and attitudes. Identifying a child's coping responses early in treatment helps to prevent escalating difficulties and informs staff about how best to guide the child towards more effective coping. Determining the child and parents' coping responses is one aspect of an overall assessment of the child's pain. As we will discuss in Chapter 4, observing, obtaining a self-report, and questioning provide added dimensions in our understanding of what is going on with the child in our care.

Chapter 4

Assessing and Measuring Pain

With Carl L. von Baeyer

"On top of the pain, I then had people coming in and prodding me and not believing that I was in pain – just because I wasn't screaming like those cry-babies down the hall."

Sixteen-year-old, later diagnosed with a painful neuromuscular disease

Assessing and measuring another person's pain is like speaking a foreign language you don't fully understand. When you are in pain, you know what is happening, even if it defies accurate expression. When someone else is in pain, you can only observe, empathize, and rely on hunches and your accumulation of clinical experience. To throw a bridge across this chasm, researchers and clinicians have designed instruments to measure some dimensions of pain and to provide some consistency and validity in better understanding another's pain. The task is a difficult one. These tools cannot tell the whole story of a child's pain. They can, however, provide health care professionals with a measure of some aspects of the pain, such as its intensity for a particular child at a specific point in time. In this chapter we'll examine how children of different ages and abilities understand pain and what to look for developmentally when determining a child's pain. Also included are some questions to ask in assessing recurrent or chronic pain. We'll cover the methods of measuring pain and the current tools used in this process.

Assessing Pain

In assessing a child's pain, the health professional makes a clinical judgment based on:

- *Taking a careful and thorough history of the pain:* its onset, duration, frequency, location, and intensity; finding out whether there are associated symptoms, what medical evaluations have been done, and what interventions have been undertaken; inquiring about events prior to the pain and the impact of the pain on the child, schooling, social life, and the family

- *Observing how the child's pain presents,* physically, emotionally, and behaviorally

- *Attending to how the child describes the nature, significance, and context* of the pain.

Assessment is broader in scope than measuring the specific intensity, frequency, or location of the child's pain with a validated reliable measure. A skilled assessment helps determine the factors that influence the child's pain, then guides the clinicians to select those interventions which would be most effective. Careful, thorough, and ongoing assessment and re-assessment is critical to the process of relieving a child's pain. Developmental considerations are pivotal, as an infant's or young child's behavior and comprehension of pain are quite different from that of a teenager.

Infants

How Infants Understand Their Pain

Infants in the first few months of life are totally dependent on their caregivers, and are exceptionally vulnerable. Infants are able to experience pain and discomfort from before birth. Babies' distress is soothed by being held, cuddled, rocked, or comforted with familiar touch and smells. Their hunger is sated by the familiar taste of milk. Through the first months of life, infants develop an emerging sense of self and separation from their mother through a variety of bodily experiences, guided by their developing senses of touch, sight, sound, smell, and taste, and by movement. Within the first six months babies have learned a great deal through their bodily experiences. We know that six-month-old babies who have previously had needle procedures as part of a medical treatment will become fearful and actively avoid the anticipated pain. The cry of an infant who sees a person in a white coat with a needle is evidence of this early learning. Over the first year of life, new faces and strange experiences, particularly those of pain, can be deeply disturbing, disrupting the infants' willingness to sleep and to eat, and their ability to feel safe and to be separated from their parents.

What to Look For with Infants in Pain

With infants, there is no single behavior that is an absolute sign of pain. However, long experience of infants is a considerable aid. The best way of judging whether a baby is in pain is to observe carefully and ask the parents. Parents usually know their infant's patterns, and when invited to report changes in eating, sleeping, moving, or crying, they are often especially helpful. Infants tend to cry and fuss when in pain and may attempt to pull a sore limb away or to protect a painful area. The facial expression of an infant in pain may look like a grimace, with open mouth, bulging brow, eyes squeezed tight shut, taut cupped tongue, and a deepening of the furrow between the nose and corner of the mouth (nasolabial furrow) (Grunau & Craig, 1987; see Figure 4.1). Note that if an infant experiences severe pain exacerbated by any movement, then after first crying, the infant may become very still, neither moving or kicking, and may even stop crying to protect the painful area and conserve energy. Assessment of pain in an infant requires skill and experience. If an infant does not look or behave normally, consult with a nursing or medical colleague, as well as the parents. Following one's clinical intuition is an important guide to provide the best care for infants.

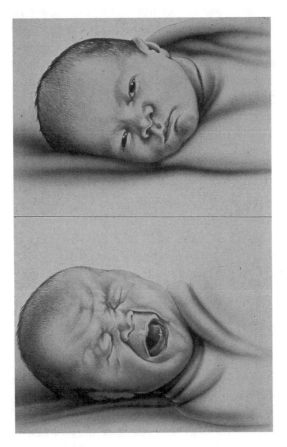

Figure 4.1 Neonatal Pain Facial Expression, Grunau & Craig, 1987 With permission from IASP.

An infant's facial expression of pain may look like a grimace, with open mouth, bulging brow, eyes squeezed tight shut, taut cupped tongue, and a deepening of the furrow between the nose and corner of the mouth, the nasolabial furrow. (Grunau & Craig, 1987)

Toddlers

How Toddlers Understand Pain

Toddlers develop an understanding of their world through their senses and body movements. From 13 months to approximately 24 months of age, it is very common for young children to regard their skin as defining 'self'. Little wonder they become terrified if their skin is punctured or scratched. "If blood came flowing out – that would be their end!" Toddlers can't articulate this fear, but pediatricians know about toddlers' pre-occupation with wounds, and how startled and fearful they become on seeing their blood. Their experiences are still strongly based on their senses: seeing is believing.

What to Look For with Toddlers in Pain

You can ask toddlers directly if they are in pain, or if a specific part of their body is hurting. Even at one year of age, toddlers can point to, or tell you if a part of their body "has a ouch". Toddlers may not be able to identify their feelings, but if you use the child's or family's words, ('owie,' 'booboo,' 'hurt'), young children can correctly identify where and how much they are hurting. Attentiveness and a little patience helps. As with infants, changes in a toddler's normal pattern of moving, behaving, eating, and sleeping are indicators of illness pain. Atypical behaviors such as whining or listlessness may indicate discomfort. Repeatedly tugging an ear could indicate an ear infection; not putting much weight on a limb or not using an arm could indicate pain or an injury.

Preschoolers

How Preschoolers Understand Pain

Preschool children, aged three to five, understand pain as "something that hurts." As with younger children, the hurting can be overwhelmingly distressing, but in contrast, preschoolers have many simple words they can use to describe their experience. They understand that there is more to their bodies than outer skin and that beneath their skin there are bones easily felt through the skin. They accept the existence of a heart, brain, and other organs. Yet preschool children's understanding of cause and effect and of how their bodies work is very different from an adult's. For example, for the preschooler the body's surface, the skin, is still more important than the interior of the body.

These are the 'Magic Years'. For preschool children the boundary between fantasy and reality are blurred. A four-year-old boy runs around the house in an imaginary world, answering to no other name than Robin Hood. A minor hurt may become a huge fear. Preschoolers will find any reason to 'explain' why there is pain, jumbling up cause and effect. Remember Clarence, the delightful four-year-old in the emergency room who had dislocated his elbow. The physician on duty examined his arm and with authority said, "This looks like a pulled elbow." Without missing a beat, the child replied, "No, it's a swollen hand!" Preschoolers are concrete in their perception of life. His hand hurt.

Preschool children don't necessarily understand why they are experiencing pain or what has caused their pain, and it is inconsequential how long it will last. The here and now is everything. They do not have an adult's concept of time. Today is still the center of the world, and a week's time is often very difficult to comprehend, ("How many sleeps is it?"). Preschool children need repeated concrete and simple explanations – and they need physical proof that pain will end. Three-year-old Hailey caught her finger in a three-ringed binder and cried inconsolably for 25 minutes until a Band-aid was found. 'A minute' does not have much meaning to a three-year-old, but holding a Band-aid while having blood drawn is proof that it will soon end. While children as young as three can reliably use some of the pain assessment tools, they experience themselves as the center of the world and may create magic explanations for why the pain is continuing – "because I was naughty". Drawings, playdough, and other creative tools are helpful to determine how a preschool child understands the pain.

What to Look For with Preschoolers in Pain

When preschoolers have the words to describe their experiences, question them about the nature, location, and intensity of their pain. You should also observe their movements and behavior, and note any changes in eating and sleeping patterns. Encourage young children to express what they are experiencing and attempt to understand how they are interpreting pain signals. Remember that children of this age often think magically (it is the age of imaginary friends, and monsters that live under the bed). Assure them that they did not get the pain because they did something wrong or are being punished, but that infections, accidents, and pain just happen, and that they can help themselves feel better by following the treatment plan. A vital part of this stage of development is gaining increased mastery and understanding of events. Evidence for this, is that preschool children are able to use coping skills that demonstrate self-control and the ability to modify their pain.

School-Aged Children

How School-Aged Children Understand Pain

Elementary school children (6–12 years of age) tend to regard pain in a general fashion. They draw on internal cues to determine whether they are sick, but they are often still naïve about external causes, such as infections. They may still think that pain is a consequence of their bad behavior or a form of punishment. School-aged children, however, are more capable of logic than pre-schoolers, even though their understanding of the link between cause and effect is still fairly concrete. With the use of books, draw-ings, and charts, school-aged children begin to conceptualize pain occurring in their bodies and learn about the nervous system and how body and brain send and receive pain signals.

Children at school are familiar with computers, which is a good analogy for how the brain functions, remembers, and makes sense of painful experiences. When health professionals take the time to discuss and explain these matters to clear up misconceptions, school-aged children understand and cope better with their pain.

What to Look For with School-Aged Children in Pain

With their more developed language skills and understanding of different situations, school-aged children are usually more con-sistent in their expressions of pain than younger children. Thus, it is much easier to identify when a school-age child is in pain. Once again, changes in eating, activity level, and ways of moving and behaving can be signs of the presence of pain. Ask a child directly and talk together over what you have observed. Note that at this age boys may have become more stoic or inexpressive of their pain than girls and therefore may require more skilled attention – as in the case of Mark in chapter 1, who had six weeks of severe back pain and said nothing.

Teenagers

How Teenagers Understand Pain

By the age of 12 or 13 years, teenagers are capable of thinking abstractly. They reflect on their own thoughts in flexible and systematic ways. Teens often show insight into the psychological factors or consequences of their pain. These are the years of becoming more of an individual, not only in clothing and looks, beliefs and attitudes, but also in the personal experiences of pain. By 11 to 14 years, teens have acquired some knowledge of how pain works and appreciate the value of pain as a protective and warning signal. But they may also have learned unhelpful responses, such as either ignoring or amplifying the pain signals. Under the stress of pain, teenagers – like all children or adults – can regress to younger ways of behaving.

What to Look For with Teens in Pain

Teenagers are reliable witnesses of their pain. They can identify the site, type, onset, history, and intensity of their pain. When in the presence of their friends, however, teenagers may adopt different behaviors and may talk very differently about their pain, than if spoken to alone. If observed by friends, teenagers tend to minimize or deny pain. To gather a true picture of a teenager's pain, it is crucial to have a private discussion so that peer pressures cannot come into play and distort the teen's reporting.

Table 4.1 presents some questions to ask about more ongoing or recurring pain. Questions like these will help you to understand the antecedents and the consequences of the pain, providing a functional analysis (von Baeyer, 2007).

Table 4.1 Developing a Functional Analysis

Characteristics of the Pain Episodes
• When did it start?
• How did it start—was there a trigger event?
• How often does it occur? Daily, several times a day or week, or ...?
• What time of day does the pain occur?
• What time is it worse? (measured 1-10) And when is it best? (measured 1-10)
• How much does it hurt right now and where?
• Describe how the pain feels.
• Are you worried that it's more serious than you've been told?

Precipitating and Relieving Factors
• What do you think is causing the pain?
• What makes it worse? What makes it better?
• Is there anything you can do that makes it better?
• Children sometimes have worries or fears—do you have any?
• What do you do when you are worried or fearful?
• What makes you happy/angry?
• What was happening when your pain first started?
• When the pain started, what was happening in your family?
• Tell me about your school? What do you enjoy most? Least?
• How did you do in your last school report?
• When the pain is over, what are you looking forward to?

Co-factors and Consequences of Pain

- How is your sleep? How long does it take to fall asleep? Approximate time?

- Do you stay asleep through the night? Time of awakening?

- How is your pain in your classroom when you're working?

- What happens if you get pain at school? What do your friends say or do?

- Are you doing less exercise since your pain started?

- What happens when you have pain at home? What do you do?

- What do your parents say or do? What do your brother or sister say or do?

- When you stay home from school, what time do you get out of bed?

- What do you like to do when you're home? Do you still do your chores?

- Do you stay in contact with your friends? How? ... text/ email/MSN/Facebook?

Measuring Pain

We face a dilemma when we attempt to measure a person's pain (or any other subjective experience). All methods of pain measurement are imperfect, but there are important reasons for making the most accurate assessment possible.

Methods of Pain Measurement

There are basically three methods of measuring pain. One method is asking a person in pain what he or she is experiencing (getting a self-report). The second is observing the person's behavior. The third is measuring the person's physiological reactions to pain. None of these gives a complete or perfectly reliable measure of the pain experience. Undoubtedly the subjective report is the most important, since the pain is within that person's body; however, each measure has its strengths and weaknesses. Especially when measuring a child's pain, using all three methods may give a fuller picture, depending on the nature of the pain.

The subjective measurement has the authenticity of inner experience. Since it is within the child's world, it is colored by those biopsychosocial factors that the brain integrates to make sense of pain: feelings, thoughts, family history, message about pain, condition or disease, and/or previous pain experiences (see Figure 3.1). As such, it is highly personal and strictly individual.

Observational measurement of pain relies on timing the duration of a child's crying, counting particular facial expressions, or noting times when the child touches an affected part of the body. These are also known as behavioral measures. Specific scales will be described later in the chapter. These fall short of perfect, for several reasons. First, overt behavior does not necessarily reflect internal experience. People change their behavior in response to social expectations and social rewards. For example, children, especially boys, are less likely to cry when their peers are watching, and more likely if they are with their mothers. Second, pain behavior lessens as pain lasts longer; a child who has had the same pain for hours, days, or weeks might show no overt signs of it even though it is intense. Third, all observers have biases based in their own previous experience, though these can be lessened by training and careful choice of measurement scales.

Sometimes the self-report and the observational measures may not seem to agree with each other and may provide two different pictures. As an example, you notice a child limping and not using his leg properly, as if his leg may be hurting. When asked about this, the child shyly denies having any leg pain. Clearly, this doesn't fit. With gentle questioning he reveals it's really his foot that hurts very badly. He lets you examine his foot, where you find red swelling on the toe mound and a deeply embedded infected splinter. You ask the child, "Is this where it hurts most?" He nods and your detective work is complete.

A third method of measuring pain is the direct measurement of the body's functions, using indices such as heart beat, perspiration, and respiration rates. We know that after an initial decrease, heart rate increases when a child is in pain. Blood pressure increases for a child in acute pain, but oxygen saturation decreases. The child's respiratory rate does change, with breathing becoming more shallow and rapid. Some research now includes the stress hormone, cortisol, to indicate the level of stress – a co-factor of pain. Unfortunately these indices do not tell us directly in a consistent and reliable way about the presence, absence, or intensity of pain. All of these signs, for example, might be a result of bodily stress from running up stairs, or mental stress from worry or fear, rather than physical pain. There are also wide individual differences in all these physiological measures. There's a further complication. Acute pain tends to increase respiration rate, heart rate, sweating, and hormonal changes. When pain persists over time, as in a chronic pain condition, the pain may be severe, but these physiological responses do not necessarily occur. Once again we are faced with the complexity of pain: pain is not one reaction or emotional response or behavior; rather, it is a multifactored, complex experience of brain and body to which our systems adapt and adjust.

A combination of all three assessment methods – self-report, observational, and physiological – can help us gain the most information about the child's pain.

Measuring pain in young, pre-verbal children or those with disabilities adds another level of challenge to the problem. Adults in pain usually speak up for themselves and describe the nature of their pain. Children who do not have the language or interpersonal skills to speak for themselves or who cannot insist on being heard, easily feel overwhelmed and fearful. As with infants and very young children, who are not yet able to use language to convey where and how much they are in pain, measurement becomes a major hurdle, requiring clinical experience and knowledge of developmental behavior. Toward the end of the first year of life, as toddlers begin to communicate with simple words and gestures such as pointing, their own report of pain, for many reasons, becomes the first and most important way of knowing that they are in pain. Thus, early on in life, self-report measures become the primary source of information about a person's pain, though other sources are still needed.

Reasons for Using Pain Measurement

There are a number of sound reasons to attempt to measure or quantify a child's pain. First, such an attempt builds a communication bridge, conveying useful details. For example, a child who has frequent headaches reports her pain is 5 on a scale of 10. When there are some changes, instead of saying, "It is worse," or "It is a little better," this child is able to say, "It's now a 7 out of 10." Health care staff can then inquire as to when it started to move up the scale and determine other factors that aggravate or ease the pain.

Second, by using an established tool, child, parent, and staff can determine the success of a pain intervention. For example, half an hour after using self-hypnosis combined with a cold cloth on his head, the child reports how the pain is. If the change is in the right direction, say a 4 out of 10, and the child feels it is helping, the intervention can be continued. If, however, the pain remains the same, decreases insignificantly, or increases, then it is clear that another intervention should be considered.

Third, when a child experiences recurring or persistent pain, the consistent use of measures becomes a finely tuned language by which the child can convey changes in pain over time. Using this language bridge provides security to the child in pain; she no longer feels so isolated when pain absorbs her energy and attention, as she knows her caregivers will appreciate the difference between a rating of a 3 and a 6 out of 10. With these increased communication skills, caregivers tend to respond more promptly and, where needed, to provide analgesic medication, physical and/or psychological treatment.

Measuring a child's pain also provides other useful information: the frequency of the pain and its duration, as well as its intensity. All three are helpful in determining whether an intervention is effective in reducing a child's pain. Noting the different levels of pain can also assist in determining the various pain triggers.

Since a pain report is private and personal, unique to that individual, comparing one child's ratings to another's has no validity and should not be done. We can only make meaningful comparisons between the same child's ratings on different occasions. For example, if a boy says his pain is 10 out of 10 and a girl says her pain is 6 out of 10, we cannot conclude that the boy's pain is more severe than the girl's. The difference might be due merely to the way each child understands and uses the pain rating scale. But if the children give us lower pain ratings after a helpful intervention, we know we are on the right track (von Baeyer, 2009).

A Caution

Children are sensitive to their environment, and this sensitivity affects how they report their pain. Some children, desiring to please the person who is asking them questions, may say what they think the person wants to hear. Others may be fearful of certain consequences, such as separation from their parents, and will under-report their pain. Under-reporting of pain frequently occurs in new and uncertain situations, like hospitals. Parents are usually very good at sensing what is really happening and may encourage the child to say what he or she is really experiencing. A useful check is to keep track of parent's non-verbal responses when you're asking the child, and follow-up on any discrepancies with the parent later. This subtle information becomes part of determining a fuller picture in an assessment of the child's pain and its impact.

Tools for a Child's Own Report of Pain

Many tools can be used with children of different ages to obtain their self-report of pain (Stinson, Yamada, Kavanagh, Gill, & Stevens, 2006). Six tools are suggested here: Pieces of Hurt Tool, a Body Map to draw in the location of pain, a Faces Scale, a Verbal Numerical Rating Scale, a Ladder Scale to measure pain severity, and a Pain Diary.

Pieces of Hurt

The Pieces of Hurt tool is ideal for young children and easy to use. It consists of four red poker chips that are shown to the child, representing "just a little hurt" (one chip); "a little more hurt" (two chips); "more hurt" (three chips); "the most hurt you could ever have" (four chips). There is no zero. Ask the child, "How many pieces of hurt do you have right now?" Clarify the child's answer by words such as, "Oh, you have a little hurt? Tell me about the hurt." Record the number of chips selected. Reportedly, children without pain will say they don't have any. There is data supporting the use of this tool with preschool age children for acute procedural and hospital-based pain (Stinson et al., 2006). Note that after use with one child, the chips require cleaning.

Body Map

Children aged five and older can use the body map tool. It is not a quantitative measure, but it assists health care professionals to see accurately where a child feels pain. Presented with a body outline, such as the one shown in Figure 4.2, the child is asked to shade or color in the places that hurt. Older children can be asked to use a different color for each different kind or severity of pain, such as mild, moderate and severe pain, but the coloring should not take more than a couple of minutes. Repeating the process over time will show changes. Using the body map, children often identify areas of pain that are not detected by other methods.

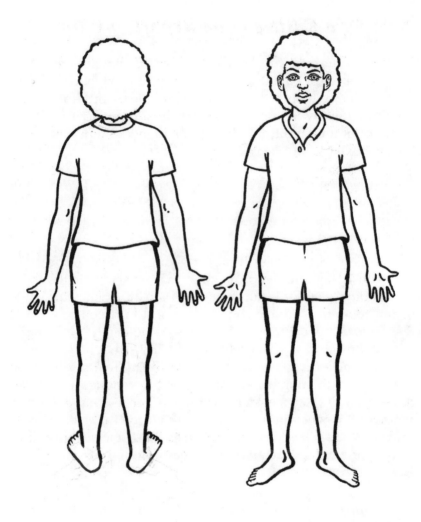

Figure 4.2. Body Map

Ask the child to shade or color in the places that hurt on both front and back body maps. Children can use a different color for each different kind or severity of pain, such as mild, moderate and severe pain. This measure can be repeated at subsequent assessments.

[The Body Map may be modified and reproduced freely.]

Faces Pain Scale – Revised

Some three-year-olds, many four-year-olds, and most children five years and older can use the Faces Pain Scale – Revised to indicate how severe their pain is (Hicks et al., 2001). In the following instructions, say 'hurt' or 'pain', whichever seems right for a particular child. The health care provider or parent shows the pictures in Figure 4.3 to the child and says, "These faces show how much something can hurt. This face (point to left-most face) shows no pain. The faces show more and more pain (point to each from left to right) up to this one (point to right-most face) – it shows very much pain. Point to the face that shows how much you hurt [right now]."

The numbers are not shown to the child. Write down the number for the chosen face, so '0' = 'no pain' and '10' = 'very much pain.' Do not use words like 'happy' and 'sad'. This scale is intended to measure how children feel inside, not how their face looks.

Verbal Numerical Rating Scale

The verbal numerical rating scale (NRS) has the great advantage of needing no paper, pencil, nor other equipment. The child can be asked for a rating, and can respond by saying a number or just holding up fingers to show the number. This scale is considered suitable for most children aged eight years and up (von Baeyer, Spagrud, McCormick, Choo, Neville, & Connelly, 2009). The parent or health care professional can say, "I'd like you to tell me a number to show how much pain you're in right now. We'll use numbers from 0 to 10. Zero would mean that you have no pain or hurt, and 10 would mean that you have the worst or most pain." Write down the number the child selects, and repeat the question at regular intervals to track the pain over time.

Note that this method requires not only the ability to count, but also some ability to estimate quantities using numbers, and sometimes may need previous experience in using a pain ladder scale (see Visual Analogue Scales Figure 4.4) to become familiar with the requirements.

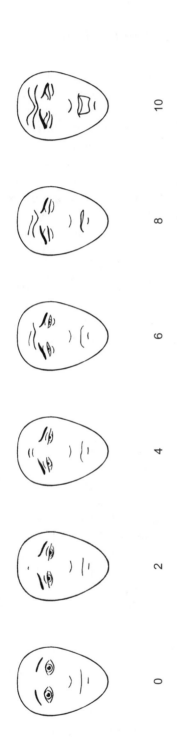

Figure 4.3 Faces Pain Scale – Revised. This figure may be copied for home, clinical and research use. The instructions are available in many languages at www.painsourcebook.ca.

From Bieri et al., 1990 & Hicks et al., Pain 2001 Copyright © 2001

[Printed with permission from IASP}

Visual Analogue Scales: Pain Ladder and Colour Analogue Scale

Visual analogue scales (VAS) appeal to children eight years and older. They indicate the extreme limits of pain intensity (no pain to the worst pain ever). A vertical ladder is one version with points 0–10, from bottom to top. The child is invited to select a point along the ladder to indicate the intensity of the pain. Another version is the Color Analogue Scale (Figure 4.4) which is well-validated (McGrath, Seifert, Speechley, Booth, Stitt, & Gibson (1996). The

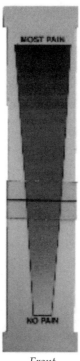

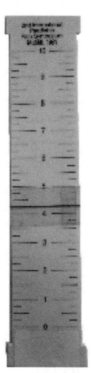

Front   *Back*

Figure 4.4 Colour Analogue Scale. Children are invited to move the marker along the scale up to the level that matches the intensity of their pain. The clinician then turns the scale over to record the corresponding number. [From, P.A. McGrath, et al., 1996, Pain. *Used with permission from IASP]*

scale, colored red, indicates an increase in intensity of colour up to 'most pain'. The reverse indicates the corresponding number and points in between. After an intervention to reduce pain, the child can readjust the marker to indicate any change in the pain. It's attractive, practical and efficient. The VAS tools are easy to create or reproduce.

Pain Diary

Pain diaries can be individually designed for a child's particular circumstance. The diary should include regular recordings of the date, the time the pain occurred, the pain intensity numerical rating, what happened before the pain started, how the pain was managed, and how successful that management was (for example, a numerical rating after treating the pain). Figure 4.5 provides a suggested format for the diary. In this version the 'Helpers'

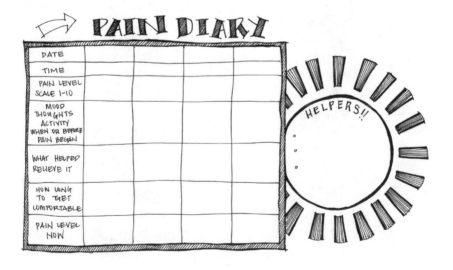

Figure 4.5 The child fills in all available helpers and takes the pain diary home to complete a column when or after the pain occurs. It is particularly useful for recurrent pain.

[The pain diary may be modified and reproduced freely.]

– which are personally identified interventions to reduce pain and increase comfort (such as, lying down, medications, massage) – are emphasized. Children in the first few years of school (six to eight years old) may need some help completing the diary. As a record, the pain diary is useful to reveal patterns of onset, frequencies over the week or months, and other events that contributed to the pain. The diary is an especially helpful tool if the child's pain is puzzling, or if it is a recurring pain that needs monitoring to determine better management.

Tools for Observational Measurement of Pain

Observational tools are useful when children are either too young (usually three years or under) or too distressed to understand and use a self-report tool (von Baeyer & Spagrud, 2007). Using an observational measure of pain is recommended when children are cognitively impaired, have communication difficulties, or are restricted by ventilation, bandages, or other physical constrictions (Oberlander & Symons, 2006); or if a child's self-report is considered unreliable because of minimization, exaggeration, or emotional or other factors.

Two tools are suggested. One can be used with children of any age, as a complement or substitute for self-report. The other is intended for children who have developmental or communication disabilities.

Face, Legs, Activity, Cry, Consolability (FLACC) Scale

The observational tool the Face, Legs, Activity, Cry, Consolability (FLACC) Scale is shown in Table 4.2. Watch the child for one to five minutes, and then pick the most appropriate number in each of the five rows, and add them up. Scores of 4 to 6 out of 10 reflect moderate pain, and 7 or higher indicates severe pain or discomfort.

FLACC scores can be used in place of self-report scores or a pain diary for children who can't provide self-reports.

Measurement of Pain Severity in Children with Developmental or Communication Disabilities

It is a special challenge for parents and health care professionals to assess pain in children who have cognitive impairment or developmental delays. Children with neurological disorders, such as cerebral palsy, and pervasive developmental disorders, such as autism, may have difficulty in expressing their pain in a way that others can understand (Oberlander & Symons, 2006).

In addition to the communication barriers these children may face, they also often have multiple medical problems, and they may have to undergo many medical procedures. Their behavior may be idiosyncratic and hard to interpret: they may laugh when in pain or moan when not in pain. However, a number of behavioral cues have been identified as indicators of pain in these children. No single cue is reliable by itself, but a child who shows several of these behaviors is likely to be in pain. The cues include facial expression; vocalizations such as moaning and screaming; sweating or flushing; and changes in posture and movement, eating and sleeping, and mood and sociability.

Table 4.2. The FLACC Scale. (Merkel et al., Pediatric Nursing 1997;23(3):293-97.

[With permission from the Regents of the University of Michigan c 2002.]

Categories	Scoring		
	0	**1**	**2**
Face	No particular expression or smile	Occasional grimace or frown, withdrawn, disinterested	Frequent to constant quivering chin, clenched jaw
Legs	Normal position or relaxed	Uneasy, restless, tense	Kicking, or legs drawn up
Activity	Lying quietly, normal position, moves easily	Squirming, shifting back and forth, tense	Arched, rigid or jerking
Cry	No cry (awake or asleep)	Moans or whimpers; occasional complaint	Crying steadily, screams or sobs, frequent complaints
Consolability	Content, relaxed	Reassured by occasional touching, hugging or being talked to, distractable	Difficult to console or comfort

Each of the five categories (F) Face; (L) Legs; (A) Activity; (C) Cry; (C) Consolability is scored from 0-2, which results in a total score between zero and ten

Several pain assessment tools help us to assess these behavioral cues of pain. The best-known is the Non-Communicating Children's Pain Checklist – Revised, NCCPC-R, (http://www.aboutkidshealth.ca/Shared/PDFs/AKH_Breau_everyday.pdf) by psychologist Lynn Breau and her colleagues (Breau, McGrath, Camfield, & Finley, 2002). There is also a postoperative version. Another instrument for these children is the Paediatric Pain Profile (Hunt, Wisbeach, Seers, et al., 2007). An advantage of the PPP is that it incorporates parents' judgments of what signs uniquely indicate pain in their own child.

Conclusion

Children in pain are commonly asked, "How is your pain today? Heard often in hospitals, this question has become a health professional's automatic social pleasantry on entering the child's room. This question is vague and of little benefit to either the child or clinician. It would be more helpful if, after a genuine hello, the child were asked: "Would you tell me about your pain? Let's measure your pain today on the number scale (or with the faces) so that I can know how much pain you still have." Or "Using those body maps again, draw where your pain is now, and using your colors show me how much pain you feel."

Using reliable and valid measures for a child's pain provides relevant information to track and treat the pain. However, we know that these responses are far from simple. The report of pain is influenced by many factors, including the child's mood, desire to please, fatigue or state of the disease, cultural and family influences, and perception of the current situation (as seen in the impact of chronic pain, Figure 1.1) The condition causing the pain is only one of the contributors to the experience of pain, as we know from the gate control theory and the neuromatrix explained in Chapter 2.

Nevertheless, the child's own report of the pain experience is regarded as the best place to start in evaluating a child's pain over time. For pain that recurs or is ongoing, children and parents can also use any of the self-report scales, the FLACC observational scale, or the pain diary, so that they can share, explore, and discuss these longer term records with a health care professional. These tools reveal important patterns of the pain – crucial evidence when considering methods to relieve pain. These methods are taken up in the chapters in Part II.

Part II

Pain Treatments – Psychological, Physical and Pharmacological

"It's not that we don't know what to do when a child is in pain. We do, but we don't always do it."

Dr. Don Tyler, Anesthesiologist and Former Pain Director, Seattle Children's Hospital

After completing a thorough history, assessment, and clinical evaluation of a child's pain, you have a clearer picture of key aspects of this pain. By selecting the most suitable therapeutic method or combination of methods, and proceeding to treat this pain, the picture will clarify further. How the child responds to the therapies often reveals more about aspects of the pain, its etiology, triggers, and other contributing factors. Once therapy has started, there is a further process of refining these interventions to optimize a positive outcome. In the process of refinement, some interventions will fall away, others will click with the child and be a good fit, and some may need further tailoring to fit and be effective. Together with the child, and sometimes parent, this is a constructive and active process to find the best-fit. The child gradually moves into the driver's seat, as the pain hopefully moves to the backseat!

Depending on the nature of the child's pain and the child's age and circumstance, the methods may be various combinations of the 3Ps – psychological, physical, and pharmacological. Psychological and physical treatments can be combined with pharmacological support, or primarily psychological treatment, with physical and occasional pharmacological support, or pharmacological analgesia, with graded physical intervention and intermittent psychological support. Sometimes these combinations shift as difficulties are encountered or progress is achieved. We need to stay attentive to emerging issues and be flexible with our treatment options, maintaining as many strings to our treatment bow as possible. For that reason I've included a broad range of treatment options of conventional and complementary techniques that are becoming increasingly integrated within our health care systems and communities.

The Therapeutic Alliance

We always work as a team with the child, and with the parent involved to one degree or another. It is important that as health care professionals we play a supportive, educative role, rather than being in charge. As the pain is in the child's body, enabling the child to become the boss of his or her body is crucial to any therapeutic endeavor. The understanding and relationship between child and clinician is central. This includes addressing what we'll do together, why this may help, how it will unfold, and the child's job and responsibilities in this process. This is the therapeutic contractual agreement for a positive outcome.

With acute pain treatment this agreement is usually fairly straight forward as there is a more predictable course of recovery. With chronic pain, however, the therapeutic journey toward recovery has a lot more variance with more complexity. The outcome can also be influenced by the quality of the therapeutic alliance that develops between the child, clinician, and parent. When the alliance is strong, the child and parents are more likely to stick with the program, despite the ups and downs in recovery, and they will draw strength and hope from the professional relationship – whatever the discipline of the clinician. When the alliance is not solid, or is broken for one reason or another, it is harder for the child and parent to trust and make their way through the disappointments or frustrations that occur in the course of persistent or complex pain.

The Interdependence of the 3P treatments

Although the pain-relieving methods in this part of the book are divided for convenience into chapters on psychological, physical, and pharmacological methods, they are synergistic and mutually interdependent. None of these methods is exclusive, and all work harmoniously with each other. When combined, they reinforce each other, providing more effective, comprehensive treatment with the potential for long-term positive outcomes. For example, if a child has severe headache pain and focuses on the image of her pain becoming smaller, while deliberately relaxing her body after taking her pain medication, she is likely to achieve more comprehensive relief from pain and suffering than from taking medication alone, or the sole use of relaxation or imagery. With more consistent use of the co-current treatment combination, her neural signature patterns that make her prone to these recurrent migraines may begin to repattern, decreasing the frequency, intensity, and duration of these migraine episodes.

The aim of treatment is to provide relief from pain, and a greater understanding and capacity of how to maintain this in everyday life. With the multi-dimensional nature of pain, methods that also attenuate anxiety, despair, or frustration and enable the child re-engage with life (social and academic) are valuable therapeutic adjuncts. Ultimately a good outcome is that the selected psychological, physical, and pharmacological treatments become a natural part of the child's coping and pain management strategy, and the pain becomes history!

Chapter 5

Psychological Methods to Relieve Pain

"Suffering children hurt us."

Dr. Joe Barber, Psychologist, Seattle, Washington

To begin this chapter on psychological interventions, let's examine the power of language and the words to use with children in pain. As mentioned before, communication is the most common of all medical or nursing or psychological procedures. Engaging with a child in pain to explain what interventions could help is an essential aspect of the therapeutic relationship – whatever the discipline of health care professional. What we say, how we say it, and how we continue the conversation to encourage the child's engagement and ownership in the process of treatment and healing, is central to the delivery of the psychological P of the 3Ps.

In this chapter we'll discuss in some depth cognitive-behavioral pain-relieving methods, such as distraction, thought-stopping, hypnosis, and imagery—as there is good evidence for their benefit to children in pain, as well as the creative therapies of music, art, and play. We'll also consider biofeedback and acceptance and commitment therapy, both useful in children's chronic pain.

Language That Helps Pain to Go Away

Language that conveys support, hope, love, courage, energy, humor, or affection, and that promises some release from suffering, is the language that helps children let go of the terror, doubt, fear, and pain that often complicate healing (Lang et al., 2005). Therapeutic language goes hand in hand with attentive listening. As you actively attend to a child's language and behavior, that focus is felt by the child. Your 'tuning-in' is often mirrored by more accurate responses to the child's messages. During this exchange your language and tone also convey your attitude. In other words: *what you say and how you say it, reflects what you think, as well as what you believe, what you teach, what you expect, and even at times what is likely to happen!* Here are some useful pointers for using language therapeutically with a child in pain (Kuttner & Kohen, 1996).

1. *Ask about and acknowledge the pain.* A child is helped by hearing validation of his or her pain: "You are in a lot of pain right now, and we are going to help you." Then, when you ask a child to precisely describe the discomfort, "Can you tell me more about it?" it helps the child to define the pain, and more important, conveys the notion that he or she is believed, that you are concerned, and that you will endeavor to help. You can say: "The more I know about your pain, the more I can understand it and the better I can help. After all, it's your pain, and you know it better than I do. Please help me understand where it is, and where it stops."

    At first glance this might seem like focusing too much on the pain, but it serves an important function. It helps the child define and compartmentalize the discomfort; to know not only where it is, but also where it is not. In this conversation the triggers of the pain, what exacerbates it, and what helps can be explored. Developing this 'cognitive mastery' is important for young children especially, so that they can begin to cope and gain some control over their discomfort. Listening to the child's description allows you to understand more clearly what the child is experiencing, to learn how he or she is conceptualizing the pain, what triggered it, what could be maintaining it. The child's language also gives you clues about what words and ideas would improve his or her mood, increase motivation, and reduce suffering.

There's a further interpersonal message. Asking about the pain at the outset, rather than taking a developmental and family history or mental status exam, indicates to the child and parent that you are accepting their foremost concern about the experience and consequences of pain, rather than trying to translate these into a mental health problem or a matter of chemistry or physiology. As my colleague Dr. Carl von Baeyer says: "It's like accepting their entry ticket instead of telling them they ought to bring you a different ticket!"

2. *Recognize the value of listening.* The other half of the therapeutic impact of language is the therapeutic benefit of listening. As you ask questions, be sure to wait patiently and with positive expectation for the child's (not the parent's!) answer, which, when given, allows you to explore further and simultaneously to convey some shift in the child's definition: for example, if a child says, "I've always get stomach pain," you can add, "Until now! But now let's talk about how it can begin to change. What would be the first thing you'd notice when the pain starts to change?" Listen to *how* the child responds, not only the words used.

3. *Pace this process respectfully.* Although we are eager to help and to 'fix it,' remember that obtaining this information should be at a pace and rhythm that works for the child. As you show that you can make the space for the child to talk, if he or she wishes, you teach not only sensitivity but also patience by your own example. Active coaching is tracking and keeping pace with the child, providing help and encouragement to get through the discomfort, so that the child doesn't experience it entirely alone.

4. *Define the child's pain by framing it with hope, not doom.* Children in pain quickly feel defeated. To counter this you could say, for example, to a child with multiple lacerations: "You're

an energetic boy. I hear you like your skateboard! It looks as if you'll need some stitches so that you heal well and continue to get even better on your skateboard." This statement is framed with hope.

5. *Avoid negative words and those that conjure up fear.* Compare the response above to this one laced with guilt, doubts, and doom, "These skateboards can be very dangerous. You'll need stitches, but I don't think you'll have scars!" Children listen carefully and watch closely. The first and most salient words, whether or not they're preceded by 'not', will be in their mind. What will the child remember? *Dangerous, stitches, scars*. Similarly, if you say, "Don't be afraid, it won't hurt much," children hear 'afraid' and 'hurt much'. Use words that inspire courage and coping, and sustain the hope that pain will ease. It is after all an electrical-chemical signal open to modulation at many sites!

6. *Reframe the child's distress.* If a child has defined the pain as a catastrophe, immediately reframe it. For example, a child says, "This pain is killing me!" A positive reframing may begin with some acknowledgement. For example: "It does hurt a lot, and your body is clearly saying it is ready for some powerful help. Let's get these pain medications into your system, and then you'll notice the comfort getting stronger." This offers an alternative without denying the child's experience.

    When a child is startled and frightened by the sight of his or her own blood, reframe it by saying, "What beautiful blood you have! It's a bright strong red. Look! I can tell it is healthy by its color. Your blood is doing a good job of cleaning the wound out. That's excellent. Once it has done the job, the bleeding will stop, soon." Using positive language is powerful and its effects are long-lasting. Take the time to think about what you say and how you say it. If the child's catastrophizing continues, the clinician needs to help the child learn more adaptive self-statements to replace the arousing, negativity of catastrophic talk.

7. *Replace pain-loaded words with more tolerable words.* What we believe and how we think and talk about pain and suffering are products of how we were brought up and the personal experiences we have had with discomfort. Did you notice the shift from the word *pain* to the word *discomfort*? The word *discomfort* holds within it the possibility of comfort, and there is even the possibility of emphasizing the *comfort* part rather than the *dis-* prefix. This kind of shift even in single words is an important step in the development of your own conceptual framework of what pain is and is not – and, more important, what you believe you can and cannot do in response to it.

   Another necessary shift, especially when talking to a child about previous or recurrent pain, is to refer to an 'episode' or 'a time you had pain' instead of an 'attack' of pain. 'Episode' is a neutral word that doesn't suggest hurt. 'Attack' is a battle word that implies being at risk, a victim, and heightens feelings of vulnerability, helplessness, and fear – clearly of no therapeutic value. Instead, you might say to the child: "Let's use 'episode' or 'event' for each time you have discomfort or when you are 'bothered'." Most children will accept the invitation to throw out the negative word.

8. *Draw on language or words that have worked for you.* How you think about pain comes from how you made sense of, and navigated uncomfortable pain experiences as a child yourself, and how the adults around you responded at those times. As you think of language that eases pain and suffering, you may draw on the phrases you remember adults saying to you that were reassuring or useful. "You *can* do it. You're helping your body get more comfortable… I can tell already how much better you're doing."

9. *Note the parts of the body that are not in pain.* If a child is preoccupied and over-focused on pain and not open to coping, use language that shifts the child's attention. Six-year-old Josh, pediatrician Dan Kohen's son who delighted in hypnosis, was on a picnic with a group of friends. Another boy about his age fell while running and banged his knee. As he sat

screaming on the ground holding his knee, Josh was the first one to reach him. As the other adults approached moments later, they heard Josh asking his playmate, "How's your other knee?" which had not been injured. In a flash his friend stopped crying, turned his attention to the other knee, and said it was fine, and then they both got up to play.

Shifting attention to where it is not hurting moves a child out of panic or shock. You can then delineate the limits of the pain. For example, if a child feels trapped by persistent pain, say: "I know your leg in traction is hurting with the pin in place, but is it sore in your hip? No! Good. How about in your back? No! Excellent! And in your ankle? No! I'm very glad to hear this, because it means that the pain is contained from the top of your leg to your calf, but it isn't in your hip, your back, or your ankle. We'll check this again, after you've had your medication in an hour and see how much it has improved."

Post-surgery require frequent assessment of the child's pain, to ensure that the child has sufficient pain medication and is not suffering needlessly.

10. *Use language that implies positive change.* One day while walking through the general clinic, pediatrician Dan Kohen overheard a little girl about five years old crying and coughing, complaining that her throat 'hurt a lot'. Her mother, embarrassed by her daughter's commotion, was reprimanding her. Dan asked if the child would tell him about her sore throat. She stopped crying and told him. She was given some acetaminophen for her discomfort and fever and told that her doctor would be in to check her over soon. Before leaving, Dan told her, "You'll probably be surprised how fast you start to get better." She calmed down. Her hurt had been acknowledged and some relief provided. Perhaps just as important was using language that was positive and supportive. Dan's final words of encouragement provided this little girl with hope for change without making false promises or denying her discomfort. Language like this provides comfort because it diminishes fear and uncertainty.

11. *Where possible, let the child know that what he or she is experiencing is normal and not life-threatening nor the result of a terrible disease.* Children have active imaginations and unless correctly informed may imagine the worst: "Your pain is strong because your arm is broken and bruised. The nerves in your arm are sending fast and strong messages to your brain so that you know not to move it. This is usual when a bone breaks. So to bring comfort and better messages back into your body, we're going to do the following…"

12. *Remind the child that the pain will come to an end.* Always truthfully provide the child with some idea of when the pain is likely to ease or go entirely. Fit this into developmentally appropriate language for the child. For a preschool child you could say, "After one sleep you'll be able to get out of bed and the 'hurt' will be gone." Here is a phrase to convey that pain will come to an end: "I'm wondering how quickly and easily you'll notice the easing of your discomfort, because children's bodies heal quickly." Note how hypnotic that sentence is in drawing one's attention to positive aspects: quickly, easily, easing, heal. Pain is rarely a steady, consistent sensation, and children's bodies do repair and heal much more quickly than those of adults.

The words you choose, and when and how you use them matter a lot. They accompany the many psychological or cognitive-behavioral pain-relieving methods described in the rest of this chapter.

Mind Skills to Relieve Pain

The skills of using distraction methods, thought stopping, imagery and hypnosis provide children with skills to reduce their pain and distress. With guidance children learn to promote pain relief and feelings of well-being. These self-administered or initially therapist guided treatment can be further sustained by the child, parents or staff. They are inexpensive and foster competency. Feeling overcome by pain or helpless is a natural consequence of having to undergo a disliked invasive procedure and the impact of pain itself on the body. Offering some self-control in situations that by custom don't lend themselves to it helps reduce these feelings. Giving control doesn't mean that the child dictates what will happen. It means the child has some choices. This can change the meaning of the pain from, "There's nothing I can do to make it different," to "Now that I have this technique that I can do, I can get through this. And, the more I do it the stronger it works to help me feel better."

In 2006 there was a Cochrane review of twenty-eight randomized controlled trials (RCTs) of psychological interventions for children and adolescents between two and nineteen years old, undergoing needle-related procedures (Uman, Chambers, McGrath, & Kisely, 2008). The outcome measures included self-report, observer report, behavioral or observational measures, and physiological correlates of pain and distress. The researchers found that distraction, combined cognitive-behavioral interventions, and hypnosis treatments produced the largest effect sizes for treatment improvement over the control conditions. There was promising but limited evidence for the other psychological interventions.

Distraction uses objects external to divert and hold attention away from the pain. As such it's easier for younger children. Thought-stopping, an inner control method, isn't developmentally suited to children under six or seven years of age.

Distraction

Age: Ten months and older.

Pain: Treatment-related, acute, and chronic pain.

Time: As needed and usually for a short duration.

Distraction is the active diverting of the child's attention – not tricking the child, but inviting the child to shift attention onto a chosen, interesting, and more pleasant physical object than the painful procedure.

The child chooses anything of interest, such as a pop-up book, a musical toy, a magic wand, bubbles, or a colorful egg timer. The rationale is that since the pain experience depends on the brain's processing of sensory and emotional signals, distraction could interrupt or interfere with this processing. Distraction is most effective with mild and short-term pain, particularly pain that is familiar to the child. The child will be more willing to shift attention away if the procedure is known, the distraction self-chosen and the situation holds no surprises. Here are some useful distracters:

- *Blowing bubbles* is a child-centered winner. After 30 years of use, it is still a hot and regular favorite of mine (see Chapter 6 for a fuller discussion of this a distracter).

- *Focus on objects in the room* is an easy but short form of distraction, such as counting the flowers on Mom's blouse or tracking a musical toy as it completes its routine.

- *Pop-up books* provide multiple choices for diversion, surprise, and humor. The child has control over which tab to pull, can feel accomplishment when identifying an object or number on the page, and can be delighted and surprised by the many and unexpected situations in these inventive and amusing books. Pop-up books have a role to play in procedure rooms. I have noticed, however, that the most spectacular of these, tend to disappear from procedure rooms. Finding a way to secure them is important for children who become reliant on this playful, interesting form of distraction.

The following case of how three-year-old Meg and her mother managed a tough week in hospital illustrates how some of the methods discussed above can be creatively combined:

Meg had a diagnosis of retinoblastoma, a rare eye cancer. In the course of treatment, she needed five consecutive days of IV therapy. Not surprisingly, by the third day she had learned what was in store for her and began kicking and crying when she was taken into the treatment room. Her mom, however, was prepared. She straddled the treatment table with Meg nestling between her legs and took out Meg's favorite book, Curious George Goes to Hospital *(Margret Rey, 1995). She read the book in a loud, confident voice, asking Meg questions and making humorous remarks. Meg became involved in the story, but every now and again looked around the room. She tensed when the IV nurse entered the room and whimpered when the nurse began looking at the veins on her foot. Mom successfully distracted Meg's attention back to the book by saying, "Hey, what is Curious George doing on the telephone? Do you remember when Mommy accidentally phoned New York instead of Aunt Elsie?"*

As the nurse began cleaning her foot, Meg's mom began blowing bubbles and then held the wand for Meg to blow. "Blow away the owies!" directed Mom firmly as Meg looked at the needle, blowing and whimpering. As the needle was inserted, her mom guided Meg's attention back to the story by saying, "Good, we'll soon have the Band-aid on. What on earth is Curious George up to now!" Her positive involvement, her physical containment of Meg, and her active direction of Meg's attention away from the source of pain to her loved story enabled Meg to finish the remaining days of that treatment with steadily diminishing anxiety and distress. The nursing staff were impressed and grateful.

Thought-Stopping

Age: Six years and older.

Pain: Anticipatory anxiety for medical and dental treatments.

Time: Brief.

A child can exert control in an internal way, such as using thought-stopping. Developed for children by Dr. Dorrie Ross (1984), this method is suited for those who catastrophize, focusing on and exaggerating the unpleasant aspects of the pain (see Chapter 3). Thought-stopping teaches children to catch themselves as they begin to catastrophize and to deliberately substitute a positive thought. Children, with a clinician's support, assemble a set of positive facts about the impending procedures (e.g., "I have good veins; having the needle put in my arm doesn't take long"). Then some reassuring facts are added, "The rest doesn't hurt once the needle is in" (Ross, 1988, p. 247). These facts are condensed, working with the child, into a positive statement all of which he knows is true and related to him. The child memorizes and repeats this every time an anxiety-arousing thought occurs. For example, Frederick, a seven-year-old boy on dialysis for his kidney condition, had an intense dislike of his dialysis machine:

If I think about it [the machine], I get real mad at myself, and I say, "Fred, you stop that thinking . . . STOP!" Then I say, "It's just two hours. My friends are here. The TV is on and I'll feel really good afterwards." And if I start thinking about the machine again, I just say, "Stop that thinking, you dumbbell", and repeat, "It's just two hours," all over again and again!

Imagery and Hypnosis

Imagery is the spontaneous or deliberate mental reconstruction of sights, sounds, smells, tastes, and feelings as if they were actually occurring. As part of our inner life, images carry personal meaning and power and undoubtedly play a central role in helping the body heal. Imagery is an active process and generates new internal experiences, unlike the passive act of relaxing. Whether images spontaneously spring to mind or are consciously created, they help to bring a desirable state closer to reality. Focusing on chosen or favorite images provides an opportunity to escape from pain and not be preoccupied with it. Even more important, focusing on altering the image or sensations of the pain may enable a child in pain gain more self-control and relief from the pain. Imagery needs to be gentle, child-centered, and energy conserving to relieve children's and adolescents' pain and suffering.

The benefit of imagery as a pain reduction technique with long-term results, were the findings in this recent pilot study. Children ages 6 to 15 years old diagnosed with functional abdominal pain who used audio recordings of guided imagery at home in addition to standard medical treatment, were almost three times as likely to reduce their abdominal pain, compared to children who received only standard treatment. Those benefits were maintained six months after the end of treatment (van Tilburg, et al., 2009).

Thirty four children recruited by pediatric gastroenterologists all received standard medical care and nineteen were randomized to receive eight weeks of guided imagery treatment. The guided imagery sessions had been developed and recorded onto CDs for the children's use at home. Their treatment consisted of four biweekly, 20-minute sessions and shorter 10-minute daily sessions. For example, in session one the CD directs children to imagine floating on a cloud and progressively relaxing. Therapeutic suggestions and imagery for reducing discomfort included letting a special shiny object melt into their hand and then placing their hand on their belly, spreading warmth and light from the hand inside their tummy to make a protective barrier to prevent anything from irritating it.

The children using guided imagery reported that they enjoyed using the CDs. Three quarters of that group reported that their abdominal pain was reduced by half or more by the end of treatment. Only a quarter of the group receiving standard medical care achieved the same level of improvement. This more than doubled when guided imagery treatment was offered later to the standard medical care group. In both groups combined, these benefits persisted for six months in over 60% percent of the children. The study concluded that guided imagery treatment plus medical care was superior to standard medical care for the treatment of functional abdominal pain. Notably, the effects of treatment were sustained over a long period.

How are imagery and hypnosis related? Both hypnosis and imagery are internal imaginal experiences requiring a shift from present reality (Olness & Kohen, 1996). They differ in the degree of absorption and focused concentration needed to experience an internally constructed reality. The difference between hypnosis and imagery is not one of kind, but of degree of absorption and consciousness alteration – and as a result, the degree in the capacity for therapeutic change. Hypnosis creates more physiological changes, more intense involvement and concentration, and therefore greater sensory, perceptual, and memory changes occur. Furthermore, imagery methods don't use direct suggestions for change, such as creating numbness in a body area. Imagery uses indirect suggestions through the creation of an imaginary pleasant experience (the indirect suggestion in that scenario is one of comfort and well-being). Hypnosis, on the other hand, uses the child's altered state of consciousness to optimize therapeutic change with many forms of hypnotic suggestion. Let's examine hypnosis in more detail, before going into the practice of Imagery.

Hypnosis

Hypnosis is a powerful method for managing many forms of pain and discomfort, and has a long, colorful, and eventful history. In 1958 the American Medical and Psychiatric Associations accredited hypnosis for use in treatment. Since its resurgence, hypnosis has become increasingly used as a therapeutic tool in many areas of health care, sport, and academic performance. It has particularly been researched and valued by health care professionals as a primary or additional pain-relief method for adults as well as children. Hypnosis requires training provided by accredited organizations with pediatric faculty. Adult methods of hypnosis are not recommended for children.

Hypnosis is an altered state of consciousness, or a trance, characterized by a temporary suspension of critical judgment, rapid assimilation of information, the capacity to alter sensation and perception, increased suggestibility, the loosening up of habitual frameworks and beliefs, and the capacity to become absorbed in feelings, sensations, or ideas even if they are unusual or out of context (Olness & Kohen, 1996).

During hypnosis for pain relief, a change in the child's perception of pain is facilitated. This change appears to bypass the child's conscious effort. The clinician invites the child to shift into an altered state of consciousness by focusing and narrowing attention. Hypnosis occurs in the relationship between patient and therapist. "The 'active agent' is not the words, but the quality of the rapport, and the hypnotic inductions, suggestions, and imagery proposed" (Wood & Bioy, 2008, p. 443). Although we still don't know the precise neurophysiological mechanisms by which hypnosis alleviates suffering and diminishes pain, we know that it is effective. As a result, clinicians and researchers in the pain field have become reliant on hypnosis for pain relief intervention (Barber, 2004; Kuttner, 1988; Liossi, 2002; Liossi et al., 2009; Vlieger et al., 2007; Zeltzer & LeBaron, 1982; Zeltzer et al., 1991).

Recent research studies on the neuroimaging of hypnosis for pain control in adults are providing more evidence and validation for the existence of a hypnotic state and ratifying its therapeutic effects. Hypnotic states are associated with higher levels of cerebral blood flow in the anterior cingulate regions and in the occipital cortical areas of the brain (Rainville et al., 1999). Increases in hypnotic relaxation were associated with cerebral blow flow increases in the occipital cortex and decreases in brainstem areas and in the right parietal lobe. In a further study when subjects reported an increase in mental absorption during hypnosis, these were associated with increases in cerebral blood flow within a connected network of brain structures involved in attention (Rainville et al., 2002).

It is now recognized that certain regions of the brain are activated by pain stimuli and that hypnosis modulates these activations. It appears that when suggested experiences are accepted without any censoring, such as can occur in a hypnotic trance, this enables suggested alternative sensations and feelings, such hypnotic analgesia, to occur. These studies enable us to better understand how hypnosis is effective on the cortical level (for further information see the review by Wood & Bioy, 2008).

In early research on how hypnosis alters pain, Dr. Ernest Hilgard, a psychologist at Stanford University, found that adult patients under hypnosis reported aloud that a normally painful sensation to the arm was not painful (Hilgard, 1977). Dr. Hilgard then asked the patients, who were still in hypnotic trance, whether a part of their consciousness had noted any pain. Hilgard learned that hypnosis created a dissociative state in the brain, a conscious part that reported no pain, and a subconscious part, which he called 'the hidden observer', responded with automatic writing that pain was indeed being experienced. The pain signal got through to the brain, but because of the hypnotic trance it was not deemed 'pain' or perceived as 'painful'. Hypnosis allows us to change or ignore the meaning, while the sensory input is still active and noted.

Children who have been trained to use self-hypnosis report the same experience. Eight-year-old Seanna, while in a light hypnotic trance when an IV catheter was placed in a vein on her hand, said: "I know the pain is there, but somehow it doesn't bother me anymore!" Clearly her brain dissociated from or altered the experience of the pain, which previously had hurt and upset her.

Hypnotherapy includes suggestions for change to occur when the child is in a trance state. Suggestions can take many forms, for example, direct suggestion: "You'll notice within the next one minute of clock time how much the pain will diminish. It may reduce by half or by three-quarters. You can let go and notice the difference in pain sensation beginning right now." Being in a trance makes it possible for a child to be open to rapid change in pain. Children in a hypnotic trance can achieve analgesia and partial anesthesia; some are able to create complete anesthesia in selected body parts, without any medication (Kuttner, 1986, 1998; Sugarman, 2006). The goal is to provide the child with some degree of control over reducing anxiety and painful sensations. It isn't always possible to remove pain entirely.

Suggestions can be very specific, as in this fine Dutch RCT on Hypnotherapy for children with functional abdominal pain or irritable bowel syndrome by Dr. Arine Vlieger and associates (Vlieger, Menko-Frankenhuis, & Wolfkamp, 2007). They used gut-directed hypnotic suggestions to reduce pain and distressing abdominal symptoms with children aged from eight to eighteen years for six sessions over a three-month period. For example, after going into a hypnotic trance the patient was invited to visualize a normal working gut using metaphors reflecting the child's interest, such as a car running at normal speed. The patients also received a standardized hypnosis session on CD and were asked to practice it daily. There were fifty-three pediatric patients. The control group received standard medical care and 6 sessions of supportive therapy. Pain intensity, pain frequency, and associated symptoms were scored in weekly standardized abdominal pain diaries at baseline, during therapy, and six and twelve months after therapy. Pain scores (pain frequency and pain intensity) at baseline to one year follow-up decreased significantly in both groups. However, hypnosis had a superior effect, with a highly significant reduction in pain scores compared with standard medical treatment. The long-term follow up at one year found that 85% of the hypnosis group and 25% of the standard medical group had retained their successful treatment outcome.

There are some powerful techniques for pain control, such as 'The Pain Switch' (see Figure 5.1) and 'The Magic Glove' both of which are taught in hypnosis training courses. It is important that the child's hypnotic experience be guided by a suitably qualified health care professional – psychologist, physician, nurse, social worker, or child-life worker – who has received training from an accredited institution. Be aware that there are people who call themselves 'hypnotherapists' but who are not health care professionals qualified to treat pain and, therefore, are not recommended to consult.

Figure 5.1 The Pain Switch at Work.

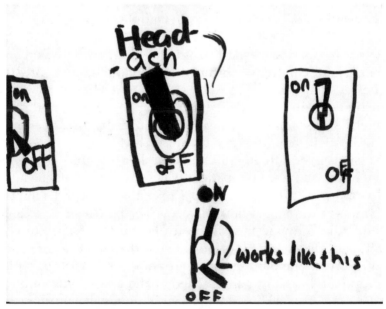

A ten year old girl depicts how the pain switches look in her head, particularly the switch that is on indicating her headache. Using the hypnotic "Pain Switch" technique with careful breathing and concentration she turns it down towards OFF.

Imagery

Imagining is a spontaneous and natural act for children. In fact, children think in images and learn to recognize objects in the world using all of their senses. The majority of children imagine primarily in pictures or sounds rather than with body sensation or smells. A child's predominant sense may be vision, nevertheless, all other senses can be called upon to reconstruct a memory or to create a new vision (see Table 5.1). Often the most primitive sensations, such as smell, evoke the strongest imagery experience.

Table 5.1 Directions to lead a child to use each of the five senses in imagining

Visual	"I wonder what you can see ..."
Auditory	"Listen closely to what sounds are here ..."
Olfactory	"I wonder what smell you may notice ..."
Gustatory	"There may be something tasty here ... As you taste it, what does it remind you of?"
Touch	"Notice what can you touch or feel right now."

Imagery can produce physiological changes. "The images we spin inwardly become the reality we spin out," writes Maureen Murdock in her useful book on guided imagery with children, *Spinning Inward* (1987). It is optimal to start imagery when pain first enters a child's life, and when used regularly, it becomes a reliable source of support and strength for the child in intermittent or chronic pain, as previously cited evidence indicates. As the child's absorption in the imagery increases, the capacity to increase comfort, diminish pain, and reduce anxiety and discomfort becomes greater.

Children's images are unique and unexpected and vary from child to child. It's recommended to select images that the child prefers and avoid disliked experiences. For example, if a child is afraid of the water, the imaginary experience of 'swimming then floating like a starfish' is more likely to create panic than relief! Whereas re-creating an activity that the child adores, like riding a horse, is more likely to provide the necessary relief. Always use the child's own spontaneous images. Here are a few stunning examples: a four year old boy's spontaneous image to increase body temperature was to 'sit on the sun!', and a fourteen-year-old hockey player who had sustained a concussion enjoyed imagining taking off the top of his skull to decrease the pressure and bring down his pain. Older children and teens can be enormously inventive in using images to change their pain perception and experience.

Seventeen-year-old Jason found one simple image that could always be counted on to help him deal with the gnawing abdominal pain from the recurring ulcerative colitis in his intestines. His method combined distancing himself from the pain and altering it. Concentrating, he imagined all his pain being put into a bag, like an intravenous bag that carries fluids and hangs from an IV pole. When he had stuffed all his pain into the bag, he would imagine deliberately taking the bag and hanging it on the far side of the IV pole, a distance away from the bed in which he lay. He would repeat this one-minute exercise whenever he needed to, with a certain mischievous glee, as he 'hung his pain out to dry!'

Monitor the child's facial expressions, position, and movements. These indicate the child's degree of involvement with the imagery and whether it is providing relief. If you note that something is amiss, ask a non-leading question: "What's happening right now?" Having a dialogue while the child is involved in the imagery can enhance its effectiveness. The child will sense the support and enter the experience more fully to obtain relief.

Some children may be reluctant at first to become involved in imagery exercises and may put up some resistance. You could tell such a child that imagery often helps the pain to ease and that you're curious about how it could help the child. Don't push it on a child. If the child isn't willing, let it go. This resistance indicates that it is not the right time or the right method for this child.

The Construction of Imagery Experiences

An imagery experience can be constructed in two ways: (1) by dissociating from the pain into a favorite place or activity; or (2) by associating the pain with a specific image and gaining some control over it by changing it or tracking how it spontaneously changes.

Dissociating from Pain

Dissociation invites the child to choose a favorite person, place, activity, or story; to leave the pain behind; and to enter the imagery, creating a rich experience using all the senses. When the present reality is fraught with pain, anxiety, fear, and tension, this dissociation helps the child to distance him or herself from the pain and escape it to some degree.

Favorite Place Imagery

Age: Five and older.

Pain: Persistent pain.

Time: 5 to 25 minutes.

Children enjoy the imaginary experience of going to a favorite place – a place of fun that's a fantasy or is familiar and has happy memories with significant people. Significant repetition to this favorite place gains potency to deliver comfort and well-being.

Here's an example:

Ten-year-old Alicia enjoyed traveling in her imagination to her favourite beach, where she could walk on the soft sand. The rhythms of the waves, like her breath, allowed the pain in her stomach to settle like the sand at the bottom of the ocean. Alicia found the pain would subside quite rapidly, despite the fact that on one occasion, to her distress, she had envisioned herself on the beach with no swimsuit on!

To guide the use of favorite place imagery, invite the child to settle into a comfortable position, ask for a favorite place where the child would like to go, and quietly begin:

Allow your eyes to close because then you can experience everything more clearly. Breathe out as your body settles down… if you like… down into this (pink/white) fluffy cloud, soft, yet strong enough to lift you up, up, and away from your bed, the pain, and discomfort. Notice how everything you no longer need remains down below; the aches, frustration, tiredness stays down, as your body on the cloud floats up, up lighter and lighter in the sky. A good feeling as the wind gently lifts the cloud, and you float effortlessly and easily across the sky, faster than any car or train taking you to your favorite place… [Mention the place the child has told you is a favorite: Disneyland/Candyland/a grandparent's home/ a holiday spot.]

Isn't it wonderful to notice how the closer you get to this place, the farther away you are from anything that used to bother you. You can probably notice it getting farther and fainter and smaller. Snuggle into the cloud, pulling it over you like a blanket, feeling warm and good. Here we come…. I wonder what you see first… (pause)… what you hear… (pause) and what you smell… (pause) [draw on the child's five senses to elaborate the experience]. Whatever you'd like to do here, you can – now. Enjoy this fun, playful imaginary experience. [If the child wishes to talk as it's unfolding, listen and support the experience.]

Soon it will be time to leave, but it's so good to know that we can come back here again, and so easily. When we reach your room, you may be surprised to notice that while we were gone the discomfort had time to dissolve, so that when you open your eyes, you'll be feeling different, maybe refreshed, or re-energized and filled with memories of your favorite place. Notice the good feelings in your body, as the pictures of your time in this, your favorite place remain clear.

The degree of pain relief will vary, depending on the child's talent to dissociate from the pain by entering the imaginary experience. Using passive language, such as 'Allow your eyes', removes volition and permits the desired change to happen without deliberate effort. A variation on this activity is to replace pain with a favorite or familiar activity, ideal for youngsters and teens who love sports.

Favorite Activity Imagery

Age: 5 and older.

Pain: Persistent pain.

Time: as long as needed.

The goal is to replace the pain with an engrossing activity that leaves no room for pain. Older children and teens can readily relive a favorite activity, such as athletic activities like skating, swimming, cycling, playing soccer, or skiing, or quieter activities like reading a book, playing a musical instrument, listening to an iPod, or sorting football or hockey cards. All can be harnessed to become an absorbing, fun-filled reality to replace the experience of pain.

Kim, a keen sportsman, was diagnosed at thirteen years of age with Crohn's disease, a disease of the small bowel. He experienced severe cramping abdominal pain and diarrhea. Since he enjoyed physical activity, when his pains began, he drew on images from sports to help him through the painful cramping spasms that characterize this disease. He would focus on becoming as comfortable as possible, though this was often hard. Then he would take himself skiing down one of his favorite runs.

In the beginning it was difficult, he said, for the pain would pull him back. But then, he told me, he would focus on the powdery snow, the sound of his skis making tracks where no one else had been. He would focus on moving, on his crouched position as he prepared to fly over a mogul, twisting and turning, and on the feeling in his legs. Then he would focus on the sights: the sun peering through the alpine trees heavy with snow, the village so small in the valley below. If this was difficult, he would conjure up smells: the crisp winter air, the smell of wet snow. He would come to the end of his run, sometimes five to seven minutes later, filled with energy and free of pain for a while.

The effect of imagery can last longer than the actual imagery experience.

Favorite Stories

Age: Two to six years.

Pain: Any mild, moderate persisting or treatment-related pain.

Time: 5 to 15 minutes.

Young children's familiar bedtime or favorite stories have a particular power (see *Annie's Stories*, Brett, 1988). Often preschoolers will ask to have their favorite story repeatedly read. Young children experience a delight in this ritual, in its predictability and its associations, anticipating what is going to happen and chiming in at the dramatic moments. Preschoolers often know their stories by heart. As a result, these favorite stories can be very helpful to utilize during scary or painful times.

Today, procedures like this one on a five-year-old would usually be carried out with conscious sedation or general anesthesia, but in the 1980s this was not the case, and we needed to rely more heavily on psychological pain control methods. We can learn a lot from how Samantha coped with just a local anesthetic for a bone marrow aspiration.

Five-year-old Samantha, diagnosed with leukemia, was referred to me for her fear of pain. I worked with her over many sessions before a dreaded painful procedure of a bone marrow aspiration, which occurred monthly as part of her cancer treatment. I asked her if she liked the story Snow White. *"I don't want that story!" she said emphatically. "I want the story of Grandma Tildy and the Elephant!" Not having heard the story, I asked her to tell it to me. She told the story vividly, complete with concrete details and sound effects.*

"Now, how about if I tell you the story of 'Grandma Tildy and the Elephant' while your bone marrow gets done?" I suggested, "I wouldn't be surprised if, by the time we got to the end of the story, the bone marrow was over and the Band-aid was on. Wouldn't that be nice?" Samantha nodded. We had a working contract.

Tightly holding her 'Kitty', she anxiously walked into the surgery room and climbed onto the table. I told the staff what we had decided to do and began the story: "Grandma Tildy lived by herself and was such a brave little lady. One day there was a knock [knocking sound effects] on the door..." Samantha's attention was glued to the details of the story. Her body moved when the sensations were uncomfortable, but her eyes were fixed, and it was striking how her concentration did not waver. I stretched out the details, increasing the intensity and excitement of the story during the more painful parts of the procedure so that the story would effectively compete with her discomfort, and hopefully mask it.

After the procedure, Samantha told me that the pain was a 5 out of 5, but her scary feelings were only a 1 out of 5. This discrepancy suggested that Samantha continued to be aware of the pain of the procedure, despite the local anesthetic, but in contrast to previous occasions when she would cry, during this time she was not anxious and the procedure did not bother her. With highly focused concentration, she had become absorbed in her favorite story, and the pain sensations while not entirely eradicated had become less relevant, supplanted by the story and therefore didn't distress her. This suggests a degree of dissociation, and indicates that Samantha was probably hypnotically absorbed. Hypnosis helps to change the meaning given to the pain so the child is less bothered by it. This is a striking example of the capacity under hypnosis of human consciousness to segment itself into different parts, as explained earlier.

The favorite story technique, like all these methods, needs to be tailored to each child's needs and temperament. The only way you'll know whether it fits is to make an educated guess and let the story unfold. There is no substitute for the telling, with the intent to transform the child's experience. This requires some dramatic flare, creativity, and interest in the child's world. Children's focus is on the novelty, so the more drama, the better! Creatively alter the tales to offer metaphors for courage, competence, and accomplishment during taxing times. Many fairy tales easily lend themselves to drama (and undergoing a medical procedure is a drama!).

With some children one can select suitable moments for a brief pause to allow the child to fill in a word or a name, making the story collaborative: "And the bear's name was...?" These tales powerfully evoke previous associations of hardship, stress, and desperate circumstances that require exceptional effort. These stories also reveal how in these times of duress, the hero – with whom our little patient will hopefully identify – draws on inner resources of courage, inventiveness, mischief, and daring. Somehow the forces for good in the universe join this conspiracy to triumph over these overwhelming difficulties. When it's a good fit, this is one of my most favorite techniques for its enduring benefit for the child.

Associating and Changing the Pain

Association is particularly useful if the pain isn't overwhelming, or is puzzling. Invite the child to focus on what the pain looks like inside his or her body. This generates a direct image of the pain, such as a red ball of fire or a dense rock. The experience is then to use the following imagery methods to alter, shrink, and change it to decrease the hurting and discomfort.

Shrinking the Pain

Age: Six years and older.

Pain: Any mild or moderate persistent or puzzling pain.

Time: 5 to 15 minutes.

With regular practice, shrinking the pain helps the child generate inner strength and greater self-reliance in working with pain.
Adapting the language for the age of the child, lead the child into
this imagery experience by gently saying the following:

*Close your eyes and breathe out. Take in a breath and again breathe out,
releasing all tension. Take one final cleansing breath as you travel inside
your body by whatever route you wish—through your nose, on your
breath, or through your ears… Travel all the way to your pain. When
you see your pain, nod your head to let me know [wait for this non-verbal
response].*

*Look at it from every angle—from top and bottom and each side… Notice
what color it is, what shape, if it is dense or not. Then take out your magnifying glass and inspect it, before it shrinks. Take out a can of shrinking
solution, spray the thick colored solution over the entire area of the pain,
on the top, on the sides, and underneath, doing a thorough job. Notice
what's happening… Tell me… Notice how your pain is changing…
shrinking, becoming less dense, perhaps more porous as the solution is
absorbed, and changing color as it becomes smaller and smaller. Take out
your magnifying glass and inspect it as shrinks. Notice it all. Give it a
final spray, allowing it to shrink away as far as it can. Now, enjoy the difference in sense and feeling. Leave your body by the route you entered…
and take a deep breath in. As you breathe out, notice the changes… and
slowly open your eyes.*

Pain can be shrunk in many ways. Develop the possibilities with
the child, assessing which works most quickly and lasts longest.

Painting the Pain

Age: 3 and older.

Pain: Mild, moderate, persistent.

Time: 5 to 25 minutes.

Painting the pain to alter the sensation is a variation on shrinking and changing the pain. Children who enjoy art enjoy this experience. The following example begins with some breathing to allow the child, whatever the nature of the pain, to relax. Invite the child to become comfortable by sitting or lying down and then to take three deep belly breaths.

Let's go to Innerland… and take yourself to a big painting tent. Let me know when you're there… [wait until the child indicates]. Inside you'll find an easel and a table filled with pots of paints in many different colors. Paint a picture of your body… Now choose a color that best shows the kind of pain you have and paint the pain into the picture of your body. Brush it over all of the areas where you hurt. If there are different kinds of pain, choose the color that best describes each kind of pain. You may use a lighter shade of the color for the areas that are not hurting as much and a more intense color for the areas that are hurting the most. Do a thorough job so that your picture shows exactly how your pain is. Check it out. After you've finished, take a pail of whitewash, and pour it all over your picture. Feel and watch how the whitewash gradually seeps down, washing out the intense colors, softening and making the light color even lighter. If you wish, you can pour even more whitewash and experience how that soothes the pain more. Guide the wash to areas that need it most. Watch how it soaks into your body picture and changes the pain. Now you can step back from the picture of your body, and if you wish, lock the picture into your mind where you can recall it whenever you want to wash new pain away.

Combining Pain Imagery with Medication

Imagery exercises that change pain also work well when combined with pain medication to minimize pain and suffering. The effects seem synergistic: the analgesics enhance the effectiveness of the imagery in altering the pain, and the brain's absorption in the imagery seems to aid the impact of the analgesic. In addition, since analgesics can take 10 to 20 minutes to be absorbed, imagery is ideal to create comfort while the medication is being absorbed.

Fifteen-year-old Jamie was having a difficult time sleeping in the hospital. Achy bone pain, IV pumps with alarms, morphine steadily infused into her system, the lights, the sounds of other children, interruptions at night, and her own highly active mind, all contributed to her discomfort and insomnia. She was wary of using imagery but agreed to discuss the possibility. After exploring several options, she agreed to listen to relaxing music to calm herself and to focus her mind and then to see what images came to her. She saw her hip as a throbbing red fireball, emitting spurts of fire down her leg and across her pelvis [this is nerve pain]. I suggested, "How about making snowballs and throwing them on the fire, one after the other?" The quenching of the pain began slowly. After about ten minutes, the combination of pain-relieving methods began to work for Jamie. The session was recorded onto a CD, with the music she had chosen in the background. Jamie used the CD at times throughout her hospitalization and at home. The hospital and its noises became irrelevant, as her 'achiness' eased and she would fall asleep.

Hypnosis and imagery can be combined with other methods, such as physiotherapy or TENS (see Chapter 6), or biofeedback (discussed later in this chapter).

The Creative Therapies of the Arts and Play

Music and other creative therapies have been used primarily for reducing distress in anticipation of procedures (Klassen, Liang, Tjosvold, et al., 2008; Malone, 1996). A recent study with adults found that both happy and sad melodies can successfully modulate pain from heat (Zhao & Chen, 2009). Music is enjoyed by everyone, not just children – and more so if the children can participate in making music or singing along. As a therapy it is particularly beneficial for young or nonverbal children.

Music

Age: All ages.

Pain: All types.

Time: As long as desired.

Music in its many forms – listening to a lullaby, singing, listening to an iPod, CD or playing an instrument – can ease suffering and tension. Music is increasingly being used in hospitals and particularly in hospices for children in palliative care. Music is a gentle, wonderful therapy that, depending on the rhythm and quality, can promote relaxation, harmony, and peace. When a child joins in playing a percussive instrument or guitar, music can become a form of self-expression and joy. Participation can be very simple, such as a child shaking a tambourine while a music therapist strums the guitar in the waiting room prior to an invasive procedure – as I've seen at Royal Children's Hospital in Melbourne Australia. Or this therapy can take the form of a wandering minstrel playing guitar to the wonder of babies and children of various nationalities in the wards of the Anna Meyer Children's Hospital in Florence, Italy. Only the visiting dogs of the pet therapy program were more popular!

Bringing an iPod or CD player into the treatment room during a painful routine medical or dental procedure can provided an increased sense of control for teenagers. Playing a favorite nursery rhyme, accompanied by the singing of a parent, during a blood transfusion or other time-consuming medical procedures may help toddlers and preschoolers get through the trying procedure. Music is a wonderful way to harmonize the child's world with a medical setting, supporting the well-being of the child and making long periods of time feel shorter – or at least more interesting.

Music therapists are popular professionals who provide a much appreciated mood change with their various and familiar sounds. Music can be used as a form of therapy to foster self-expression or as encouragement during rehabilitation or a graduated physical exercise program. Singing along with a child, playfully creating new verses, encouraging the teen or child to create his or her own verses, or writing a song together can be therapeutic. Music aids in shifting attention away from pain and onto a very pleasant experience. Music needs to be included more often in the treatment and recovery process for children. Any worry that the child's music will be intrusive in the clinic or hospital is generally unfounded. Most staff members welcome the music and are reminded of the pleasures of working in pediatrics. However, a meta study indicated that guidelines for music-based interventions are needed to improve reporting in order to advance evidence-based practice in this area (Robb & Carpenter, 2009).

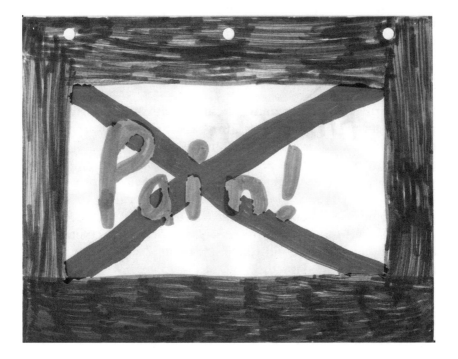

Figure 5.2 No Pain

A 9 year-old girl struggling with the pain of a Juvenile Idiopathic Arthritis flare-up, declares in this drawing how she wants her life to be: Pain is forbidden to enter!

Play and Art

Age: 15 months and older.

Pain: Pain that has upset the child, particularly treatment-related or persistent pain.

Time: 10 to 45 minutes.

Play is a natural part of every child's life. When we pay attention to a child's play, we learn about the child's way of understanding the world, of coming to terms with puzzling and complex occurrences, and of mitigating traumatic experiences. Play provides the child with an opportunity to assimilate these experiences into his growing sense of the world. Play therapy with a trained professional provides the child with a safe opportunity to express a range of emotions, and reveal the child's understanding of recent or distressing experiences (Bandstra, Skinner, Leblanc, et al., 2008).

Medical play provides young children with an opportunity to come to terms with the distressing experiences and separations of hospital life (Moore & Russ, 2006). Both medical play and art therapy are of particular benefit for children undergoing recurring intensive treatments that involve multiple painful procedures, as these treatments can be traumatic and undermine the child's psychological well-being and safety. Trained child-life specialists, psychologists, and social workers can provide many therapeutic opportunities for the child (Bandstra et al., 2008), including the following:

- Playing with a doctor's kit or with some of the medical equipment, such as putting a tourniquet on and off a non-favorite toy (so that the favourite toy isn't hurt) to gain an understanding of procedural details.

- Using playdough to make little figures that 'need to have a painful procedures' and talking to them. Using imagination invites the child to take on other roles, such as that of the nurse or doctor, and reveals the child's perception of them and fantasy or concept of their motives.

- Drawing – children's graphic drawings powerfully reveal their inner world, their concerns, suffering, perceptions, and misunderstandings (as in Figure 5.2).With such visual information on hand, the issues can be explored, providing some relief, and misconceptions can be corrected and clarified.

- Playing with puppets to help children articulate more details of their experiences and to provide them with an opportunity to work through distressing experiences.

- Keeping a journal or writing a blog or Facebook entries for older children during convalescence, with personal commentary, and comments from others. Later, children can look back to their journal to make sense of their experience.

- Joining with a group of teens on a website for kids with chronic pain, which can be validating and supportive during difficult painful times.

In a safe context even within a hospital, children will spontaneously express through play and talk, what has been bottled up inside and is troubling them – information that may be helpful for the child's physician, psychologist and team in order to provide better care. Play is a child's natural medium of communication and is a means to recovery. Being sick and in pain must not remove the child's right to have access to this source of pleasure, well-being, and therapeutic benefit.

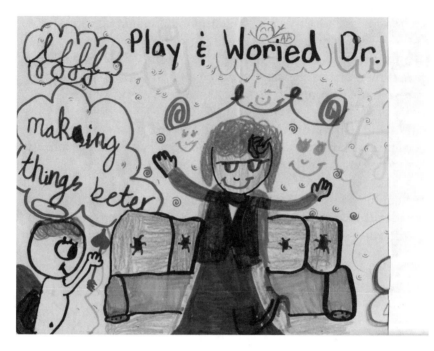

Figure 5.3 "Play and Worry Doctor"

In treatment I sometimes introduce myself as a 'Play and Worry Doctor' to provide the child with the opportunity to play and work through the fears and worries that accompanies pain. This drawing was presented to me by a child at the end of a session.

Biofeedback

Biofeedback is the monitoring and altering of a biological function usually not thought to be under voluntary control. It is a well-documented and effective therapy for adults and children (Gertz & Culbert, 2009), but it is important that it be guided by a trained professional. Unlike the previous methods, biofeedback allows the child to experience objective feedback of his or her physiological functions. A body signal, such as peripheral body temperature, heart rate, electrical brain activity, or muscle tension, is continuously fed back as a sound or in a visual form by computer so that the child can attempt to change the signal in the desired direction, such as decreasing muscle tension. Without this continual computer feedback, the person would have no awareness of these changes. Children and teenagers are usually interested in and enthusiastic about this method and quickly learn it. Training consists of learning to recognize the body's signal and then training to produce the desired change.

The clinical application of biofeedback has been for chronic pain. A study (Holden et al., 1999) has recommended it for children's recurrent tension-type and migraine headache, and this was further endorsed by Cochrane systematic reviews (Eccleston et al., 2003, 2009). Emphasizing the child's control and the development of self-regulation, biofeedback is evidence of the continual interaction of body and brain and demonstrates to children and teens how emotion and stress impact physiological functioning and plays a part in creating or maintaining pain.

Eighteen-year-old Jonathan, diagnosed with tension headaches that had recurred over three years, described his pain as a tight band across his forehead. A clinical assessment and interview revealed that Jonathan tended to keep quiet about matters that worried him and to avoid problems rather than deal with them directly. In conversation, Jonathan said it was unlikely that his difficulties, particularly those with a group of peers at school, were contributing to his headache.

Since he was intrigued by the notion of biofeedback, we placed self-stick electrodes from the machine on his forehead and temples (the frontalis muscle) to monitor the tension levels as we discussed aspects of his life. This made the brain-body interaction more evident. When the muscle tension increased, the beeps got progressively faster, but when he began to relax the muscle, the beeping sounds slowed down. When they reached below the desired level, and his forehead was relaxed, the beeps turned off completely. Jonathan was fascinated to note that his muscle activity changed depending on the issues discussed. He realized that his body, not only his mind and his feelings, were responding to his problem situations. It was a profound experience for him. This immediate audio feedback motivated Jonathan to learn more productive problem-solving skills to use with friends at school, spilling over, as these technique can do, to empower him in other areas of his life!

Biofeedback teaches children that they can control aspects of their own behavior that they previously thought they could not influence. Thus, it increases children's autonomy, self-efficacy, and self-sufficiency. Biofeedback requires specialized equipment and a trained health professional; the cost of both can restrict its use. However, there are some simple feedback devices for ascertaining temperature, such as biobands, temperature-sensitive strips that are attached to a child's finger or forehead. These change color as the peripheral temperature changes, giving immediate feedback about the degree of success of focused concentration and relaxation. It enables the child to practice the self-regulation routine at home, as a preventative pain and stress measure. Biobands can be helpful to children with migraine headaches who experience the accompanying temperature dysregulation of cold hands.

Acceptance and Commitment Therapy

Acceptance and commitment therapy (ACT) is a recent, exciting development that extends from traditional cognitive-behavioral therapy and mindfulness meditation – and from the need for interventions that will increase severely disabled patients' functioning. The focus in ACT is on improving the patient's quality of life and function by "increasing the patient's ability to act effectively in concordance with personal values, also in the presence of pain and distress" (Wicksell, Melin, Lekander, & Olsson, 2009, p. 248). This therapy deals with learning to live a valued life while in pain and accepting it as a sensation that may or may not diminish. It is based on the notion that persistent attempts to 'fight' pain produce disability (one of the 'mixed messages' about pain discussed in Chapter 1).

"Commonly patients believe that pain and discomfort prevent them from behaving in accordance with values (i.e. 'I can't do it because I'm in pain')" (Wicksell, 2007, p. 14). The therapist helps the patient identify personal values, that suggest "an important direction in life (e.g., 'being a supportive friend')," and helps the patient "to direct his or her efforts to achieve this" (p. 14). Implicit in this therapeutic process is a movement to accept what cannot be changed, and to change that which can be. The patient's inner experiences are explored and defused through teaching the patient how to be more 'mindful' of private, previously avoided thoughts. This practice requires the patient to learn to be non-judgmental, non-controlling, and to allow the thought to just be a thought without getting emotionally caught up in it. This is the detachment that mindfulness meditation teaches. With this skill they can pursue their goals. The key here is promoting this psychological flexibility, rather than a focus on symptom reduction (Wicksell, 2007).

ACT has evolved from treating adults with chronic debilitating pain. The ACT model of longstanding disabling pain recognizes "the patient's unwillingness to have pain." This is manifested by patients not engaging in their valued activities so that they can avoid experiencing fear of pain, a sense of failure, disappointments, and other experiences that they associate with pain (Robinson, Wicksell, & Olsson, 2004). It recognizes that therapies to date have focused on controlling pain and distress to improve the patient's quality of life. Yet a number of patients have not been helped by this approach. As we've discussed before, there is often no concordance between the nature of an injury and the amount of pain felt. So too, pain in itself is not sufficient to explain disability.

Adult chronic pain studies have shown that acceptance accounts for more of the change than does coping (Wicksell, 2007). With an acceptance of pain and a willingness to experience it and any other interfering personal experiences, rather than attempting to control or reduce these distressing symptoms, patients experienced less pain, less disability, anxiety, and depression and a willingness to return to work (McCracken & Eccleston, 2003). In a recent child study Wicksell and colleagues in Sweden (Wickell et al., 2009) evaluated the efficacy of 10 weeks of ACT compared to multi-disciplinary treatment including amitriptyline with 32 children with long standing pain syndromes. Their results were very encouraging for long-term positive outcome at six-and-a-half months, and an increase in perceived function and reduction in pain frequency and intensity. ACT holds promise as a treatment for children and teens with disabling longstanding pain.

Conclusion

Children naturally think in images and love to hear their favorite stories or visit a familiar favorite place in their imagination. Most children know the difference between helpful thoughts and the kind of thinking that aggravates pain and anxiety. Furthermore children like to have some choice in what happens to them. When offered psychological techniques to make their medical or pain experiences easier, they will willingly divert their attention to something more interesting – if they trust that it will help them through the pain. The methods described in this chapter are respectful, effective ways of joining with children to help them to better manage, accept and relieve pain. When used frequently, they become a coping repertoire for recurring or ongoing pain, and forge strong bonds between child, parent and pediatric staff. Learning some physical therapeutic tools can further increase the efficacy of this repertoire – the focus of Chapter 6.

Chapter 6

Physical Methods to Relieve Pain

"In humans, touch is the first sense to develop.
Over the centuries, human touch has been shown to be
emotionally and physically healing."

Beider, Mahrer, & Gold (2007, p. 1025)

Physical intervention is a mainstay of comprehensive pain management, addressing a wide range of acute and chronic pain conditions. Massage, acupuncture, and heat are centuries-old techniques of providing pain relief. Today's methods include a wider acceptance of yoga, TENS, and regular exercise in the management of chronic pain and mood regulation. These and other physical interventions provide a direct and immediate response to children's pain – and children respond both to the touch and the caring that it conveys. In focusing on physical methods to relieve pain, this chapter is divided into five parts:

- Self-directed biobehavioral methods, that children can be taught to use on their own, such as breathing, blowing bubbles, and relaxation methods. Obviously, these require the simultaneous interaction of both psychological and physical processes, but I consider them best placed in this chapter. Over the years I've noticed that the physical components of these processes tend to be minimized at the expense of the psychological aspects – and I want to redress that balance.

- Physical methods that use water, warmth and cold such as hydrotherapy, heat-packs, ice, and warm or cool showers.

- Those methods requiring a professional's skilled technique such as acupuncture, acupressure, TENS, and massage, in which the child can relax and passively absorb the effects. Specific manipulative techniques for pain relief practiced by physical therapists are briefly mentioned, and while valued, are beyond the scope of this chapter.

- Informal methods involving touch that clinicians can encourage parents to use.

- An overview of the special physical methods for pain control and relief for newborns and infants.

Self-Directed Methods

A good place to start is to give children an experience of control over their bodies. Starting with breathing – which allows this self-control to be immediately experienced. Breathing methods are taken for granted, underestimated, and as a result infrequently utilized! Perhaps because of their elemental connection to being alive, when breathing methods are well used, they have profound impact and long-term benefit, especially when relaxation, imagery, or hypnosis techniques are added to the breathing. Breathing methods have been central to yoga practice for hundreds of years: controlling the breath calms the nerves and is a prerequisite to controlling the mind and the body (Swami Rama et al., 1979).

Breathing

Have you noticed how your breathing changes when you are feeling angry or afraid? The breath becomes deep and often trembling when angry, and suspended or extremely shallow when afraid. How we feel immediately affects our breathing. The reverse is also true: breathing affects how you feel and behave – as many practitioners of the martial arts, actors, and other performers well know. By changing breathing patterns, the karate practitioner is able to concentrate, focus energy, and break a thick plank of wood with the back of his hand, or with a deep belly breath change fear into effective action. Physiological states, heart rate, respiration rate, perspiration, and blood pressure change as a function of different breathing patterns. Breathing has a profound effect on our physical and psychological functioning (Bradley, 1991). In essence, it is a crucial connection between brain and body.

The Physiological Benefits of Controlled Breathing

Each time a long deep breath is drawn into the body, a number of very important physical changes occur in the spine, the diaphragm, the rib cage, and even the stomach. The biomechanics of breathing are rather complex (S. Tupper, personal communication 21 October, 2009), since there are many moving parts in the upper body. In general, the spinal column will slightly extend stretching some of the muscles around the vertebrae. The ribs do different things at different levels depending on the depth of the breath. There is generally a contraction of the intercostal muscles between the ribs. Because of their orientation this causes an increase in the distance between some ribs, and the abdominal muscles will stretch because of distention. Within a few deep breaths, another physiological effect, bronchodilation occurs, making subsequent breaths more efficient and increasing oxygen in the body. This, and the musculoskeletal release produces a feeling of well-being.

Despite the beneficial effect of breathing deeply, our instinctive reaction when in pain is to stop or restrict our breath, so as not to cause any more pain by deep breathing. This is a protective reaction, but does not relieve pain. When breathing is shut down in this manner, contraction in the muscle fiber increases and tension builds, a common pattern with persistent pain. In contrast, each time you exhale, you release muscle tension and rigidity, and pain can more easily disperse. With a series of generous, deep exhalations, the resulting neuromuscular release promotes relaxation in those muscles, may ease pain, and release pressure in the sensory nervous system.

If this release does not occur and the muscles remain protective, overactive, and tense around the pain site, neuromuscular fatigue

185

builds up, heightening the pain. Over time the neuromuscular pathways confuse the messages of pain and muscle tension and a peripheral and central sensitization may develops (discussed in Chapter 2). A cycle of myofascial pain and fatigue escalates. Massage therapy can be therapeutic. The muscles are manually softened and encouraged to release, and in the restful state, repair themselves. Many a patient has fallen asleep on a massage table, or at the end of a yoga class!

Since pain and anxiety intertwine, mastering the breath during pain also controls anxiety. Exhalation is the key to breaking the pain cycle. By first emptying the lungs and relaxing the diaphragm and intercostal muscles, inhalation, a reflexive muscle contraction occurs, which draws fresh air into the lungs. Breathing in a regular, easy, deepening rhythm releases pain. This rhythmic action is comforting and predictable, like a regular heart beat, and so enables the body's homeostatic physiological balance to be re-established. Protective fear, the need to hold tight, can then be repatterned. Rhythmic breathing can be a valuable asset when pain, distress, or anxiety is a part of life.

Learning to recognize when children in pain are breathing shallowly or restricting their breath requires attention. If it is shallow, light, rapid, or only upper lobe breathing, then the child is good candidate for this method. When their patterns are identified, children find it easy to learn to repattern and regulate their breathing. School-aged children, in particular, find this mastery rewarding whenever they are in pain or anxious. Breathing methods are subtle and easy to use at school, and they bolster self-confidence and coping, while helping to diminish pain and distress (Powers, 1999). Following is a description of two breathing techniques that can be used from toddlers to teens.

Blowing Away the Pain, or the 'Red Cloud Technique'

Age: Ten months and older.

Pain: Acute, brief pain from scrapes, falls, or injections; anticipatory anxiety and pain associated with medical treatments.

Time: 2 to 10 minutes or for the duration of the pain.

Tell the child to 'blow out the pain', or alternatively, pretend that the pain is a big red cloud and blow it out! Demonstrate this by blowing out in a steady, slow, long breath, adding that pain leaves the body this way. Encourage the child to blow out with you over several deep breaths with a good pause after three or five breathes to ensure the child does not hyperventilate.

"Breathe out as if you're blowing candles out and empty your lungs. Now you'll find yourself breathing in… and let's blow the red cloud out! This gives your body the immediately instruction to let go the pain on each out breath. It feels good, and you start feeling better. Continue with this breathing until you start feeling the tension leave your body. Good!"

Provide the child with information on how breathing this way benefits the body:

"When you breathe more deeply and regularly, your muscles stretch and this expands your ribs. Your spine lengthens, easing tension and stretching and helping the pain to release and tightness to go. Let's do it. Close your eyes and after five cycles of breath when you feel some change you can tell me about it."

This simple method can be used for many types of pain and can even be taught to pre-verbal young toddlers as young as ten to twelve months. Most one-year-olds adore blowing out candles! Toddlers and younger children depend heavily on their parents' involvement to engage and sustain any breathing technique. For this reason, have the parents join in so that they mirror and support their children's efforts. Children aged six and older can easily learn to regulate their breathing. Children with recurrent pain report that blowing away the pain when it recurs helps to contain their anxiety as well as settle their pain. "It helped to cool the pain," said a nine-year-old. Breathing methods can be used during procedures when a child has to remain still for two to ten minutes (Power, Liossi, & Franck, 2007), such as, for an injection, intravenous access, laceration repair, or a cast setting. Children can use breathing to stay calm during X-ray, CT, a bone scan, and other assessments, or during more prolonged achy pain. When analgesics are given prior to the procedure, blowing away worries and fears will help settle the child until they take effect. Breathing techniques give the child a constructive job to do while the procedure takes place – being still is not a natural state for most awake children!

Nine-year-old Seanna had mastered blowing out as her preferred way of ridding herself of scary feelings and distress during spinal taps, part of her treatment for leukemia. After she was discharged from hospital, she feared that she might forget how to do her blowing, her mainstay. So she practiced daily, in case she had to return into hospital. She was determined to ensure that she could cope. "All I need to do is to return to my blowing, and I know I'll get through!"

Blowing Bubbles

Age: One year and older.

Pain: Acute, brief pain, as from a scrape, fall, injections, or IV starts.

Time: Before and for the duration of the pain.

This is an all-time favorite simple pain and anxiety reducer. It's versatile, entertaining, a great tension breaker and the child feels back in charge – you can't lose! Bubbles, party blowers, or pinwheels are all eligible, as they can be used to sustain and regulate the child's breathing to reduce pain and anxiety, while adding an element of fun. Children love to blow colorful bubbles of different sizes and watch them travel across the room. In an otherwise anxious or uncertain situation, children will respond to an inviting challenge: "See how far you can blow this bubble!" "I wonder how many twin bubbles you will blow this time while I look at your veins," or "Can you catch a bubble and blow even more bubbles from it while I wash your skin clean? I wonder how many more it'll make?" Throughout this purposeful activity, instead of being gripped by fear and pain, the child has a job to do – breathe and produce bubbles – and so gains a sense of success and competence.

Children are individuals. Some children become totally absorbed in this task, find relief with bubble blowing, and want to continue blowing long after the acute pain has ceased. Others may refuse to blow, may reject the bubble wand, or choose to blow out without bubbles. It is the child's pain, and the child should decide what works and how to participate in the process. Do not feel defeated and throw the method out just because it hasn't worked on the first occasion – remain flexible. At the next procedure the child may surprise everyone by spontaneously blowing or requesting the bubbles – I've seen this happen on more than one occasion. Give children the opportunity to learn and to choose the method they want. (When bubbles aren't handy, an inventive colleague shows the child how to blow gently on a pretend candle, first on his finger and then on the child's finger to make the flame flicker but not go out!)

Relaxation

There is considerable evidence for the benefit of relaxation for children's pain management for abdominal pain (Brent, Lobato, & LeLeiko, 2009) and for painful procedures (Power, Liossi, & Franck 2007; Uman et al., 2008). Children who experience pain enjoy relaxation. Twelve-year-old Kevin trained himself to relax 'by becoming a wet noodle!' for his recurrent medical procedures. Once begun, the relaxation process will lead the child into a gradually deepening state of rest characterized by increased feelings of warmth and comfort. Many physiological changes naturally occur when one is relaxing. Pain, such as gastrointestinal pain, may lessen and achy muscles may soften as the relaxation progresses.

It's a great skill for teens to use if shutting off the day and getting to sleep is difficult. For older children and teens, breathing techniques can easily be combined with lying down, closing eyes, and going into a relaxation. When combined with an analgesic, breathing-relaxation significantly relieves anxiety and pain.

School-aged children and teens can become proficient using relaxation and breathing methods, independent of an adult. Children with persistent or recurrent pain find that 10 to 15 minutes of daily or regular practice of breathing relaxation or relaxation combined with imagery (see Chapter 5) has long-term benefits. To support this, make a digital audio recording of the relaxation imagery for use at home on a CD or MP3 player or an iPod. A few hints for success before you begin a session:

- Ensure that you will not be interrupted. Put a sign on the door 'Work in progress' or 'Do not disturb', and unplug the telephone.

- Ensure that both you and the child or teen are comfortable. The child should lie in a recliner or on his or her back on a couch or bed, without crossing legs or arms. Cover the child with a light blanket if you have one, since warmth promotes muscle relaxation and the child will feel more secure.

- You too need to feel as easy and relaxed as possible so that you can convey this calm and comfort in your voice, pacing, and style. Talk slowly and calmly as you guide the child through breathing-relaxation.

Breathing-Relaxation

Age: Six years and older.

Pain: Non-acute, persistent achy pain, abdominal or limb pain, and disease-related pain such as Crohn's disease, and syndromes such as irritable bowel and chronic fatigue.

Time: 10 to 30 minutes.

"Make yourself as comfortable as you can be... let all of your breath out of your body... now it's easy to let your lungs fill up all by themselves. Notice how your lungs know exactly how much air to take in, how long to hold, and how to automatically let your breath out. Follow your breath. Track how each breath has its own timing and rhythm. Your body knows how to breathe automatically. Keep your attention following your breath and observe how your body breathes all by itself. It's an effortless, natural, easy, wonderful process.

"Notice also, with your attention on your breath, how the tension is beginning to leave your body. Your muscles release, becoming softer, looser, more and more comfortable. Notice how some parts of your body may feel heavier and other parts may feel lighter – it's very interesting. Notice it all. Notice how your body is becoming warmer, and pleasant sensations are getting stronger. You may notice that one part of your body is feeling particularly warm and another part feels particularly heavy. Another part feels very good. It's so nice to just let go and go with the flow of your breath, as the relaxation eases your pain farther and farther away."

Breathing relaxation uses the focus on breath to lead the child into greater relaxation. Here are some other ways of achieving physical relaxation:

Relaxing from Head to Toe. Encourage a child to focus attention systematically on each part of the body, starting from the head and scalp working downwards, soothing eyes, relaxing jaw, back of neck, through the shoulders, torso, arms, softening the belly, inviting the child to release tension from every part of the body down to knees, calves, ankles, feet, and finally releasing tension out the toes.

Alternatively, some clinicians prefer to reverse the sequence, from toe to head, maintaining that it's easier to let go of tension in the toes first and children may even find thinking about their toes humorous. This sequence would be most helpful for children with headaches, where creating and experiencing relaxation gradually progresses to the child's painful head. Relaxation is a useful self-regulation method for children who find it hard to 'turn off their brains' when going to sleep at night. As a nightly ritual, it becomes more effective with regular practice.

3 × 3 Breathing Cycle. This method I adapted as a routine to induce relaxation and sleep from one of Hatha Yoga's *pranayama cycles*. These cycles deepen breathing in a controlled way, creating a rapid and profound relaxation effect. Count the exhalations and inhalations initially aloud for the child in the following way, so that in time the child counts inwardly, while lying down with eyes closed.

Count to three during an exhalation, suspend breathing and drift for the count of three, then inhale for the count of three, and hold the breath for a count of three (3 × 3 × 3 × 3). The pauses to three between inhalation and exhalation and its reverse, trigger the sleep response. If the child can't hold it for three, count a little quicker until the child relaxes and can suspend breath for three. It's deeply relaxing! As the 3 × 3 cycles progress, sleep is induced. As a result I playfully called this *Slinky-Sleep!* If the child's breathing significantly slows as you repeat the cycles, you can, if it's advantageous, move to a counting cycle of four, 4 × 4 × 4 × 4. This technique is more suited to older school-aged children and teenagers than younger children.

Jacobson's Relaxation Technique. Certain muscles in the limbs and trunk can be selectively tensed and then released. Children who are not aware of carrying tension in their muscles or who have trouble relaxing may find this method beneficial, as it builds somatic awareness. This should not be used with children who are prone to muscle spasms. Here's how to guide a child through this:

"Lying down comfortably, close your eyes and let your breath out fully. Take a deep breath in and exhale slowly. Focus all your attention on your right arm. Squeeze your right hand into a fist, hold it tight for the count of five, and now relax your hand. Feel the difference in your hand. Now bend your arm, making a bicep muscle, hold it tight for five seconds, and relax it completely. Feel the change in sensation and comfort and notice what has changed. Push your arm into the bed, feel the tension, hold it for five seconds, and let it go. Enjoy the release as your arm relaxes fully into the bed. Pay attention to how your whole arm feels now and how different the other arm feels. Repeat this process on the left side."

You can follow this with tensing and relaxing the toes, feet, calves, and thighs on one leg, drawing the child's attention to changes in sensation, and then repeat with the other limb. Whatever permutation or creative variation of relaxation you develop with the child, making it fit for the child will ensure it's more likely to be practiced.

Raggedy-Ann/Andy

Age: Six years and younger.

Pain: Non-acute, persistent achy pain, abdominal or limb pain.

Time: 4 to 6 minutes.

Relaxation in the form already discussed is not ideal for children six years and younger. They find the concept of relaxing difficult to grasp and associate it with sleep, and find it hard to keep their eyes closed. *Raggedy-Ann/Andy* is a playful favorite relaxation variant developmentally suitable for younger children. Introduce the child to a rag doll that is floppy. Invite the preschooler to flop in a chair "like a Raggedy Ann or Andy" and demonstrate the floppiness with your own wrist. Play enters as you 'test' how very Raggedy Ann or Andy, the child has become, by lifting an arm to ensure it flops down again to the chair or lifting a foot to check that it is properly floppy. Pre-school children engage, giggle, and love this game. A playful colleague told of lifting a strand of the child's hair if the child has long enough hair adding, "Even your hair is relaxed!"

Methods Using Cold, Water, and Heat

Heat and cold in their many various forms can soothe, provide comfort and relaxation, and increase function and mobility, even though the mechanism of action for this relief is not well understood (McCaffery & Pasero, 1999).

Cold

Age: Five years and older, or old enough to report poor sensation and move the cold away if they don't like it.

Pain: Pain related to acute injury (without an open wound), bruising, or muscle sprains.

Time: As long as needed before skin becomes numb, or to a maximum of 15 minutes. Application can be repeated after a 15 minute break. If there is any question about sensory loss, test prior to applying any cold.

Ice is the cheapest and safest form of treatment to use immediately after sustaining bruises, spraining a wrist or ankle, pulling a muscle, or being bitten by an insect. It is effective as a mild local anesthetic; the cooling effect of the ice may reduce the conduction of pain signals. Physical therapists recommend that cold be used within the first 24–48 hours of an injury to control the inflammation and prevent swelling (McCarthy, Shea, & Sullivan, 2003). Cooling is especially beneficial when combined with mild to moderate pressure, such as firm application of a tensor bandage. Cooling and compression together slow blood flow and reduce muscle spasm and inflammation, limiting tissue damage and speeding the healing process. Some children report that the sensation of coolness on a recent injury feels good. Younger children can use cold packs that have been wrapped with more layers of dry towel to prevent freezing or tissue damage.

It is commonly recommended to apply a compression bandage after icing an injury, a swelling, or a chronic recurring muscle or tendon pain for up to 10 to 15 minutes with a 15 minute break for the first 24 to 48 hours. Then regularly check the affected area for adequate blood flow or until the inflammation has subsided. Resting and elevating the painful limb seem to help reduce inflammation and bleeding. Children are tolerant of cold for brief periods and say that ice soothes immediate, sharp pain. However, in a randomized controlled study using an ice pack placed on an injection site 15 minutes prior to injection, children aged from ten to eighteen years did not show any significant reduction in their procedural pain (Ebner, 1996). Ice is not advisable for babies or toddlers as they are more sensitive and susceptible to cold and ice than older children. It is also not recommended for non-communicative children or those unable to remove the cold pack to prevent tissue damage. Some very general guidelines for using ice are listed below.

How to Use Ice
Use ice cubes crushed or shaved, or frozen peas or corn in a plastic bag and wrapped in a thin towel; or gel ice packs.

- Frozen corn or peas in a plastic bag wrapped in a towel have a distinct advantage over ice, since they conform much more easily to the shape of the injured area and are convenient for mobile children.

- Be cautious with gel packs, which contain refreezable chemical gels and may cause frostbite. Ensure there is no puncture in the pack, as chemicals can burn.

- Icing can be more fun for younger children by using commercially available gel cubes in terry cloth shapes, such as the Ouch Mouse distributed by Discovery Toys. Alternately, cut colored sponges into favorite animal shapes, soak them in water, freeze, and store these in the freezer for easy access. This is useful in the emergency room or a busy pediatric practice. You can then give the child a choice: "You've bumped yourself! Do you want a cold bunny or a freezing giraffe to help the pain go?"

Caution: Do not use ice
- on an open or bleeding wound, or if the child is in shock, shivering, and cold

- directly on the skin; wrap the ice in a towel, so that it doesn't burn, cause frostbite, or damage nerves

- for longer than fifteen minutes on one place, and monitor its effects every five minutes

- if the child has any circulatory problems or lacks normal skin sensation, or cannot identify that the cold is burning, or physically protect the site by removing the ice.

Vapocoolant

Vapocoolant is an inexpensive, quick-acting cold spray, consisting of either ethyl chloride and fluoro-ethyl or other chemical formulations. With adults it was found to reduce vaccine-associated pain (Mawhorter, Daugherty, Ford, et al., 2004). Given that young children have many immunizations, and that early pain is associated with increased sensitivity to later pain events, researchers investigated the use of vapocoolant for pain relief during preschool immunization injections (Cohen et al., 2009). Their results were surprising and important. They found that vapocoolant alone showed a stronger increase in observed pain from baseline scores during the injection, when compared to typical care. They concluded that for children, vapocoolant is not an effective pain management intervention for intramuscular injections. They wondered if distraction had been added whether it may have controlled the children's anxiety, and speculated that children might be more sensitive to the chemical spray. Nevertheless they urge that we need to put our efforts onto more effective interventions for children during painful medical procedures. Other studies of the use of vapocoolants with children have had mixed results, with some showing reduction of pain and others not.

Water (Warm or Cool)

Age: From Birth.

Pain: Muscle aches, headache, abdominal or fatigue-related pain, arthritis pain, or sickle-cell disease pain.

Time: Limited to 15 to 20 minutes for full-body immersion for children younger than twelve years – see below for details.

Hydrotherapy is soothing for painful conditions and is particularly valued for gaining mobility and function. The warm water action increases circulation and provides gentle tactile stimulation and muscle relaxation. Children find it enjoyable, decreasing their weight-bearing forces and providing buoyancy. Techniques include whole-or-part-body submersion in warm whirlpools (McCarthy et al., 2003). Since younger children don't have mature thermal regulation and can't dissipate heat as well as adults, full-bodied immersion longer than 5–10 minutes in a whirlpool should be avoided for children younger than twelve years. Younger children can partially immerse for longer, 15–20 minutes (S. Tupper, personal communication, October 2009).

Warm baths are helpful for children with achy musculoskeletal pains, fibromyalgia, or juvenile idiopathic arthritis and increases the nutritional supply to joint surfaces and surrounding tissue (Walsh, 1996). Regular warm baths in the morning and evening can help mobilize stiff joints and reduce ache, but if too hot it can induce fatigue. Heat packs and hot baths have been found helpful for sickle cell disease pain (Dampier & Shapiro, 2003). Warm showers with running or pulsing water over the head and down the neck and shoulders can ease the build-up of tension and muscular pain associated with tension headaches.

Michel, a seventeen-year-old six-footer, experienced recurrent severe tension headaches that wiped him out for a day. His severe headaches made concentrating and keeping up with school difficult. Smoking and occasional drinking only added to his feelings of physical discomfort. He experienced the tension build up in his neck muscles 'like a tight band' across his head. Occasionally he smoked marijuana to alleviate the pain, even though it didn't give much relief. His resulting lack of motivation and lassitude added to his difficulty in picking up his life after each episode of headaches. He was willing to try other options – physical and pharmacological – in his pain management program.

When he felt the headache tension start, Michel immediately took two acetaminophen extra-strength and would massage his neck and temples while standing in a shower, as the soothing action of warm, cascading water washed away his tension. (His showers were lengthy events.) He would lie down and rest afterwards. He reported that altering his posture in this way released the various strains and tensions in his neck and head. The shower, analgesic, and rest brought his headaches from a rating of seven or eight out of ten down to around a three, within half an hour. The combination of physical strategies was just a beginning, yet a crucial first step for Michel to get a grip on the headaches that were 'wrecking his life'.

Cool water, in contrast, doesn't have as strong an efficacy for pain relief (French, Cameron, Walker, Reggars, & Esterman, 2006). Anecdotally, using cold water cools the burning pain that often accompanies injury; the sensation and sound of the water can be soothing for children; a cool cloth is often soothing for a child with a headache or fever. In a Cochrane review of nine studies, there was moderate evidence that heat provides short-term pain reduction for low back pain, but no good evidence was found as to whether cold therapy has an effect (French et al., 2006).

Heat

Age: Six months and older.

Pain: Achy persistent muscle or stomach pain, pain related to acute injury with closed wounds, bruising, sprains, or muscle strains, and 'growing pains'.

Time: Dependent upon the heat source. If the temperature remains constant limit to 15 to 20 minutes – see below for details.

The application of superficial heat is preferred after the first 24 to 48 hours (McCarthy, 2003). Heat in the form of a microwavable hot pack, hot water bottle, warm blanket, helps to improve circulation, promote pain relief, reduce joint stiffness, relax muscles, and ease spasms. Heat is soothing for abdominal pains, menstrual cramps, and general muscle aches, since it encourages relaxation.

Using heat increases the blood flow to the painful area and helps disperse the build-up of muscle waste products (Walsh, 1996). Note that electric blankets that keep a steady temperatures are not recommended as a safe way to deliver heat. Most hot-packs will lose their heat over time and can be left on longer. A warm water bottle provides comfort that can be managed by the child, who can move it onto achy muscles or to relieve menstrual cramps, and the warmth relaxes spasms and provides some relief.

Precautions
• Since heat increases the blood flow, it can dislodge a newly formed blood clot that is repairing after injury, causing bleeding to recur.

• An electric heating pad should not be used. Children fall asleep and parents forget.

• If using a hot compress, remove it when it becomes cool.

Ice and Heat

Age: Six months and older.

Pain: Acute painful and inflamed injury, a muscle spasm, or sore joints.

Time: See below for icing and heat time and limits.

Alternating ice and heat promotes pain relief: the ice tends to reduce inflammation, and the heat eases the muscular pain and tension. This technique works by alternating the constriction and dilatation of blood vessels and acts as a mild analgesic (McCaffery & Pasero, 1999). Using both ice and heat can be effective for a child's sore joints. For small joints, such as finger joints, apply cold for 15 seconds, followed by warmth for 45 seconds; repeat for 10 minutes. For larger joints, such as elbow or knee, apply cold for one minute, followed by heat for one minute. Check with the pain team to ensure that these methods will aid in healing the child's particular pain condition. For children with cancer or nerve damage (neuropathy), conditions in which nerve fibers are not reliable in communicating pain, extra caution must be exercised and frequent checking the skin, to prevent burns or frostbite.

Methods Requiring a Trained Professional

The physical treatments covered in this section require a trained health professional. Acupuncture and acupressure are ancient Chinese medical practices that have been evaluated, are gaining acceptance, and are being incorporated into children's hospitals. Physical therapy, also known as physiotherapy, is a standard part of all children's hospitals, and uses manual and electrical techniques and exercise programs to address pain. TENS is an electrical technique that initially requires a physical therapist's guidance before parents or children can use it for relief at home. Yoga is gaining popularity for stress relief, and is beginning to be studied for its effect on pain. Massage is another ancient and cross-cultural practice, with many diverse forms of touch.

Acupuncture

Age: All ages.

Pain: Acute, recurrent and particularly chronic pain.

Time: Determined by the Acupuncturist.

Acupuncture has been developed and practiced in China for more than 5,000 years to relieve many medical conditions, including pain. Special fine needles are inserted through the skin into underlying tissue at very specific acupuncture points that often correspond to a nerve plexus on the body. With younger children a laser can be used instead of needles (Kundu & Berman, 2007). If a laser is not available, the needles are very briefly inserted and then removed.

Acupuncture is one of the treatment modalities in Chinese Medicine. In this practice the body is viewed as a dynamic system of organs connected by the flow of Qi (vital energy) within a complex system of energy lines in the body known as meridians. Pain and illness result from the blockage, improper flow, or balance of Qi along the meridians. Proper flow may be restored by needling or manually twirling needles in specified and established combinations of the 365 classical acupuncture points. We don't as yet understand precisely how acupuncture relieves pain. It is thought to work through the central, not the peripheral, nervous system by activating the body's own pain-inhibiting system, which either raises the pain threshold or modulates the response to pain.

Acupressure may be more useful in predictable situations, such as post-operative pain or dental procedures, and for recurring pains such as sickle cell or recurring abdominal pains in children, rather than for accidents or injuries (Lin, 2003). Acupuncture seems to have a particular value for chronic pain in children. In a study with a large sample of children (n=243), Lin et al., (2002) found that using acupuncture to treat chronic pain over a six week period significantly decreased pain intensity scores. The children reported an overall improvement of well-being and no side-effects or complications.

This finding of 'overall improvement of well-being' may be a function of the broader framework of understanding and practice within which Acupuncture operates. In this framework, improving the flow of Qi, (energy) throughout the body is the primary aim. The reduction of pain would be regarded as a function of improved flow of Qi. Consequently, in chronic painful conditions where existing treatments are less than effective or if there are unacceptable side-effects, acupuncture may be a valuable therapy, either as an adjunct to existing therapies or in some cases as the sole treatment (Lin, 2003).

In a phase I feasibility and acceptability study Zeltzer and colleagues (2002) examined a combination of Acupuncture and Hypnosis for chronic pain treatment with children. Ninety percent of the children completed the six-week treatment package reporting significant improvements in their pain and function. Parents' reports were in accordance with this, and no adverse effects were reported. The findings are consistent that children in chronic pain find acupuncture an acceptable and helpful treatment.

Eight-year-old Corey's initial complaint of back and leg pain and progressive walking difficulties, was diagnosed as a spinal cord neuroblastoma. He had multiple interventions including surgeries, chemotherapy, spine and brain radiation. Two years later with uncontrollable tumor spread, escalating pain, and failing neurological function, his death was thought to be imminent. With a palliative treatment plan in effect, Corey was discharged home with an intravenous fentanyl infusion pump. His neurosurgeon had little more to offer and so referred him for acupuncture hoping to improve his quality of life.

Corey's mother was initially skeptical that acupuncture offered her son any relief where Western medicine had failed. On his initial visit, Corey was in considerable pain, crying that his leg pain was unbearable and he had not slept in 3 days. His fentanyl infusion pump had been increased to deliver 975 µg per hour, but was not controlling his pain. Acupuncture began with two 40-gauge acupuncture needles (the width of a strand of hair) placed in two key analgesic points, and Corey fell asleep within 2 minutes, remaining asleep for 90 minutes. When he awoke, he report that his pain was significantly lower, and he was hungry. With treatments scheduled for twice a week Corey received acupuncture, acupressure, Tui Na medical massage, moxibustion, herbal therapy, and a five-point auricular (ear) acupuncture treatment utilized for addiction, tolerance, and pain – all with the goal of improving his quality of life.

Corey responded surprisingly well. After six acupuncture treatments his fentanyl dose was reduced to less than 200 µg per hour. By week five he was rotated to 50 µg per hour fentanyl patches. He was now able to interact with family and participate in their daily activities, and his pain was well-controlled. With this change his physicians recommended that physical and occupational therapy be reinitiated, and by the 4th month of treatment Corey was able to stand and walk down the hall wearing leg braces. Due to his illness, he had spent little time in school with other children but his wish was to be like other eight-year-olds and attend third grade. Corey started third grade and attended school for the first half of the year until a reoccurrence of spinal tumors led to his death. Corey died peacefully with his family by his side. (Ruth McCarthy, personal communication, 2007.)

Acupuncture therapy in the hands of a trained acupuncturist is acknowledged to be a safe and effective way of treating pain, and the insertion of needles need not be painful. Since children generally dislike needles, special skill is required to treat children and build up trust. Despite children's fear of needles, the studies indicate acupuncture treatment was a positive experience, and children's pain lessened and function improved (Zeltzer et al., 2002). The handful of studies indicate that acupuncture can be effective for children's chronic pain, such as recurrent migraines (Kundu & Berman, 2007). More than one session is usually necessary, and one study cited an average of 8.4 sessions (Lin et al., 2002).

Acupressure

Age: One year and older.

Pain: Headaches, dental pain, shoulder and back pain.

Time: Brief and as required (can be repeated every two to three hours) or as determined by a physiotherapist, acupuncturist, or massage therapist.

Acupressure is derived from acupuncture and is an adjunct therapy. Specific acupuncture points are stimulated using finger pressure or rubbing. One of the most powerful analgesic points is known as Hoku, a highly sensitive acupuncture point located in the web of skin in the muscle between the thumb and forefinger. Hoku, also known as Large Intestine 4 (LI 4) because it is on the large intestine meridian, is the second most important point in acupuncture because of its major influence on the upper section of the body.

For upper body pains such as tension headaches, or dental pain, strong (and not always pleasant) pressure is delivered to the point with finger or thumb on both hands for 30 to 40 seconds. This procedure can be repeated every two to three hours. When the point is stimulated correctly, a red ring, associated with endorphin release, appears around it. Pressure on the point can be painful, but the subsequent pain relief in the other areas can be quite marked. When combined with pressure on additional points identified by an acupuncturist, physiotherapist, or massage therapist as helpful to a specific pain, the analgesic effects for the child or teen can be enhanced. Children can learn to do their own acupressure on accessible points, empowering them to cope more independently.

Physical Therapy/Physiotherapy

The goal of Physical therapy (PT) is to use the science and art of exercise and physical modalities to restore physical well-being, nerve-muscle function, balance, posture, and strength to the structural body (McCarthy et al., 2003). A range of physical techniques are used including manipulation, mobilization, and massage, as well as electrotherapeutic techniques such as electrical nerve stimulation (TENS described later in this section), ultra-sound, short-wave therapy, and low-level laser therapy. Active exercise is considered one of the most important of all physical therapy treatments, particularly for pain. As a teacher of motor skills, the physical therapist on the pediatric pain team advises on exercise regimens for children. The goal is to improve daily function and decrease disability as a result of disuse and persistent pain. Here is an example of PT:

Ten year old Kaylee had an inherited musculoskeletal pain syndrome from her mother's side of the family. Both she and her mother are very tall, lean, and prone to achy muscles. Her mother found that her achy pains responded well to exercise and stretching – and she became a popular gym school teacher. Kaylee found that when she skated twice a week and played hockey and baseball the other days, her 'restless' legs felt better and the pain didn't escalate (see her drawings in Figures 6.1 & 6.2). However, the mornings were tough. She would awake with an achy back and sore legs, and she found it very hard to sit in her seat at school. Her physiotherapist gave her a series of morning stretches that included leg lunges to open her hips; lying on her back and rocking side to side with

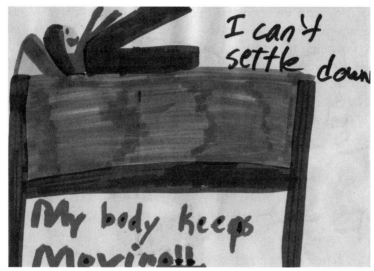

Figure 6.1. 'Restless Legs'

Kaylee's drawing reveals how uncomfortable and restless her legs are when she has to lie down in her bed to go to sleep.

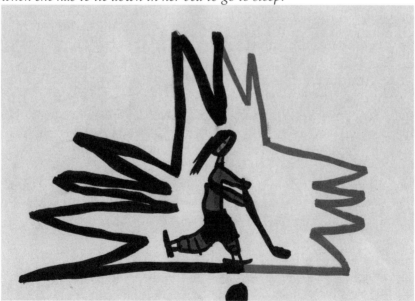

Figure 6.2: Skating within a Maple Leaf.

Kaylee draws what helps best for her leg pains – skating, with her Canadian maple leaf.

her legs curled onto her chest and breathing deeply to lengthen her back muscles and lumbar spine. Her physiotherapist then arranged for permission for her to stand, move around the room, or go for a walk. (It helped that she was one of the best students in the class.) Kaylee learned the 'the pain switch' hypnosis technique and belly breathing to use in her classroom breaks, so that she could remain at school and feel more in control of the pain. Given that she is likely to have this condition throughout her life, it was important for her to develop effective coping skills now.

TENS

Age: Three years and older.

Pain: Various pains, including burn pain, muscle aches and spasms, incision pain, bone metastasis, neuropathy, shingles, phantom limb pains.

Time: 30 minutes, two to three times per day, or as advised by the physiotherapist.

TENS (transcutaneous electrical nerve stimulation) is a safe, non-invasive pain relieving technique for blocking pain sensation, partially or completely (McCarthy et al., 2003). Traditionally TENS has been viewed as a device to relieve muscle pains and pain from surgery incisions; however, it also relieves pain associated with headaches, burns, damaged nerves, the spread of cancer to ribs and other bones, phantom limb pain, painful IVs, intramuscular injections, arthritis, and painful wounds. Precautions need to be taken for children who have epilepsy or cardiac problems.

TENS combines well with other pain-relieving methods and can be used on its own for acute and chronic pain relief with no serious side effects or complications (Smith & Madsen, 2003). It is relatively inexpensive and widely used to manage children's pain in clinics and at home, even though its efficacy has not been adequately studied. Lander and Fowler-Kerry (1993) have undertaken the only study on the use of TENS for children's acute pain management. In a blinded placebo-controlled study with children from five to seventeen years, TENS was found to be effective in relieving pain for venepuncture.

What Is TENS? TENS units are battery-powered, pager-sized plastic boxes, with attached wires and black rubber electrodes, which are attached to the patient's skin's surface with gels and gum karaya at selected sites. The unit delivers electrical impulses through the surface of the skin. The electrodes come in many shapes and sizes, and most can be cut with scissors to fit a specific body part, a property that makes it useful for children's smaller bodies. Three types of TENS can be selected: conventional, brief intense, and acupuncture-like. Each type has several settings that can be modified to improve pain control. Children who do not react well to acupuncture are more likely to accept TENS and tolerate the brief intense TENS and conventional TENS.

How Does TENS Work? TENS transmits electrical impulses along the nerves and competes with pain signals, and acts as a pain inhibitor. In addition, the stimulation helps the brain release endorphins, our naturally occurring form of morphine. How can electricity be helpful in relieving pain? The amount of energy delivered through the TENS electrodes is very small. In fact, every time your heart beats it puts out more electricity than a TENS unit!

Most TENS units have three basic controls that can be selected and adjusted by the person in pain: rate, pulse width, and amplitude.

- The rate determines the number of electrical impulses delivered through the skin. A low rate is experienced as a pulse; a faster rate, as vibrations.

- The pulse width, or the duration of the pulse, controls how deeply the pain-relieving signal goes into the tissue. A low pulse width keeps the electrical sensation on the surface of the skin, which is helpful in relieving the pain of wounds, such as an incision or skin lesion. A higher pulse width sends the signal more deeply into the tissue.

- The amplitude settings are highly individualized, controlling how many milliamps are delivered to the skin surface. Settings need to be fine-tuned to determine which are most pleasant and provide the greatest pain relief. A higher amplitude is not necessarily better for relieving pain than a lower amplitude, and TENS should never cause pain or make existing pain worse.

- Additional controls can provide a massage-like sensation or alternate six seconds of the electrical signal with a six-second pause. This latter use is thought to prevent the area from becoming accustomed to the stimulation, an important factor for relieving some types of pain.

The duration of use of TENS must be individually assessed by a trained therapist for both the child and the type of pain. For example, to control pain during burn treatment, TENS is used for 5 to 15 minutes. If applied for at least 30 minutes, there is a longer-lasting analgesic effect.

Sixteen-year-old Enrico was driving home one day when a car ran a stop sign in front of him, causing him to smash into the side of an old pick-up truck. In the sudden impact, he sustained a concussion, and in the emergency room, it was discovered that his retina was also significantly detached. He had a variety of treatments, including laser therapy. As a result of the injury, however, his trigeminal nerve (the nerve that supplies the forehead, upper cheek, and eye; see Figure 2.7) had become terribly bruised. This pain was neuropathic, it was hot stabbing pain. His eye hurt terribly, and he was seeing double and feeling quite desperate. It was difficult to control the pain of his damaged nerve using medication, so the nurse recommended TENS. One electrode was placed above his eye and one below, and with the controls in his own hands, he adjusted them to a pulse that felt good. After 15 minutes of continual TENS, he was pain-free. TENS became Enrico's primary method of pain control for the following year until he had healed enough not to have to use it regularly. (Jo Eland, in Kuttner, 1996.)

TENS can help minimize or relieve many types of pain, even short-term needle pain, when other alternatives don't work or are not available.

Amy, aged four, had leukemia. As part of her treatment, she had to have an intramuscular injection every day for six weeks. The injection of chemotherapy hurt, so Amy and her parents were keen to use anything that would help. Since topical anesthetic solutions were not yet available at their clinic, they chose a TENS unit.

Every morning after breakfast Amy's mother put the TENS unit on her daughter. One electrode went across Amy's leg above the knee cap and the other up her leg at her panty line. With the unit working, Amy watched her favorite TV show Reading Rainbow *after which she and her mother went to the clinic with the TENS unit still on and working. After two days Amy became so at ease with the routine that she would skip down the hall to the treatment room ahead of her mother and allow the nurse to give the injection. Only then did Amy take the TENS unit off, handing it to her mom. With her pain well controlled, Amy no longer had to be carried, clinging and crying, from her house to the car to the clinic. Instead she became willing to make the injection part of her daily routine.* (Jo Eland, in Kuttner, 1996).

Benefits of TENS for Children. The dearth of data on the use of TENS with children is unfortunate, for it has many features that are highly desirable for children: in particular, it is non-invasive requiring no needles; it is a neat little device that a school-aged child can apply, control, and wear to school as it provides a fairly steady reduction or relief of pain (McCarthy et al., 2003).

Yoga

Yoga is a 5,000-year-old practice developed in Ayurvedic medicine (an indigenous medicine practiced in ancient India) that combines breathing exercises, physical postures, and meditation. It is intended to calm the nervous system and balance the body, mind, and spirit. Now widely practiced in classes across many western countries for its relaxation and physical benefits, yoga's physiological benefits include reduced heart rate, blood pressure, and modulation of the parasympathetic nervous system.

In a pilot study of yoga to treat teenagers with recurrent abdominal pain and irritable bowel syndrome, the teens were led through a yoga routine designed for abdominal pain relief. They were then given a DVD of a ten minute daily yoga routine for home use. Results showed a significantly lower functional disability, and reduction in anxiety compared to a control group (Kuttner et al., 2006). The conclusion was that yoga holds promise for reducing gastrointestinal symptoms. There are, however, few studies to determine its efficacy to reduce pain in children. The UCLA Pediatric Pain Clinic is studying the impact of Iyengar yoga classes as one of the treatments in their integrated pain program. To date they have found that it is accepted and attractive to children and teens in chronic pain (Evans, Tsao, & Zeltzer, 2009). Iyengar Yoga is noted for its discipline, precise alignment of poses and its use of props to support the practice.

Massage

Age: Birth to adult.

Pain: Achy muscles, tension headaches, spasms, 'growing pains'.

Time: 15 minutes or as long as needed.

Massage therapy is a universal technique practiced for thousands of years in various forms. It combines tactile and kinesthetic stimulation to relax muscles, fascia and to ease spasms and aches. A therapist trained in massage primarily uses his or her hands, but sometimes elbows to press, knead, or manipulate the body's skin, soft tissue, underlying muscles, tendons, and ligaments in a purposeful sequential approach (Tsao et al, 2006). When muscles are tired, in spasm, or over-worked, lactic acids and other waste products accumulate causing aches and tightness. Massage can relieve pain and spasm, mobilize contracted muscle through techniques that assist the return flow and increased circulation of blood. (For a comprehensive perspective on pediatric massage, see Beider, Mahrer, & Gold, 2007; Beider, O'Callaghan, & Gold 2009.)

While the precise mechanism of action of pain relief due to massage is not known (Ireland & Olson, 2000), there are a number of theories. These include the gate control theory, in which pressure from massage on the more rapidly transmitting A delta fibers closes the gates on the slower pain C fibers; and there is an increase in serotonin release from being massaged, which modulates pain control. Massage is thought to work by increasing parasympathetic activity and a slowing of physiological processes. Massaging can improve circulation, eliminate waste products, promote relaxation, and increase access to nutrients with the increased blood flow.

There are many different forms of massage such as Swedish massage; Rolfing, which is a deep tissue massage; and Craniosacral therapy, a gentle technique that works with the body's rhythms to address subtle body disturbances, such as persistent dizziness from a mild head injury or concussion (Upledger & Vredevoogd, 1983). Research into these methods has been limited and Swedish massage has been predominantly studied (Beider et al., 2009). All need to be evaluated to better understand and determine their efficacy in pain relief.

Research is just beginning to examine the benefits, physiological and psychological, of pediatric massage, and is limited to date. In one study (Field, Hernandez-Reif, Seligman, et al., 1997) children with juvenile arthritis were randomized to either massage or relaxation groups. In the massage group the children were given daily 15 minutes massages by their parents for a month. Both children and parents reported less pain at follow-up than those in the relaxation group. In 2001 researchers (Hernandez-Reif, Field, Largie, et al., 2001) studied whether 15 minutes of massage prior to burns-dressing changes could effect change in indicators of behavioral distress for children with severe burns, in comparison to attention-control. They found those receiving massage therapy demonstrated minimal distress indicators in contrast to the control group's demonstration of multiple distress indicators. It seems that providing simple massage as part of pain treatment may be both helpful to children and appreciated.

Registered massage therapists undergo training in physiology and anatomy and different massage techniques. As yet, few hospitals or clinics have massage therapists on staff. Often a referral is required to an outside massage therapist.

Here are some basics steps in massage: With the child's or teen's consent, warm a little lotion or oil in your hands and rub with light, easy, circular sweeps over the requested areas of the child's body. Physiotherapists and massage therapists recommend the use of the fleshy palm of your hand rather than your fingers for better contact with the child's body. Your hand should not leave the child's body until the massage ends so that the child always knows where you are and the contact remains unbroken. As you finish a sweep, allow your fingers to trail gently back up so that your fingertips don't leave the child's skin. Be careful to avoid tickling the child. Allow your hand to flow around bony points. When massaging a child's back, a preferred movement is up the muscle along the spine and then to the sides of the body, avoiding the ticklish ribs! Have the child guide you in degree of pressure and location. Teenagers may want firmer pressure. Start off gently until the muscles relax; then increase the intensity to soften the muscles further. Be guided by the child at all times.

Sometimes a warm hand lightly resting on an achy stomach can help the muscles relax and soften. Gentle massage in this location can also be helpful. You can lightly stroke the stomach in concentric circles, going from small to large, or vice versa, from large circles to small ones. Deeper massage of the stomach is seldom helpful and can induce pain.

Seven-year-old Christopher had a few episodes of severe stomach pains characterized by spasms that made him double over crying. He began walking around with his arms protectively over his stomach area. Over a two-month period he had been thoroughly investigated by his family doctor and a pediatric gastrointestinal specialist, who found no underlying medical cause. Christopher's pain continued, as did his reluctance to eat anything solid, apart from oatmeal cereal. I used a number of methods to help Christopher ease his stomach pain, including asking him to draw what he thought was going on inside his stomach, and my drawing how the brain and belly communicate through nerves to one another; imagery-relaxation; gradually extending his range of foods; and massage. Tolerating and relaxing into the daily massage his Mom provided became proof for Christopher that his tummy was getting better. Previously he had been so scared that anything might start the pain up again that he had not been able to tolerate anyone touching his stomach, let alone massage it. Gradually, over three weeks of using the different pain-reduction methods, and slowly increasing his foods to include full range of nutritious meals, Christopher began to trust that he did not need to fear the pain. He learned that he and his mom could help the pain subside. He became stronger and more playful, and his parents reported that he smiled more often. With the reduction in stomach pain, his massages became transformed into an animal recognition game: his Mom drew patterns of different animals on his stomach, which he would name or guess!

Massage can create a competing sensation in a pain-free area that will comfort and distract the child from the pain. While waiting for wounds to heal after surgery, you can massage head, feet, toes (if the child is not too ticklish), or any other area unaffected by pain. When a child is having mild bowel pain, tenderness, constipation, or gassy pains, light or slightly deeper small circular motions from the right of the bowel across the belly button to the left may be helpful. Older children often prefer massaging themselves, since it enables them to do what feels best. For children and teenagers who are very ill and don't have the energy or inclination to talk, massage is a wonderful method of staying connected and providing comfort. Here is how I used it with Jessica when she was in isolation to protect her from infection, following a bone-marrow transplantation.

Jessica, a spunky teenager with leukemia, was struggling to recover. Her entire body ached from the effects of the treatment. She had developed complications secondary to the transplant of graft-versus-host disease. Her skin was sloughing off. It hurt to move. Her mouth was filled with ulcers as a result of her weakened immune system. It hurt to talk. Even her eyes were sore. But her feet were OK. She wanted company but no conversation. She softly nodded when I suggested a foot massage. Using peppermint foot cream, I gently rubbed and kneaded her feet, massaging her heels and around her ankles, down over the front of her foot to her toes, and gently between each toe, for about ten minutes. On each visit she requested and I repeated the foot massage. After her release from isolation, she said that the foot massage had helped her to concentrate on one good feeling in her body, while the rest of her felt so weak and sore. Thereafter she would request a foot massage from her nurse when she felt weak or despairing, as it supported her will to recover.

Informal Methods Involving Touch for Parents

Given that in humans touch is the first sense to develop (Beider et al., 2007), being held, touched, or correctly positioned and supported when in pain, cuts through the isolation of experiencing pain. It is a reminder of love, security, and human comfort and potentially can shift, distract, and/or ease the suffering for children in pain. Parents know this intuitively. However, the unfamiliar clinic or hospital environments often inhibits them from responding in a way they may wish, or the child needs. Family members need to be told by staff that they have the right to hold, massage, or stroke their hurting child. Sometimes older children's feelings of self-consciousness prevent them from asking for or from accepting the comfort of touch. Health care professionals can do a great deal to change this perception by addressing its acceptability as a valid response to providing comfort. Unfortunately, too, clinic or hospital pressures and protocol often prevents staff from taking the time to touch, soothe, or physically comfort a child in pain.

Touching the Non-Hurting Area

This is in essence a form of physical distraction: when part of the body is in pain, there are usually other areas that are not hurting. If the child wants to be touched, parents can stroke, pat, tickle, or massage a non-hurting area of the child's body. If the child finds the sensation pleasant, it will compete with the painful one, and close the gate, modulating the child's perception of pain.

In day surgery, post tonsillectomy, Tammy felt groggy and had pain in her throat. Tammy's mom tickled the sensitive inside of her arm. The familiar sensation informed Tammy that she was not alone: Mom was there. That soothing tickling feeling had a long history and evoked memories of their nightly bedtime routine, lying in bed, with her mom at her side, tickling her arm, as she would fall asleep.

Patting, Stroking, and Rubbing

By asking parents what touch the child likes, health care practitioners help parents to become more effective caregivers, and this information can make the clinicians' therapy more effective. If the child chooses to be touched even when in severe pain, we know that touch will comfort, support, and provide some relief. Children report that holding a familiar loving hand while being in pain was a lifeline. Here are some simple options for health care practitioners to encourage parents to use with their children.

Patting is soothing for infants, toddlers, and fearful young children. A baby whose parents routinely comfort him by patting his back in a particular way will recognize that distinctive style and respond – a reminder of their attachment. A stranger patting him with hesitancy or too much vigor will be less successful! Patting at a rate of about twice a second is a natural cadence that stimulates the large movement fibers and inhibits the small pain fibers, providing some relief. Be guided by your knowledge of the child. Older children in pain may feel infantilized if patted. Or, if older children regress because of pain and distress, the distraction of patting may be soothing and settling, providing an alternative focus and sensation – a reminder that the pain isn't completely overwhelming and has not isolated the child from parental care.

Stroking can be a favorite touch used by many parents to sooth and provide comfort. These ritual 'creature comforts', which are a natural part of family life, have a place in the clinic or ward too. Children love to have their faces stroked or their hair played with, brushed, or repetitively stroked. This rhythmic motion becomes a physical distraction from the insistent and unwelcome presence of a needle or gnawing and draining pain. I've heard a child instruct a parent, "Dad, stroke me here. No, higher!" to break the tedium of lying in a hospital bed.

Rubbing can provide physiological benefits. Rubbing a mild injury stimulates the large muscle and nerve fibers, which in turn inhibit the smaller pain fibers at the spinal cord level (see Figure 2.5). Teach a young child when superficially injured, to rub the sore area in the way that feels best, as it helps the pain to recede. Children learn quickly what works. Rubbing and simultaneously blowing out make a good combination for reducing pain and distress.

Methods of Pain Relief for Newborns and Infants

Newborn infants, born either at term or preterm, and older infants up to one year of age, require special care to wherever possible prevent pain, and to control and minimize pain. Pain is commonly from medical procedures for diagnosis or treatment purposes, some are invasive, and many are planned interventions. Therefore, ensuring that the infant's pain is prevented or well-controlled is a primary responsibility of the health care team. As explained previously, the impact of unrelieved pain in early infancy has the potential to change the physiology of the infant's developing nervous system. We know from research studies that when infants are not provided with pain relief, they become stressed, their cortisol levels increase (Anand & Aynsley-Green, 1988; Anand, Sippel, &

Aynsley-Green,1987), and they learn to recognize and fear future procedures (Taddio et al., 1997).

Infants need to be positioned as normally as possible for procedures. Despite monitors or other attachments, the infants can be positioned, for example, side lying and swaddled in blankets in a midline position with knees flexed towards the chest and hands placed so that they can self-sooth through sucking. Here are some simple and effective interventions for relief from pain during procedures such as heel sticks and immunizations. These techniques can also be used when newborns and older infants exhibit colic or incessant crying.

Swaddling, Containment and Kangaroo Care

We know that close body contact and being carried reduces an infant's distress and crying. Infants are soothed and feel more secure when swaddled (wrapped in a blanket or cloth), held by facilitative tucking (placing a cloth over the newborn and holding the infant so that their limbs are closer to their trunk), or placed bare skin to bare skin of their mother or father (kangaroo care).

Studies have shown that swaddling a preterm (31 weeks and older) reduced the pulse rate (a physiological pain indicator) in response to procedural pain (Fearon, Kisilevsky, Hains, et al., 1997). The more reliable behavior indicators of pain reduction were also reduced – grimacing, crying, and flailing of limbs.

Kangaroo care has become an accepted practice in many NICUs and has been found to be effective in diminishing preterm infants pain response to heelsticks (Johnston et al., 2003). Mothers and fathers are encouraged to have skin to skin contact with their infants to optimize their well-being and ability to self-soothe and to settle. Furthermore, sucking from the mother's breast, a pacifier, or a bottle helps regulates an infant's breathing and often enables an infant to settle when distressed or in pain. The combination of being swaddled, moving with a parent's body with skin-to-skin contact, sucking, and hearing a familiar voice helps newborns and infants re-regulate themselves.

Sucrose Solution

There has been extensive research into the use of non-nutritive sucking of a pacifier and sucrose solution as a short-acting analgesic for painful procedures to newborns and infants up to the age of 6 months (Gradin, Ericksson, & Holmqvist, 2002; Johnston, Stevens, & Franck, 1999; Stevens, Yamada, & Ohlsson, 1998). The analgesic effect of these interventions is thought to be mediated by the release of endogenous opioids, the body's own analgesic process. A 24% solution of sucrose is given with an oral dropper, nipple, or dipping a pacifier in the solution. Therapeutic effects are maximized by giving sucrose solutions of 24%, and are most effective when sucrose is given two minutes before the painful procedure. The peak effect is at two minutes and some data suggest that the effect is gone by seven minutes.

Many protocols recommend giving the sucrose solution two minutes prior to the painful procedure, and again right at the beginning of the procedure. If the procedure continues beyond two minutes, the sucrose dose can be divided into smaller portions and given throughout the procedure. The recommended dose for a full-term newborn or older infant is approximately 2ml; for premature and small infants the dose will be smaller. If sucrose is given for multiple, sequential painful procedures, there is concern that hyperglycemia and feeding intolerance can develop – but this is not well supported by research evidence (Stevens et al., 1998). Many hospitals have developed protocols which allow for either a total number of times sucrose can be administered in one 24-hour period (for example, from two to four) or a total volume (4–10ml). If an infant is expected to have more painful events than will fit within these guidelines, other pharmacologic strategies should be considered.

Pacifier and Non-nutritive Sucking

Non-nutritive sucking refers to the use of a pacifier to promote infants sucking without receiving any milk. To introduce this intervention, gently stroke the infant's cheek very close to the infant's lips with an appropriate size pacifier. This prompts the infant's desire to suck the pacifier. The act itself of sucking is calming. Studies have shown that this calming effect does reduce observed pain scores during painful procedures (Stevens, Johnston, & Franck, 1999). Using sucrose appears to be more effective than non-nutritive sucking in reducing pain. However, combining both sucrose and a pacifier appears to be cumulative and is the most effective strategy. In very preterm infants or infants at risk for neurologic impairment, health care professionals need to carefully observe for any side effects such as choking or oxygen desaturation. Since infants learn rapidly, there was concern that they may develop an aversion to sucking if this method is used frequently with their painful procedures. The prevailing approach is that these concerns should not impede using sucrose and a pacifier for painful procedures.

Rapid Rocking

Rapid rocking is a practical technique for infants suffering from colic, incessantly crying, or distressed after a minor medical procedure. There appears to be no research evidence on this method for pain relief in infants, with the exception of one study using a oscillating mattress (Johnston, Stremler, Stevens, & Horton, 1997), Johnston and colleagues investigated the effectiveness of sucrose and simulated rocking, alone and in combination, on the pain response of preterm neonates during a routine heelstick procedure in the neonatal intensive care unit. The groups that received sucrose alone or in combination with simulated rocking showed fewer facial actions indicative of pain than the rocking alone or control group. Adding rocking to the sucrose condition further blunted the facial expression of pain, but this did not reach significance. They found that simulated rocking did promote quiet sleep. They found no difference between the simulated rocking and control groups in either facial expressions indicative of pain or heart rate. These results indicate that sucrose, not simulated rocking, may be the method to reduce pain from minor procedures in preterm infants. The researchers recommend further research to examine the contact component of natural rocking, as opposed to simulated rocking.

The practice of natural rocking is commonly used in traditional cultures, where babies are carried on mother's back or in pouches, while the mother works. The infant is swaddled and rapidly rocked (50 beats or more per minute). With the infant's head well supported, rapid rocking can be combined with rhythmic patting, and the regulated rhythm will re-regulate the crying infant's disorganized respiration into a more harmonized synchronistic pattern. Used in this way, rapid rocking can set a regular pace that guides the infant's erratic crying breaths into settling. Large, smooth movements, rather than tight, abrupt ones, create a steady, powerful pattern that soothes both infant and caregiver – especially if the rocking is combined with rhythmic singing. Although this method requires energy on the part of the caregiver, after five to ten minutes of rapid rocking, the baby tends to fall asleep.

Conclusion

Physical methods are an integral part of pain management for children. There is a vast array of effective physical techniques for relieving the many types of pain, for all ages and stages of the children. These include simple methods like breathing, relaxation, hot packs, or massage to self-directed methods such as daily physical stretches and yoga exercises, and more sophisticated professionally-directed treatments like ultra-sound, TENS, and acupuncture. Given this generous selection, health care professionals can be versatile and select good combinations of treatments, both for their efficacy for that particular pain and that child, but also for the fit with other methods, psychological and pharmacologic – the topic of Chapter 7.

Chapter 7

Pharmacological Methods to Relieve Pain

By Stefan Friedrichsdorf, MD, Leora Kuttner, PhD, & Helen Karl, MD

"When I hear a baby's cry of pain change to a normal cry of hunger, to my ears, that is the most beautiful music…"

Albert Schweitzer, 1903

Pharmacologic treatment is often needed to control severe acute or chronic persistent pain in children. Relieving pain can begin the process of healing. Fortunately medicine has progressed in understanding the physiology, impact, assessment, and measurement of pain, and new analgesic medications to interrupt and treat pain have been developed. Yet a sole reliance on medication can be counterproductive to children's health and well-being. Analgesic medications should be used as a bridge to enhance the child's capacity to function. As emphasized in this book, the 3Ps mnemonic – Psychological, Physical, and Pharmacological – provides a useful treatment principle for pain relief. This chapter takes up the third P, pharmacological treatment, and provides an overview of the best analgesics currently in use for acute and chronic pain. We discuss their safe use for greatest efficacy, and how best to administer them and enhance compliance.

Children in pain must be comfortable asking for and taking analgesics. When talking to children and their parents about pain relief, the terms *medicine* or *medication* are more useful than the term *drug*. Many people associate the use of drugs with street life and addiction. Children and parents, especially those of teenagers, need to be assured that medications taken for pain are a world apart from drugs taken for a high or for psychological addiction. Remember while talking about medications, what you say and how you say it sets up expectations. You want to invite the child's and parent's compliance with the regimen, and maintain their hope and positive expectation for pain relief.

The way pain medicines are used depends on the nature of the underlying painful condition. If the pain is only intermittent or short-lived, such as after a minor injury or incident, medication could be taken on an 'as needed' basis only, abbreviated as PRN (Latin: *pro re nata*). However, prescribing PRN pain medications (without scheduled analgesia) for all other cases remains a common mistake. For more than a decade, the World Health Organization (WHO) has recommended a By the Clock analgesic medication schedule. This is a finer way to control pain and often prevents it altogether: for instance, long-acting morphine is often scheduled every 12 hours to control the pain. If the pain breaks through, then 10% of the daily morphine dose can be used as a rescue prescribed treatment PRN.

The importance of the WHO By the Clock principle cannot be underestimated. Its implementation would reduce the needless suffering of a very large number of infants and children in acute pain. The prescription and administration of PRN (as needed) medication delays pain relief by several hours and ultimately requires higher opioid doses. PRN has been translated into 'Patient Receives Nothing' (or 'as little as possible') as an ironic comment on this method of administration. This practice unfortunately results in cycles of under-medication and pain, alternating with periods of over-medication and drug toxicity. The regular scheduling of pain medication ensures a steady level in the blood, reducing the peaks and troughs related to PRN dosing.

If you are in doubt about a child's need for medication, it often helps to put yourself in the child's situation, such as: "Would I be in pain with a chest tube?" Since the answer here is affirmative, you can be certain that it is equally painful for an infant, and hence this baby will require scheduled strong pain medication. When it is clear that medication is needed, give it as soon as possible. The sooner it is administered, the faster the relief, and the buildup of pain and its sequelae is prevented. It has been noted that less medication is required when pain medication is given to prevent pain, such as pre-emptive analgesia prior to painful physiotherapy for a child with CRPS, as opposed to giving medication only to relieve pain (Vetter & Heiner, 1994). Giving analgesics around the clock will keep a child comfortable and pain-free, allowing the child's energy to be used for healing and recovery instead of dealing with pain.

In this chapter we will cover some broad groups of analgesics: the non-opioids and opioids for acute pain. We will also discuss routes of administration, topical medications, and nitrous oxide for pain prevention, and briefly antidepressants and anticonvulsants for managing chronic complex pain. A full discussion on anesthetics and sedatives is beyond the scope of this chapter. However, it's important to state that since the early 1990s the planned and skilled use of these agents (such as, propofol, ketamine and midazolam) have revolutionized procedural pain management, making extremely taxing, distressing, and painful experiences more humane for children, their parents and for health care professionals. The primary concern in using anesthetics and sedatives must be safety. Injuries and deaths have occurred (Coté, Karl, Notterman, Weinberg, & McCloskey, 2000), so following sedation guidelines closely is mandatory when using these agents (Cote, Wilson, et al., 2006).

Common Medications for Acute Pain

The choice of an analgesic for the management of acute pain should follow the WHO-pain ladder (see Figure 7.1 & 7.2). For mild pain use acetaminophen (paracetamol) and/or ibuprofen; for medium pain, tramadol; and for strong acute pain, strong opioids such as morphine. In the figures the term *adjuvants* refers to medications, such as anticonvulsants or antidepressants, with a primary indication other than pain that have analgesic properties in some painful conditions (as we discuss later in the chapter).

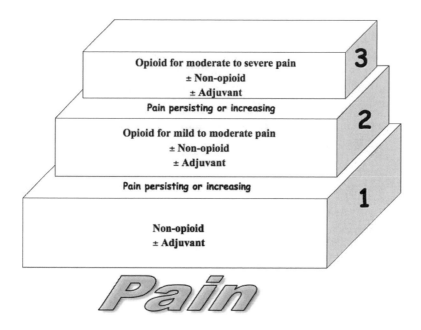

Figure 7.1 The WHO recommendation is to adopt a step-wise approach to administration of pain medications. First step for mild pain use acetaminophen (paracetamol) and/or ibuprofen; for medium pain, tramadol; and for strong acute pain, strong opioids such as morphine. [Reprinted with permission of the WHO]

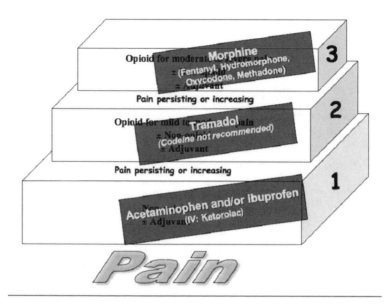

Figure 7.2 This graphically depicts the WHO recommendations

Non-Opioids

The most frequently used non-prescription medications in pediatric pain management are acetaminophen and the nonsteroidal anti-inflammatory drug (NSAID) ibuprofen. These medications are used most commonly alone or in combination for mild to moderate pain. They can also be effective for moderate to severe pain in combination with opioids or antidepressant or anticonvulsants.

Acetaminophen (Paracetamol)

Brand names: Tylenol®, Panadol®, Perfalgan®.

Dosage: 10–15 mg/kg by mouth/per rectum Q4–6h

Dose limit: <2 years: 60mg/kg/day, >2 years: 90mg/kg/day

Acetaminophen is generally well tolerated by children and lacks gastrointestinal and hematological side-effects. Significant hepatotoxicity is rare, but careful attention to dosing is paramount.

Benefits

- Acetaminophen reduces fever and relieves pain from a wide variety of causes including toothaches, teething, ear infections, sore throats, mild menstrual pain, and some headaches.

- There is a great deal of experience with this medication in pediatric patients.

- Acetaminophen has very few undesired side-effects when not taken in excess.

- Routes of administration are oral (liquid and tablets) and rectal (suppository). In several European countries and Australia it is also available in a novel intravenous form (Perfalgan®). It can also be given in a G-tube.

- A big plus is that it does not need to be taken with food. Acetaminophen is therefore suitable for infants and children unable to tolerate food by mouth or feeding tube.

Drawbacks

- Acetaminophen has no anti-inflammatory properties, so if inflammation is causing the pain or adding to it, acetaminophen may not be the most useful choice, unless combined with an anti-inflammatory medication. Inflammation may be present in muscle pain, sprained joints, arthritis, toothaches, menstrual cramps and other kinds of tissue injury.

- If too much acetaminophen is taken, as in acute or chronic overdose, it may lead to serious, life-threatening complications, particularly damage to the liver.

Cautions

- Acetaminophen is a component of many over-the-counter and prescription medicines, so check the labels carefully to make sure the total DAILY (not per administration) acetaminophen dose does not exceed the daily recommended amount. Use of acetaminophen in pre-formulated combinations, such as with codeine (Tylenol No. 1®, Tylenol No. 2®, 3®, 4® and elixir®), hydrocodone (Vicodin®, Lortab®), or oxycodone (Percocet®, Endocet®, Tylox®), can be problematic, as explained later in the chapter. The parents of children may not be aware of the presence of acetaminophen in these combinations, and administer additional acetaminophen leading to overdose. Furthermore, fixed combinations limit the ability to change the dose of opioid.

- If liquid acetaminophen is chosen, carefully measure each dose using an oral syringe or medicine spoon. Never use a household teaspoon to measure the dose of any medication. If the measuring device that came with the product is not available, get dosing syringes, a medicine dropper, a medicine spoon, or dosing cup from the pharmacy. If it is a suspension, shake the bottle well before withdrawing the dose.

- Double check the strength of the acetaminophen product. Because there are so many dosage forms, it is easy to make a mistake. Do the math; if you are not sure of your answer, check with a pharmacist.

Ibuprofen

Brand names: Advil®, Motrin®, Nurofen®

Dosage: 10mg/kg PO every 6 hours

Dose limit: 2400mg/day for children weighing more than 50 kg (110 lbs)

Ibuprofen is a nonsteroidal anti-inflammatory drug pain reliever which, as the name implies, has anti-inflammatory properties. It has the least gastrointestinal side effects among the NSAIDs. However, it should be used with caution with hepatic or renal impairment, or a history of GI bleeding or ulcers, and it may inhibit platelet aggregation.

Six-year-old Amy (15 kg) reported right knee pain after a minor injury at gym. An X-ray revealed no fracture, but she showed clinical signs of a mild tendonitis. Her knee was locked in a straight position, and she could or would not bend her knee while walking or at physical therapy, although she could do so when asleep. Scheduled ibuprofen 150 mg every 6 hours plus acetaminophen 300 mg as needed every six hours (usually only before physical therapy once daily), plus teaching her breathing and a self-hypnosis technique, helped her significantly. She was able to walk normally on the following day and pain free after three days.

Benefits

- Available in liquid, tablet, and chewtab forms.

- Ibuprofen is effective for pain associated with inflammation, including

- pain from juvenile rheumatoid arthritis, post-surgery recovery, muscle and tendon injuries, headaches, and menstrual pain.

- Ibuprofen, like acetaminophen, may also be used to treat fever.

- Teens can learn to use this medication properly at home or at school if they have a tendency to headaches or menstrual cramps.

Drawbacks

- This medication can cause stomach mucosal damage, and as a result is best taken with food or milk. A few crackers or other small amounts of food are all that is needed. It is also best for the child to take a full glass of water with this medication, decreasing any potential for stomach upset.

- It may worsen asthma and may reduce kidney function which is not a significant clinical effect, except for children with compromised kidney function.

Cautions

- All NSAIDs may induce an asthma attack, hence children with diagnosed asthma should be carefully watched after administration.

- Ibuprofen has the rare potential to cause bleeding problems, much like aspirin. Avoid pre- and intra-operative NSAID if a child is going for surgery, and stop ibuprofen two days before surgery.

- If bloody or dark, tarry emesis or stools are noted, the medication must be stopped. This may indicate internal bleeding, and the child's physician should be notified.

Other NSAIDs

At recommended analgesic doses, all NSAIDs provide the same analgesia (equianalgesic). However, as mentioned above ibuprofen seems to provide the best safety profile for children, and other NSAIDs, such as naproxen, diclofenac, indomethacin, and ketorolac, should only be used if ibuprofen causes adverse effects. For children with juvenile rheumatoid arthritis, the twice daily administration of naproxen may improve compliance compared to the three or four times daily administration of ibuprofen. Intravenous ketorolac can be administered for a maximum of five days, if a child is not taking oral medication, but should be switched to oral ibuprofen as soon as tolerable. Intravenous or rectal administration still has the same gastric side-effects, as the systemic anti-prostaglandin will remove the protection in the stomach.

Aspirin

The use of aspirin for children or teenagers cannot be recommended. Aspirin may rarely cause Reye's syndrome, resulting in liver and brain damage, and possibly coma and death.

Cox-2 Inhibitors

After some medication-recalls, the only remaining Cox-2 inhibitor on the North-American market is celecoxib (Celebrex®). The pharmaceutical company unfortunately has decided not to perform any pediatric studies, and its use has not been approved for children. However, especially in pediatric oncology, where NSAIDs are contraindicated because of chemotherapy-induced thrombocytopenia and its associated bleeding risk, some pediatric cancer centers do use celecoxib successfully. Its pediatric side-effect profile, however, is yet unknown.

Opioids

The benefits, physiological and psychological, and the toxicity of opium have been known for centuries. For many years derivates of opium, such as morphine, have been used for the treatment of pain (Yaster, Kost-Byerly, & Maxwell, 2003). As a class, opioids are used to treat moderate to severe nociceptive pain, the temporary pain that results from damage to previously normal tissues (see Chapter 2). This is the most common kind of pain in children – the pain from broken bones, cancer, inflammation, and surgery. When children's pain becomes chronic and is maintained by changes in the nervous system, it has become our daily experience that opioids become ineffective and their drawbacks become increasingly prominent (Friedrichsdorf, 2008). This includes musculoskeletal pain (juvenile fibromyalgia), back pain, tension headaches, migraines, functional abdominal pain (chronic recurrent abdominal pain), and irritable bowel syndrome. Self-coping skills for chronic pain in part rely on endogenous opioid production in the paraequaductal grey in the brain, which stimulates the descending inhibiting pathways (Solomon, 2002). Opioid administration conversely possibly inhibits the endogenous opioid production, reducing the ability to self-regulate pain, requiring ever higher opioid doses and carrying the risk of opioid-induced hyperalgesia (a lower sensory threshold and therefore an increased sensitivity to pain).

Some professionals may underestimate the amount of pain relief that can be achieved with acetaminophen and/or other NSAIDs, and tend to overuse opioids. Generally comfort (adequate pain relief with few side effects) is best achieved by titrating opioids to effect; that is, begin with a safe 'starting dose', then increase the dose, for instance, by 50% in each step to effect. Only the amount prescribed should be taken, and the next dose should not be given if the child seems too sleepy. All patients taking opioids should be cautioned not to cycle or drive until they have been on a stable dose and know how it will affect their balance and judgment.

Remind parents that all medications, particularly opioids, should be stored safely out of reach of infants and children.

Drawbacks

All the medications in this class have the potential to cause decreased breathing, sedation, dizziness, nausea, itching, and constipation. Opioid side effects generally depend on the dose used and on each individual's response to each medication. Because constipation is an expected side effect, a scheduled bowel regime (stool softener alone or in combination with a stimulant) must be commenced if a child takes more than one opioid dose per day. Nausea is also very common. When opioids are taken as a pill or liquid, a meal or snack may help to minimize nausea and stomach ache. Otherwise, anti-nausea medication should be considered with oral opioids and should be given together with IV opioids.

Tolerance

If opioids are needed to treat a longstanding painful condition, increasing doses may be required to achieve the same relief. This is called 'tolerance'. It is completely different from 'addiction', which is the result of using these medications for psychological reasons or to get high. Using the term 'opioid' instead of 'narcotic' (from the Greek *narco* to deaden) emphasizes the difference between pain treatment and addiction. Children with strong acute pain need strong pain medications (i.e., opioids), and when administered appropriately for acute pain, there is no risk of addiction.

Opioid Rotation

No matter which opioid is chosen to treat a child's acute pain, some children will display dose-limiting side effects, such as itching, nausea, sedation, or respiratory depression. These dose limiting side-effects must be expected, vital signs must be frequently assessed, and these children will require switching to another opioid ('opioid rotation') at equianalgesic doses. This is necessary in more than 10 per cent of the children provided with opioids by the Pain & Palliative Care Team at the Children's Hospitals and

Clinics of Minnesota in Minneapolis/St. Paul. When one opioid is switched to another, this is often accompanied by a change in the balance between analgesia and side effects. If changing between opioids with a short duration of action, start the new opioid– because of incomplete cross-tolerance – usually at 50% of equianalgesic dose and titrate to effect.

'Weak' Opioids

Codeine and tramadol are frequently used for mild-moderate pain and are so called 'weak opioids' due to their ceiling effect; that is, increasing above the recommended dosing does not increase analgesia, but does increase adverse effects.

Codeine

Codeine is no longer recommended in pediatric analgesia (Williams, Patel & Howard, 2002). First, codeine is a weaker analgesic than commonly believed: a standard dose of many NSAIDs produces more effective analgesia than 30 to 60 mg of codeine in adults after surgery (Moore, Collins, Carroll, et al., 1997). More important, codeine is not a reliable analgesic as its analgesic effect is produced only through its metabolite morphine. This pathway depends on the activity of a liver enzyme (CYP 2D6). However, a large percentage of children, estimated at one third, are so-called 'poor' or 'intermediate' metabolizers and show remarkably inefficient hepatic conversion of codeine to morphine (Williams et al., 2002). Furthermore, approximately 5% of the general population have multiple copies of the enzyme CYP 2D6 and are 'ultra rapid metabolizers', and therefore metabolize unusually high doses of morphine. We had a recent case of a ten-year old girl who, after receiving an appropriate dose of 1mg/kg codeine for post surgical pain, displayed significant respiratory depression (rate 6/minute) and required several doses of the opioid-antagonist naloxone to respond. And rarely, unfortunately, children have died after the administration of codeine (Koren, 2009).

Table 7.1 Opoid analgesics: usual starting doses (Friedrichsdorf & Kang, 2007).

Drug (Route of administration)	Equianalgesic dose (parenteral)	Starting dose IV	IV:PO ratio	Starting dose PO (transdermal)	Starting dose cotrolled release
Morphine (PO, SL, IV, SC, PR)	10 mg	Bolus dose: 50-100 mcg/kg every 2-4 h Continuous Infusion: 10-30 mcg/kg/h	1:3	0.15-0.3 mg/kg every 4 h	0.45-0.9 mg every 12 hours
Fentanyl (IV, SC, SL, transdermal, buccal)	100-250 mcg	Bolus dose: 1-3 mcg/kg (slowly over 3-5 minutes – fast bolus may cause thorax rigidity) Continuous Infusion: 1-2 mcg/kg/h	1:1 (IV to Transdermal)	12 mcg/h patch (must be on the equivalent of at least 30 mg oral morphine / 24 hours, before switched to patch)	n/a
Hydromorphone (PO, SL, IV, SC, PR)	1.5 mg	Bolus dose: 15-20mcg/kg every 4 h Continuous Infusion: 5 mcg/kg/h	1:5	60 mcg/kg every 3-4 h	180mcg/kg every 12 h – currently not available in USA

Drug					
Oxycodone (PO, SL, PR)	5-10 mg	n/a	n/a	0.1-0.2 mg/kg every 4-6 h	0.3-0.9 mg/kg every 12 h
Codeine (not recommended)	120 mg	n/a	n/a	0.5-1 mg/kg every 3-4 h	n/a
Tramadol (PO, PR)	100 mg	IV not available in USA/ Canada [Bolus dose: 1 mg/kg every 3-4 h Continuous Infusion: 0.25 mg/kg/h]	1:1	1-2 mg/kg every 3-4 h, max. of 8 mg/kg/day (> 50kg; max. of 400 mg/day)	2-4 mg/ kg every 12 hours

Calculated rescue (breakthrough) dose: 10-16 % of 24-hour opioid dose to be given every 1-2 hours as needed

IV	= intravenous
PO	= by mouth
SL	= sublingual
SC	= subcutaneous
PR	= rectal
n/a	= not applicable

Tramadol

A better pediatric choice of a 'weak' opioid is tramadol (Ultram®), which is a synthetic analgesic for mild to moderate pain and has been used in pediatrics in Europe since the 1970s. It been trialed in neonates and children (mainly postoperative) and shown to be safe and effective (Bamigbade & Langford, 1998; Rose et al., 2003). (For recommended starting doses, see Table 7.1).

Benefits

- The analgesic strength of tramadol (a weak mu-opioid-receptor agonist) is augmented by an additional effect in inhibiting monoamine neurotransmitter (norepinephrine/serotonin) reuptake.

- Although tramadol is metabolized by CYP 2D6 into a more potent metabolite (O-desmethyltramadol), tramadol is a potent analgesic on its own.

- For poor CYP 2D6 metabolizers, the parent compound (tramadol) remains active, hence those individuals experience no decrease or only a slightly diminished effect on their analgesia.

- Tramadol appears to impair gastrointestinal function less than other opioids and is fairly safe regarding respiratory depression with overdose. In the United States no symptoms were noted in children younger than 6 years who ingested 10/mg/kg or less, and in 87 adult patients with overdose, only two demonstrated respiratory depression (Marquardt, Alsop, & Albertson, 2005).

- In the United States tramadol is available in tablets only, however pharmacies can easily compound it into a stable liquid.

Drawbacks

- As expected from an opioid, common adverse effects include nausea, vomiting, dizziness, constipation, and sedation.

- A rare, but severe side effect is the serotonergic syndrome, which presents with mental status changes (confusion, hypomania), agitation, myoclonus, hyperreflexia, diaphoresis, shivering, tremor, diarrhoea, incoordination, and fever.

- Tramadol appears not to increase the risk of ideopathic seizures; but patients with seizure tendency or who are taking medication that lowers seizure threshold (tricyclic antidepressents, SSRI, antipsychotics) may be at increased risk (Bozkurt, 2005).

Caution

'Weak' and 'strong' opioids should not be combined due to an unfavorable side effect profile.

'Strong' Opioids

Morphine

Morphine remains the most frequently used opioid in pediatrics for moderate to severe pain. Therefore a lot is known about its action in children. Morphine also exists as an oral extended-release form, allowing twice daily dosing, which increases compliance and effectiveness. (For recommended starting doses for morphine and other strong opioids, see Table 7.1). Opioid-associated side effects, such as constipation, pruritus, nausea, have to be expected and treated accordingly.

Oral morphine undergoes a strong first-pass metabolism, which means it is metabolized by liver enzymes (glucuronyl transferase) into Morphine-6 glucuronide (M6G) and Morphine-3 glucuronide (M3G). This is why there is an oral to intravenous conversion rate of 3:1 – 1mg intravenous equals 3mg oral morphine. M6G is a much stronger analgesic, resulting in the adverse effects including nausea, vomiting, sedation, and respiratory depression. M3G has no analgesic effect and is an opioid-antagonist causing hyper-excitability and other neurotoxic effects. The ratio of M6G/M3G therefore in parts defines its analgesia to adverse effect profile. All opioid metabolites can accumulate in patients receiving long-term infusions. Since both metabolites need to be excreted by the kidney, it is not be suitable for children with kidney impairment. Fentanyl or methadone are not excreted renally, and are preferable for these children.

Oxycodone

The potency of oral Oxycodone to oral Morphine is usually estimated around 1:1.5; that is, 3mg morphine equals 2mg oxycodone (Kalso, 2007). One advantage of oxycodone over morphine is the slightly longer half-life, which often allows a once-every-6-hour dosing, in contrast to once every four hours with morphine. Renal and hepatic impairment increases the oxycodone serum level. It also exists in oral extended-release form, allowing twice daily dosing.

Hydromorphone

Unlike morphine metabolism, in Hydromorphone metabolism there is no hydromorphone-6-glucoronide (H6G), but there is hydromorphone-3-glucoronide (H3G), similar to morphine metabolism. Opioid neurotoxic effects can occur particularly with patients with renal impairment.

Fentanyl

Fentanyl is a popular opioid for analgesia prior to painful procedures because of its rapid onset of about 1 to 3 minutes, and the brief duration of action of a single dose (30–45 minutes). When fentanyl is used chronically, it has a much longer elimination. It is also used in the pain management of children with cancer, for intra- and post-operative analgesia, in palliative care, and in sedation analgesia for ventilated children on the intensive care unit. Fentanyl provides a good alternative to morphine when dose-limiting side effects of the latter require a rotation of opioid drug. Fentanyl is also available in patch form for opioid tolerant patients, which is discussed later in this chapter.

Methadone

Methadone is an excellent opioid choice in the management of long-term acute pain, such as cancer pain, or in pediatric palliative care. Its use requires experience and it remains underutilized. It has unique pharmacological properties: opioid receptor agonist, a NMDA-receptor antagonist, and presynaptic blocker of serotonin and norepinephrine reuptake.

Benefits

- Long half-life.

- High effectiveness in chronic and neuropathic pain.

- NMDA receptor antagonist mechanism which helps prevent tolerance.

- Lower incidence of constipation.

- Absent active metabolites.

- Safe usage in renal failure and in stable liver disease.

- Inexpensive!

Drawbacks

- Wide dosing variation.

- Variation in half-life in different children because of individual metabolism variability. This can lead to opioid accumulation, making quick titration difficult.

- More complex equianalgesic conversion, which requires a much longer and closer patient observation than with other opioids.

Cautions

Methadone should not be prescribed by those unfamiliar with its use! Its effects should be closely monitored, particularly when it is first started and after dose changes. It is very long acting and has variable metabolism.

Brian was a twelve-year-old (37 kg) boy with bone cancer in his right femur. When he developed severe pain, he was started on oral morphine, 11mg every 4 hours plus 7mg oral morphine every hour as needed. The dose was titrated to effect by 50% for the scheduled and the rescue dose; and 2 days later, by going up 3 titration steps (step 1: 16.5mg; step 2: 25mg). At step 3 he was using 37.5mg morphine every 4 hours plus 22.5mg morphine every 1 hour for rescue dose as needed. Once he was comfortable, his morphine was switched to 110mg extended-release morphine every 12 hours with the same as needed rescue dose of 22.5mg morphine. He practiced self-hypnosis and underwent regular physical therapy and remained fairly comfortable.

About four weeks later he developed right hip pain, and imaging revealed a growing metastasis. The morphine dose was increased by about 50% to 160mg sustained-release morphine twice per day, which reduced the pain from severe to medium. However, the next 50% increase caused some over-sedation. Since he experienced a dose-limiting side-effect, the opioid had to be switched. He was rotated to oral oxycodone 60mg extended-release twice per day plus 35mg rescue dose, once every hour as needed. A 50% increase for scheduled and rescue dose 2 days later provided excellent analgesia. (At this stage hydromorphone or fentanyl might also have been chosen.)

About two months later he developed increasing bone pain at the site of several metastases. When he also developed nerve pain as well as constipation, despite an aggressive bowel regime, he and his parents agreed to switch to methadone. Oxycodone 40mg was used for breakthrough pain. He received good analgesia and constipation management for the next 2 months, requiring only 1 increase of methadone. Brian died peacefully at home, receiving pediatric palliative home care.

Meperidine (Pethidine)

Brand name: Demerol®

One of its metabolites causes seizures, occasionally even after single dosing, so meperidine should not be used in children or teens for pain management at all.

Combination Analgesia

Fixed combination analgesia, usually acetaminophen plus an opioid, should not be used in pediatric analgesia. Examples include Acetaminophen/Hydrocodone (e.g., Vicodin®), Acetaminophen/ Oxycodone (e.g., Percocet®, Roxicet®), or Acetaminophen/ Codeine (e.g., Tylenol No3®). The fixed ratio of acetaminophen to the opioid leaves poor or dangerous choices – either using suboptimal opioid doses, or when using adequate opioid doses, administering a liver-toxic dose of acetaminophen. Also it is unclear, if a child takes a scheduled combination formulation, which medication to choose for a rescue dose. Also, can we be certain that a caregiver will not administer additional doses of the drug if the child remains in pain, increasing the risk of an acetaminophen overdose? How can the opioid be increased and titrated to effect?

Furthermore, parents and patients may be unsure which of their several medications actually contains acetaminophen, and by combining them administer a possible dangerous dose of acetaminophen. For these reasons a U.S. government advisory panel voted in June 2009 to recommend that the FDA eliminate prescription drugs that combine acetaminophen with opioids in the United States. State of the art pediatric analgesia thus requires the individual administration of stand-alone acetaminophen with a single opioid, the latter titrated to effect.

Administration Of Medications

Medications can be given to children by mouth, by rectum, through the skin, and other routes, such as liquids through a G-tube. Whatever the route, children need an explanation of why the medication is being given, what it is intended to do, and how long it may take to work. The older the child, the more information you should convey. Be positive and clear. Do not let anxieties about whether or not a child will take the medication cause you to lie or mislead the child. For example, do not state that it doesn't taste bad when it does. Instead, discuss options and give children choices as to where and how to take the medication, what they would like to drink afterward, and what rewards they may have immediately afterward, such as hearing a story. You could say, "Susie, it is now time to take your medication. Would you like to follow it with a glass of juice or a popsicle?" Or, "It is now time to take your ibuprofen, would you like to swallow it with a small amount of peanut butter or applesauce? While you are swallowing it, I'll read the rest of the story to you."

Another WHO guiding principle in pediatric pain management reads, "By the appropriate route." If possible, the least invasive route of administration and one chosen by the child should be used, making painful intramuscular injections of pain medication unnecessary and obsolete.

By Mouth

The *oral route* is convenient, non-invasive, and usually preferred by the children and their caregivers. This is the best way for children to take medication in the form of tablets, capsules, and liquids.

Liquids

Children under 6 years of age are often not willing to swallow pills; they manage liquids much better. These are usually sweetened and flavored to make them taste better. Liquid oral syringes, available at most pharmacies, facilitate taking liquid medications. The tip fits into the bottle, allowing easy aspiration of the required dose. Be careful not to squirt the liquid into the child's mouth, which will cause spluttering or choking. Slowly push the liquid into the side of the child's cheek so that it is easily swallowed. As children become familiar with the oral syringe, they sometimes prefer to give themselves the medication, and do so with pride.

Some children resist swallowing liquid medicine. Here are some considerations and alternative methods:

- Liquid medications are more likely to taste bitter than tablets, since the liquid covers more surface area of the mouth and tongue than does the tablet.

- Chilling the liquid medicine may weaken its taste, making it more tolerable. Mixing the medication with syrup (chocolate or cherry) can disguise the taste.

- Immediately follow the 'bad'-tasting medication with a carbonated drink, which helps to get the taste out of the child's mouth more quickly, and serves as a reward.

- If a child enjoys sucking ice, numb the tongue with ice before and/or after taking the medication. Similarly, allow the child to suck on a popsicle before and/or after giving the medication so that the treat becomes the highlight.

- Do not mix medication in a bottle of milk or liquid. When medication is placed in a bottle, there is no way of ensuring that the baby or toddler will get the adequate dose. He or she may not finish the bottle, or it may take 15 or 20 minutes to finish the bottle, delaying and possibly reducing the effect of the medication. Instead, use an oral syringe and place it in the infant or toddler's cheek, followed immediately by a bottle or breast to ensure that the medication is swallowed.

- With frequent use of medication, children should brush their teeth or have them brushed. It is well recognized that children taking liquid medications long-term have an increased incidence of dental cavities because of the sugar content and acidity of most medications.

Pills

Toddlers and preschool-aged children (aged one to four) generally put up the most resistance; therefore, crushing and disguising the medication in a small amount of food works best for this age group. Older children (aged five to eight) can more easily be reasoned with, are usually able to swallow tablets and capsules, and can be involved in how best to take the tablet. Capsules are usually easier to swallow because they are narrow and designed to shoot down the throat. Here are some tips and precautions:

- Teach children to pop the tablet on the back of their tongue and swallow it while drinking a full glass of water. Usually after the second or third swallow the tablet will go down.

- Some children may find it easier to swallow the pill with a favorite cookie. Follow up with a drink to dissolve the analgesic tablet and promote its absorption.

- As long as the tablet isn't bitter or a slow-release formulation, for children older than one year, crush the tablet finely and mix it in a half teaspoon of honey, which helps the medicine go down.

- Bury the tablet in a teaspoon of jelly or ice cream, applesauce, peanut butter, or even a softened piece of chocolate.

Cautions

- If the child resists taking medication and needs to regularly, burying the medication in the child's favorite food may backfire. It could become associated with the medication, and the child may start to dislike that food. This is particularly applicable to children with chronic pain. Avoid using their favorite food since it is often a source of comfort, and jointly choose an acceptable alternative.

- Oral medications can cause stomach upset. Taking the medication with a small amount of food will ease the discomfort. In general, most pain medications can be taken with food, although some medications may require being taken on an empty stomach if they are not well absorbed when taken with food.

- With tablets and capsules, the child should drink a full glass of water, or another liquid, to ensure that the medication does not get stuck going down the throat; the liquid will also enhance the dissolving and absorption of the medication.

- Some medications come in 'slow-release' or 'extended-release' form. They need to be taken whole and not broken or chewed in order to maintain their longer activity, making them very difficult for younger children to take. Slow-release medications are not available in liquid form in North America yet, as they are in Europe and Australia (morphine-sachets).

Sublingual

Sublingual application is when medication is placed under the tongue from where it is absorbed straight into the blood stream, bypassing the liver. This means that it acts very quickly and it is highly effective. Sublingual opioids (morphine, fentanyl, oxycodone, hydromorphone, and methadone) appear safe and well liked by children and their caregivers. This is a smart option if oral administration is not feasible and there is no intravenous access. The data for sublingual morphine are somewhat confusing because it has been shown to have variable absorption. Despite this, sublingual morphine in high-concentration is used frequently, especially in infants and toddlers. Oxycodone, hydromorphone, methadone and fentanyl can be given sublingually and are effective.

Buccal

Like the sublingual route, medication is similarly rapidly absorbed across the oral mucosa of the child's cheek (buccal) directly into the blood stream. It has been used with children 3 years of age and older. Oral transmucosal fentanyl (Aqtic®) in the form of a fentanyl lozenge (the term 'lollipop' should be avoided) is a solid drug matrix with a berry flavor. Currently the fentanyl lozenge in indicated exclusively for the treatment of breakthrough pain in cancer patients and is no longer used for sedation or pre-medication. If used for this purpose, certain guidelines should be followed by the experienced provider only. Children need to be on the equivalent of 60mg oral morphine/day in order to use the smallest fentanyl lozenge (200mcg).

Intranasal

Intranasal application of opioids is pain free and safe when appropriate doses are used, though many children find this route unpleasant (Karl, Rosenberger, Larach, & Ruffle, 1993). Fentanyl can be diluted in normal saline solution (0.9%) and may be applied as a nasal spray or in drops. The pharmacokinetic profile of intranasal fentanyl seems to be similar to intravenous fentanyl. Intranasal fentanyl does not irritate the nasal mucous membrane. Reported intranasal fentanyl doses in children (1–1.5mcg/kg) are equal to or only slightly above suggested intravenous doses (refer to Table 7.1).

Transdermal

Transdermal administration (absorbed through the skin) of anesthetics is a versatile route to manage both acute and chronic pain and easily accepted by children. Transdermal fentanyl has a role only in stable acute pain. It is **contraindicated** for the management of new onset or escalating pain because of a long onset time (it may take more than 60 hours to reach peak concentrations in children), inability to rapidly titrate drug delivery, and long elimination half-life (up to 24 hours). Patches can be applied on intact, healthy skin every 48–72 hours. The smallest patch delivers 12 mcg/hour. Note that the Duragesic® patch contains a selective semi-permeable membrane with a fentanyl reservoir, hence it cannot be divided or cut as this would result in 'dose dumping' with potential overdosing. In addition to the stable analgesia provided by the patch, immediate release rescue opioid needs to be available. Lidocaine patches for ongoing chronic pain are discussed later in this chapter.

Intravenous Route

The intravenous administration of opioid is a good option, especially when there is a central line in place. Patient-controlled-analgesia

(PCA) pumps can deliver morphine, fentanyl or hydromorphone with a continuous background and an as-needed bolus, and often provide excellent management of acute pain. As a rule of thumb, the PCA dose (every 5–10 minutes, maximum of 4–6 boluses/hour) is the equivalent of the hourly dose, and should not be less. Alternatively the opioid analgesics can be applied subcutaneously (just beneath the skin) in the same dose as an IV.

Rectal Route

Although rectal administration of medications is a common practice in many parts of Europe, in North America this route is disliked by many parents and older pediatric patients, who find it uncomfortable and embarrassing. Because of variable absorption, however therapeutic blood levels may be unpredictable. Experience shows that good analgesia can be achieved in children when suppositories, or liquid opioids via a small rectal catheter, are administered. Giving medication rectally should be reserved for children who are nauseated or vomiting, or who refuse or are unable to take their medications by swallowing. Be sure that the child understands the procedure and why you are giving the medication this way. One way of explaining it to a preschool-or school-aged child is as follows:

"Your tummy is upset and has been throwing everything up. If you swallow your pain medication, it's not going to stay down and help your pain go away. We want you to feel better and not be in this pain, so we need to use a suppository. It goes inside your bottom, and your body will absorb it and it will ease the pain. At first it may feel rather strange, but this feeling will quickly go away, and you can help by blowing out some deep breaths to get more comfortable, and your bottom will be OK."

Suppositories need to be stored in a cool, dry place, such as the refrigerator, to keep them firm. To put in a suppository, wash your hands, and remove the foil wrapper. Moisten the suppository with cool water or vaseline to help it enter the rectum easily. Have the child lie down on his or her side with the top leg bent. Talk all the time to the child and explain what you are doing. Use your finger to gently push the suppository up into the rectum until it disappears. It does not have to be placed very high, just beyond the tight sphincter muscle of the rectum. Once it is in place, the child is free to move about. For smaller infants and toddlers, however, hold the buttocks for a few minutes, as they tend to 'poop out' the suppository immediately otherwise.

G-tube route

A gastric feeding tube, or G-tube, is a tube inserted through a small incision in the abdomen into the stomach. Hospitalized children will have a G-tube in for a variety of reasons. With oncology children it is usually because they are not eating well. One of the advantages of having a G-tube is that they do not need to swallow medications. Most liquids are not a problem but you have to stop feeds when you give medication so that it is well absorbed. One needs to be cautious using this route for pills, as crushed pills and powder can clog the G-tube.

Medications to Prevent Procedural Pain

Healthcare professionals can cause pain in the course of their diagnostic and therapeutic interventions. This is an important source of pain to prevent or if not possible, to address in order to minimize, particularly as safe and effective interventions are available. Procedural pain must be avoided, especially for young children and infants (see Chapter 1).

Topical Anesthetics

A few pain medications, primarily local anesthetics, are given transdermally. Children tolerate and manage this application well. EMLA® cream or patches (described in detail on the following pages) and other topical anesthetics are increasingly being used for pain associated with invasive procedures such as injections and placement of intravenous lines. They can be applied at home to prepare for clinical care. They also work indirectly on anxiety by reducing the fear and anticipation of the pain. Topical anesthetic creams and patches usually do not have troublesome side effects.

EMLA® was the original local anesthetic cream. Other topical agents include Maxilene, ELA-Max, L.M.X.4, and Ametop. Current available data cannot support a clear recommendation of one topical anesthetic over another (Koh, Harrison, Myers, et al., 2004). EMLA®'s major detraction is its long time to take effect. Ela-Max LMX is quicker at 30 minutes and its duration of action is 1 hour. EMLA® is effective only *after* 60 minutes application and the effect continues for 1-2 hours. Because of the time required for EMLA® to become effective, its vasoconstricting properties, sometimes making it more difficult to see a vein (waiting for 15 minutes is sufficient for the vein size to return to normal), and concern for methemoglobinemia in young infants, other topical anesthetic creams have been developed.

Children who have recurrent blood draws or an IV will benefit greatly from a topical anesthetic, with a significant easing of anticipatory anxiety. EMLA® is used below as an example of how to implement these important pre-emptive pain and anxiety relieving interventions for children's acute procedures.

EMLA®

EMLA® is a mixture of two local anesthetics, prilocaine (2.5%) and lidocaine (2.5%), blended into a white cream base. It was developed to provide local anesthesia in small areas of intact skin. A thick coating of EMLA® is applied to the skin in the area where a puncture or procedure will occur, and it is then covered with an occlusive dressing such as a Tegaderm®. Parents can learn to place these on the recommended sites an hour before coming to the clinic. When the child arrives with the Tegaderm® on, ready for the procedure, the child has some assurance that with 'the magic cream' that he or she won't be bothered by pain. This is a 'win-win' situation for child, parent, and busy staff – and parents and the child spend less time in the clinic. In Canada and the United States, EMLA ® is available without a prescription, but it should not be used for infants under six months without advice from a physician.

What Is It Used For

- EMLA® as been approved by the FDA to minimize pain during the following: needle sticks for blood drawing, IV starts, split skin graft harvesting, and genital mucosa as an adjunct to local anesthesia infiltration. EMLA® or other topical anesthetics alone are clearly insufficient for circumcision, a very painful procedure, which either requires a penile block or general anesthesia.

- Non-FDA approved indications that have been used in children include: anal fissures, IM Immunizations, lumbar punctures, access for dialysis, superficial surgical procedures, such as the cryotherapy removal of small warts, and laser treatment for the removal of port wine stains commonly known as birth marks.

- EMLA ® is a helpful and effective medication for children who must undergo many painful procedures as it has a wide safety margin.

How It Is Used

- To be effective, EMLA® must be applied to the child's skin for a minimum of 60 minutes to a maximum of four hours.

- For term infants less than three months the maximum time is 1 hour. In neonates, EMLA® reduces the behavioral pain response to venipuncture but not heelsticks (Taddio, Ohlsson, Einarson, et al., 1998). Single doses have not been associated with methemoglobinemia (Taddio et al., 1998). Data shows its effective for neonates >34 weeks gestation for lumbar puncture (Kaur, Gupta, & Kumar, 2003).

- For minor procedures, leave the cream in place for at least one hour, and for deeper procedures, such as mole or wart removal, leave it for two hours.

Four-year-old Cathy required an intravenous access, because she needed antibiotics and analgesics to treat her pyelonephritis (painful kidney infection). "Cathy, you'll need to have an IV today for the medication to make you better and take this silly pain away. Would it be OK to use this magic cream on your hand to put the nerves to sleep. Many children have told me that with this cream they didn't feel the poke at all, and others told me they felt just a little bit. I wonder how it's going to be with you?" Once Cathy answered all the questions she was given the choice where she wanted the EMLA® patch applied (back of hands or cubital [inner elbow] area are commonly used). An hour later she herself wanted to remove the patch, and chose, as the majority of young children do, to sit on her mum's lap during the procedure. While Cathy was blowing bubbles during the IV access, she revealed no verbal or non-verbal sign of pain, and she was immediately rewarded with a little toy of her choice from the 'Treasure Box'.

Liposomal Lidocaine 4% Cream (Maxilene, ELA-Max, L.M.X.4)

Lidocaine creams are an alternative to EMLA® cream and also well tolerated by children (Koh et al., 2004).

- Application time, 30–60 minutes; duration, approximately 60 minutes after removal.

- No prescription required.

- May cause redness, irritation, itching, rash.

- Not associated with methemoglobinemia.

- Minimal vasoactive properties that minimize potential interference with cannulation/IV access.

The J-Tip is an inexpensive (if refilled by in-house pharmacy) single use, disposable syringe containing its own high pressure CO_2 power source. It can be loaded with lidocaine buffered by adding 1 part sodium bicarbonate to 10 parts of 1% lidocaine to raise the pH of the lidocaine and to decrease the pain associated with anesthetic infiltration. The medication is forced into subcutaneous tissue by the gas with minimal discomfort. The needleless injector virtually eliminates the risk of blood borne pathogens cross-contamination to patients and health care providers. Be sure to warn the child that "it will pop like the sound of opening a can of warm soda" because the sudden loud noise can be startling.

Amethocaine (tetracaine 4%) (Ametop)

This is a fine standby for emergency medicine. Its shorter application time and its use in open wounds such as playground accidents that require suturing, make it reliably helpful. Once again it's important to tell a child that this 'magic gel' will numb or put the nerves to sleep, so that the child will understand the process while the laceration is stitched.

- Application time, 30 minutes; duration, 4 hours.

- Low risk for methemoglobinemia so it can be used safely in neonatal period.

- Studied in premature infants during the first week of life.

- May cause vasodilatation resulting in some skin erythema.

Nitrous Oxide (Entonox®)

First used as a dental and surgical anesthetic by Horace Wells in 1844, nitrous oxide is one of the easier and safer agents to manage procedural pain of short duration in children (Gall et al., 2001). It has also been known as 'laughing gas' for its disinhibiting effect on some children and adults. Nitrous oxide is odorless, quite effective, acts quickly, and wears off rapidly once administration ends. As such, it has many characteristics of an ideal medication to relieve pain and anxiety in children undergoing procedures.

There are several factors that must be considered when deciding how nitrous oxide should be used:

- *Absolute contraindications.* Intracranial hypertension, disorders involving accumulation of gas in closed body spaces (for example, pneumothorax, ileus, sinusitis), and unconsciousness due to other drugs or disease.

- *Patient age.* Patients under one year of age are often more distressed by the mask itself, receive less analgesia, and experience more side effects than toddlers and older children. Infants are thus generally not good candidates for nitrous oxide.

- *Dosage.* For safety reasons, all nitrous oxide administration devices must ensure that at least 30% oxygen is delivered; that is, maximum of 70% nitrous oxide. Continuous flow circuits that allow variable nitrous oxide concentrations permit flexibility in the dose delivered, though concentrations below 50% have limited efficacy. Entonox® is a pre-mixed 50:50 combination of nitrous oxide and oxygen; the disadvantage of the fixed combination is that many patients receive better analgesia/sedation if they receive up to 70% nitrous oxide during a painful procedure. Entonox® is sometimes administered via a demand apparatus. This device has one safeguard against overdose, since when the child becomes sleepy, the mask or mouthpiece drops away and the flow of gas ceases. On the other hand, younger children and those who are crying will not be able to use a demand device effectively. A better option is to use a simple, well-maintained portable apparatus equipped with a scavenging system to minimize occupational exposure of nearby personnel.

- *Adjuncts.* The best medications to add to nitrous oxide are local and/or topical anesthetics that can increase pain relief without increasing sedation. These should always be maximized as should age-appropriate non-pharmacologic comfort techniques. Nitrous oxide can be used alone or in conjunction with other analgesics, but great care must be taken that appropriate standards are always met (Coté, Wilson, et al., 2006). When opioids and/or sedatives are added to high concentrations of nitrous oxide, moderate sedation can progress to deep sedation or general anesthesia and a rapid increase in the risks of its use.

- *Personnel.* As with any kind of sedation for procedures, appropriately trained personnel must be matched to the pharmacologic approach. Successful administration of nitrous oxide is a learned skill, and nurses and physicians require training in its use. In addition, for sedation of younger patients and situations in which greater doses of nitrous oxide and/or adjunctive sedative-analgesics are planned, more extensive training in rescue techniques is essential. That being said, nitrous oxide administration by non-physician providers is routine in the U.S. (particularly in dental offices) and around the world.

- *Adverse events.* The most common untoward effect of nitrous oxide is nausea and/or vomiting; this has been reported to occur in up to 26% of patients (Luhmann et al., 2006). Aspiration of gastric contents into the lung is a clear possibility, though reports of this occurring are exceedingly rare, despite the fact that most patients have fasted for very short times prior to nitrous oxide administration.

The need to scavenge the excess and exhaled gas from the room in order to minimize staff exposure is an additional concern which has limited implementation (Annequin et al., 2000). Although nitrous oxide is currently used in 88% of U.S. pediatric dental offices, most North-American children's hospitals have yet to employ this agent for procedural pain management. In France, Italy, and parts of the Middle East, rooms have been fully equipped to scavenge the excess gas, and nitrous oxide is routinely and successfully used for many painful procedures (Annequin et al., 2000; F. Barrometti, personal communication, 2009).

At Sheffield Children's Hospital in the UK,, Entonox® has been used on the general wards and in the out-patient department for reducing procedural pain of short duration (Pickup & Goddard, 1996). Nursing staff were trained by a Pediatric Anesthetist and Clinical Nurse Specialist to supervise the self administration of Entonox® following hospital protocol, without a medical prescription. They report that children have found it easy to use and beneficial in reducing procedural pain. The children enjoy the control they have with it, and parents are relieved at their children's reduced discomfort. Nursing staff report it to be an excellent analgesic, an anxiety-reducing agent, and a distraction strategy. The fact that it does not require a medical prescription enabled specially trained nurses to efficiently use Entonox® for procedures, whenever needed.

At multiple sites in the Children's Hospitals and Clinics of Minnesota in Minneapolis/St. Paul, more than 6,000 children have undergone nitrous oxide sedation for a wide variety of procedures in the last three years (Zier et al., 2007). The side effects in less than 3% of the children include nausea, vomiting, diaphoresis and rarely hallucinations or euphoria/dysphoria. During the procedure the children breathe 50–70% nitrous oxide in oxygen. Afterwards they breathe 100% oxygen for 2–3 minutes and rapidly return to a normal state of consciousness, ready to leave the hospital, or go and play.

In Summary

Today we have enough options so that procedural pain can and must be avoided every time. Topical anesthesia, such as EMLA® or LMX, or appropriate analgesia administered by a non-painful route, such as intranasal fentanyl, can be used. If good analgesia is not feasible, nitrous oxide for mild sedation, or general anesthesia including ketamine or propofol (not discussed in this chapter) for moderate to deep sedation, must be utilized. Other useful strategies to relieve children's pain include the psychological and physical methods described in Chapters 5 and 6.

Medications for Complex/Chronic Pain

In the management of complex/chronic pain in children, medication often plays a supportive role, as relying on pharmacology alone will usually not resolve chronic pain. Effective pain management usually includes regular physical therapy with daily home exercise, support to attend school full time, individual psychotherapy, parental coaching, and integrative therapies such as acupressure, self-hypnosis, biofeedback, or yoga.

Currently the most commonly used medications in pediatric chronic pain are the antidepressant amitriptyline (Elavil®, alternative: nortriptylin) and the anticonvulsant gabapentin (Neurontin®, alternative: pregabaline [Lyrica®]). As mentioned earlier, opioids are usually contraindicated in chronic/complex pain disorders in children, although there has been some controversy and this contraindication doesn't apply to all neuropathic pain (Berde, Lebel, & Olsson, 2003).

Antidepressants

Developed to treat mood disorders and depression, in clinical practice this group of medications (Tricyclics, and to a far lesser degree Selective Serotonin Reuptake Inhibitors [SSRIs]) have been found helpful in controlling a range of different pains, such as recurrent abdominal pain, complex regional pain syndrome, and chronic daily headaches. The mechanism can be partly explained by the stimulation of the descending inhibiting pathways. Antidepressants are usually prescribed at lower dose for pain management and may be combined with analgesics to provide a wider therapeutic window.

Tricyclic Antidepressants

Amitriptyline

Dosage: initial 0.1mg/kg p.o., slowly increasing to max. of 20-25mg (rarely up to 1-2mg/kg/day) once at night

Low-dose Tricyclic antidepressants (TCAs) are commonly used in children and adolescents for the treatment of chronic pain, although there is little pediatric evidence of effectiveness. The single daily dose is usually given at bedtime to avoid daytime sedation. The analgesic effect may take days to weeks to be effective. However, amitriptyline is quite sedating, so the dose once at night often helps to induce sleep. When discontinued, it should be decreased gradually over at least a week.

Benefits

TCAs are potentially helpful in many chronic pain entities, including chemotherapy-induced neuropathy, complex regional pain syndrome, infiltrative tumor pain, phantom pain post amputation, burns, and functional abdominal pain.

Drawbacks

Adverse effects include arrhythmia (an EKG to rule out QTc-prolongation or a Wolff-Parkinson-White syndrome is recommended) and anticholinergic and antihistaminic effects, such as dry mouth, constipation, blurred vision, and sedation. These effects can usually be managed by lowering the dose, then slowly titrating up again. If it is not possible to manage side effects, one can switch to nortriptyline. Some large pediatric pain centers use nortriptyline as the first line TCA.

Alternatives

As mentioned above, these include the secondary amine TCAs (nortriptyline) with less anticholinergic side effects, and the tertiary amine TCAs imipramine. Desipramine (a secondary amine TCA) cannot be recommended because of anecdotal evidence of sudden death in children.

Selective Serotonin Reuptake Inhibitors

Although Selective Serotonin Reuptake Inhibitors (SSRIs) are typically used to treat anxiety and depression, the efficacy of SSRI's for the treatment of complex or chronic pain has not been established. SSRIs' mechanism of action is to block the reuptake of the neurotransmittor serotonin throughout the body. Only fluoxetine (Prozac®) and escitalopram (Cipralex® in Canada and Lexapro® in US) have been approved for use in depression by the U.S. FDA. Others are nonapproved, but some are selectively used such as citalopram (Celexa®), sertraline (Zoloft®), and venlafaxine (Effexor®).

Drawbacks

The most common side effects of the SSRIs include headaches, gastro-intestinal upset, agitation, insomnia/hypersomia, and sweating. These side effects usually go away after several days if low doses are initially used and titrated slowly. Research evidence suggests that SSRIs are far less effective pain relievers than tricyclics (Finnerup, 2005). SSRIs take up to four to six weeks to achieve their maximal efficacy.

Caution

Many pediatric-drug randomized controlled trials for treatment of major depressive disorder and for bipolar disorder have been negative. There remains a strong concern about positive publication bias in industry-funded trials. The numbers needed to treat (NNT) – meaning: "how many children or teenagers do I have to treat to make one patient 50% better" – for a major depression using an SSRI is 10 (Tsapakis, Soldani, Tondo, & Baldessarini, 2008). Hence 9 out of 10 children will not receive any benefit from a single SSRI (the data for individual psychotherapy and especially cognitive behavioral therapy is far better). For treating anxiety with an SSRI in children and teenagers, the NNT is still only 3; that is, 2 out of 3 will not receive a benefit (Tsapakis, et al., 2008).

Anticonvulsants

Anticonvulsants are considered first-line agents for many forms of neuropathic pain. Gabapentin is the most widely used for neuropathic pain, because of its relatively low side effects, its experience in pediatrics (it has been extensively used with children with epilepsy) and its effectiveness (Berde, Lebel, & Olsson, 2003).

Gabapentinoids

Dosage: For Gabapentin gradually (usually over weeks) increasing from 2mg/kg/dose three times per day to 10–20mg/kg/dose three times per day, to a maximum 1,200mg/dose three times per day.

Benefits

The two members of this class, gabapentin (Neurontin®) and pregabalin (Lyrica®) are calcium-channel ligands. That is, they reduce the release of pain transmitters, such as glutamate and substance-P from the presynaptic nerve terminal at the dorsal horn of the spinal cord (see Figure 2.2). This reduces the excitation of the postsynaptic nerve terminal in the spinothalamic tract, creating the potential for pain reduction. The analgesic effect may take days to weeks to occur, depending on length of symptoms. When gabapentin is weaned, the dose should be decreased gradually over 1–2 weeks.

Drawbacks

Adverse side effects occur usually if dose is started too high or escalated too fast, but even with slow dose escalation worrisome side effects may occur. These include ataxia, nystagmus, myalgia, hallucination, dizziness, somnolence, aggressive behaviors, hyperactivity, thought disorder, peripheral edema.

Alternatives

If gabapentin fails once the dose limit is reached, or because of dose limiting side effects, one may switch to pregabalin at a conversion rate of 6:1 (i.e., 600mg gabapentin equals 100mg pregabalin).

Patients who fail to benefit from gabapentin may benefit from pregabalin and the other way around. No data exist to suggest that either drug is better than the other one. Other less commonly used anticonvulsants in pediatric chronic pain include topiramate (Topamax®) and oxcarbazepine (Trileptal®).

Topical Anesthetic Patch

The local anesthetic lidocaine 5% patch (Lidoderm®) is effective for diverse peripheral neuropathic pain conditions and allodynia. It may be used for localized pain only. The patch is a matrix, that is, it can be cut to fit. The pharmaceutical manufacturer recommends 12 hours on/12 hours off to avoid tolerance, however a systemic lidocaine level is very unlikely and many patients wear it 24 hours/day. It should not be used in patients with severe hepatic dysfunction. When used at home, parents need to be cautioned to carefully dispose of the patch so that they are not chewed by young children or pets.

Adjuvants

These are additional medications added to extend the analgesic or therapeutic effects, or to act as coanalgesics:

- NMDA-receptor antagonists, such as low-dose ketamine.

- Muscle relaxants, such as baclofen or cyclobenzaprine (Flexaril®).

- Low-dose benzodiazepines, such as diazepam (Valium®), lorazepam (Ativan®), MIDAZOLAM (Versed®).

- Bisphosphonates (for bone pain due to metastatic cancer or severe osteopenia, for example, associated with cystic fibrosis), such as pamidronate.

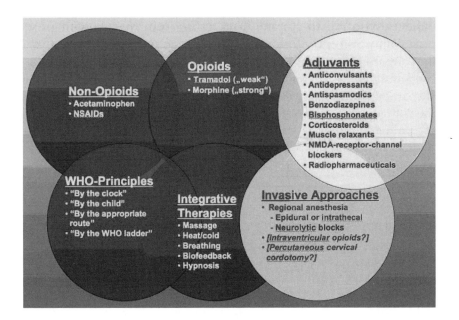

Figure 7.3: Managing Children in Acute Pain: Broad-Band Analgesia
The circles to the left and middle show the standard analgesic approach.
The lighter circles on the right show options available for further pain
management.
(Friedrichsdorf, 2008, http://www.nhpco.org/files/public/ChiPPS/
ChiPPS_November_2008.pdf)

- Antispasmodics, such as hyoscyamine (Levsin®); oxybutynin (Ditropan®), or glycopyrrolate (Robinul®).

- Botolinum toxin A or other (e.g., phenol) nerve blocks, especially in treating cerebral palsy and spasticity.

Conclusion

Guided by the WHO principles of pain management, there is an increased recognition of the importance of pain prevention, prompt acute pain intervention and more options to minimize the deleterious effects of ongoing pain in children. We are fortunate to have a wide range of analgesics, anesthetics, and other medications to draw on to prevent and control acute and to manage chronic/ complex pain. Pharmacological management has been the mainstay in pediatric practice. Combining its therapeutic impact with the contribution of physical and psychological therapies can make the pain and anxiety experienced by children in clinic visits, at the dentist, or in the hospital even more effectively managed, as discussed in the chapters in Part III.

Part III

Pain and Anxiety Management in Pediatric Practice

"The first time I go to a doctor or dentist for anything I get them
to tell me all about it first.
Then I check and find out if they're lying. It's best to know."

Twelve-year-old boy. From D. M. Ross, 1988

Children of all ages can be on the alert, vigilant or actively fearful when going to a practitioner for care. How to manage fear and anxiety during these consultations, particularly when pain is involved, is a important challenge for clinicians and a major theme of the following three chapters. First, it's important to distinguish between fear and anxiety (Dr. Bernie Whitaker, personal communication, Melbourne, December 2005). Fear is a reaction to a clearly identifiable threat, a strong motivation to avoid a threatening object or situation, often with a rational component such as a fear of needles, heights, or death – even though experiencing this fear can be self-defeating. Anxiety, on the other hand, is inherent within the person. It is a disposition, largely irrational, and sometimes psychopathological, as in an anxiety state or panic attack or 'anxiety disorder'.

When it comes to children who are fearful of painful procedures and chronic pain, even if some also have anxiety or anxiety disorders, we can be more helpful to them in the moment if we focus more on their specific fears. How effectively these are addressed will influence how readily the child's pain resolves. This is particularly true for chronic pain – remember the neuromatrix (Figure 2.8) and how pain itself and the fear of the pain serve as a mechanism through which chronic pain is maintained over time. As a result, an emphasis will be placed in the chapters in Part III on how to recognize, engage with and relieve the child's fears and anxiety in the different pediatric practice areas: at the pediatrician's or physician's office, at the dentist, and in the hospital. What follows is information that applies to all three settings.

Fear and Anxiety Co-factors with Pain

Uncertainty breeds vigilance and vigilance may develop into anxiety. Children and their parents look to the pediatric professionals to define what's going on and to provide an explanation, direction, comfort, and relief. If this doesn't occur, trust won't develop. When there's little trust in a situation or a professional, the child can become fearful. Too often this fear is regarded as a side issue, one that requires a placating word or two to dismiss. But fear is not easily dismissed. Specific fears related to medical events and non-specific anxiety are universal survival responses to threat – and children experience threat when in pain or expecting pain. We know that both fear and anxiety have a sizable impact on the child's perception of pain. Pain-related fear and anxiety are now receiving considerable attention in the adult literature as central variables in maintaining pain disability (Asmundson, Vlaeyen, & Crombez, 2004). Since it is generally agreed that anxiety involves both a psychological and a physiological response to a perceived danger, let's look closer at how this may play out with a child awaiting care in a medical or dental office.

Our limbic systems are hard-wired through our senses to perceive threat and immediately respond by mobilizing hormonal, metabolic, and autonomic nervous systems to deal with threat. What may happen when a child, sitting or lying awaiting care, sees the traditional 'white coat'? How is a learned response to this triggered? As the health professional enters the room, there is an assembly of cortical and subcortical information in the active flow of the child's brain that leads to a response. Seeing the white coat alerts the child's attention and induces perceptual orienting: "Look – I've seen this before!" If the amygdala (in the subcortical limbic system near the forebrain) registers the white coat as 'dangerous!' the child's cognitive systems, appraising the situation, arouses a fear response. "All of this occurs within seconds and does not depend on conscious awareness. Nonconsciously, the brain is wired, at least with regard to the fear response to create a 'self-fulfilling prophecy'. If the amygdala is excessively sensitive and fires off a Danger! signal, it will automatically alter ongoing perceptions to appear to the individual as threatening" (Siegal, 1999, p. 133). The amygdala activates arousal centres, which through the release of noradrenaline and adrenaline arouse a generalized excitability.

The child becomes aroused, vigilant or distressed at the recognition of the danger of imminent pain that the white coat represents. Such learned experiences of fear may also become emotional memories with lasting effects (von Baeyer, et al., 2004). The white coat together with the needle, or the prodding that causes pain, become established into a feedback loop. The child learns to anticipate the rush of adrenaline, fear and anxiety on seeing a white coat. This may be the neurobiological basis for phobias and other anxiety disorders (Siegal, 1999) that children in pain seem very easily to develop.

In a study that now for ethical reasons could not be replicated, results revealed that children require only one aversive painful experience to alter their perception and experience of pain for subsequent procedures (Weisman, Bernstein, & Schechter, 1998). In this study the small placebo group experienced their first lumbar puncture with inadequate analgesia. On their second to the fifth procedures they were given adequate analgesia. Despite this, their self-reported pain scores remained significantly higher on all subsequent procedures than the children who had received adequate analgesia at their first procedure. Learned fear is tenacious.

Rachman (1977) explains that there are three pathways for fear to be acquired. They are direct conditioning, modeling, or instructions/information. Of these, direct conditioning is the most powerful. Experiencing direct exposure to distress caused by the feared stimulus produces the most rapid and thorough learning and the greatest resistance to extinction. The study by Weisman et al. (1998) is consistent with Rachman's theory of how fear is learned. The children who received the placebo for their first procedure, and real medication after that, were undoubtedly told on the subsequent procedures that the medication would relieve their pain, but this information was not very effective in the face of direct conditioning.

This rapid learning to fear painful events applies to children's dental procedures (Locker, Liddell, Dempster, & Shapiro, 1999) and immunizations following an earlier painful experience (Taddio et al., 1997). Fear and anxiety play a powerful role in learning, particularly learning from negative experience – such as pain. As our example of the child's learned anxiety reaction to a white coat illustrates, fear and anxiety, as states of vigilance, apprehension and uncertainty, can result from the anticipation of a realistic, or even a fantasized threat. There is a lot of evidence that children who catastrophize, imagining that the anticipated medical event will have far-reaching negative consequences, suffer greater distress than those who don't (Jaaniste, Hayes, & von Baeyer, 2007). These children, some traumatized and others with a sensitive temperament, need special practical and psychological intervention to help them approach coping with less anxiety. We know that children facing recurrent pain episodes or living with chronic pain report elevated levels of anxiety and depression (Palermo, 2000), although these may not be at clinical levels (Larsson, 1991). As seasoned pediatric clinicians know, whether in general pediatric, dental, or hospital practice, the child's pain-related fear and anxiety is an essential component of the experience of pain and needs to be therapeutically addressed and followed through as part of optimal pain treatment.

The translation of pediatric research findings into standard clinical practice is an ongoing process. It requires practitioners' thoughtful reflection on their practice, and their considered action to improve the quality of care and clinical outcome for their patients. Some researchers maintain that the gap between science and practice is of a startling magnitude, and that if research findings were systematically implemented clinically, this would significantly improve children's quality of care, including in pain management (MacLaren & Kain, 2008). With a better understanding of how pain presents in the lives of children, how to assess it, and how to use a biopsychosocial approach of the 3Ps of pain interventions, in the following three chapters we'll examine how to apply these interventions to bring comfort when children in pain visit the family physician, pediatrician, or dentist, or when they go to hospital. What are the responsibilities of those in pediatric practice? What are the treatment options available and how effective are these for the common acute, recurrent, and persisting pain problems of childhood?

Chapter 8

Managing Pain and Anxiety at the Doctor's Office

"Creating a 'pain-friendly' office can relieve anxiety in the children and their parents, and lower the stress level for all involved. Office staff can learn simple techniques to help children cope with potentially painful aspects of their visit."

Neil Schechter (2008b, p. 55)

When children are reluctant to visit their physician, they may have explained that they fear experiencing pain or the surprise of having an injection (Ross & Ross, 1988). Generally, physicians don't want children to experience pain in their consulting rooms and strive to make them feel comfortable and relaxed. To achieve this, family doctors and pediatricians can make their office consultations as pain-free as possible. Immunizations and blood collection can be done by a nurse in a designated treatment room using distraction and other behavioral interventions (Sugarman, 2006) and minor surgeries may be done in the hospital.

Pain is, nevertheless, one of the most common reasons for parents to bring children to a physician's office. Many physicians, especially in small communities, must stitch lacerations, treat fractures and other injuries, or give inoculations in the surgery room attached to their consulting room. If children experience their pain, distress, and concerns as neither effectively or sensitively handled, the doctor's office becomes a place where children learn fear, lose faith in the medical system, and avoid returning for care. Eight-year-old Jason, on returning from his pediatrician, emphatically stated, "He said... he didn't believe my pain... He thought my pain wasn't like I was saying... I don't feel good about it... I don't feel like going back to him."(*"Why?"*) "Because it's no use!"

The topics of pain and anxiety management are often not well covered during medical school or residency. At best, medical students and residents are taught using a few patient cases accompanied by sporadic lectures during training. Thus the schism between the child's utmost concern and the physician's training can be the source of clinical difficulties, patient disappointments, and rifts in the doctor-patient relationship, as the physician learns by experience.

In this chapter we'll look at the value of the doctor as teacher/educator and explore the practical aspects of how to examine a child in pain. Maintaining the child-centered perspective, we'll discuss some fears children have in visiting the doctor, and the enduring importance of a trusted doctor-patient relationship in which pain complaints are heeded. Given the large number of pain-related office visits that a child has over the developing years, the physician can have a significant impact on the child's pain and capacity to understand and cope with pain.

There are many types of children's pain that present in a physician's office, the majority of which are minor or transitory. Those that are not, such as pain that accompanies a medical illness or chronic or recurring pain, tend to demand more time, skill, patience, and alliance with the child, and knowledge and understanding of pain. We'll review some common minor pains in this chapter and provide an overview of two common but complex conditions – headaches and recurrent/functional abdominal pain.

Doctor as Educator

The term 'doctor' comes from the Latin *docere* and means 'teacher'. Visiting the doctor's office is a learning opportunity for the patient. It is a place to bring concerns and explore ways of maintaining one's well-being and good health. For children, a visit to their pediatrician or family physician provides an opportunity to learn about themselves and develop greater mastery over the mysteries of their bodies.

The learning starts early. From birth most infants are given a full examination. Research mentioned before suggests that memory may start at birth and by 4 to 6 months a child appears to remember the experience of pain (Taddio et al.,1997). Boys circumcised at birth, when given immunizations at age 4 to 6 months evidenced increased crying and distress (an indication of a learned fear response), compared to those infants where the pain of circumcision was well-controlled.

As children get older, their visits to the doctor become a forum for receiving information about how they are growing and developing. They learn over successive visits not only that their bodies show signs when something isn't well, but that there is someone apart from their parents who can be trusted to look at these signs, diagnose what they mean, and tell them what to do to get well again. This doctor-child relationship is an important one when it comes to pain. Interview studies on children's concepts of pain have shown consistently that they seldom mention any beneficial aspects of pain, such as pain's diagnostic value, its warning function, or its role in evaluating treatment (Abu-Saad, 1984a, b, c; Ross & Ross,1984a, b; Savedra et al., 1982). Of the very small group of children who recognized that pain could be of value, a nine-year old child said: "Pain is a way of telling you *not* to do it in a way that you don't like. If something in your head just said, 'Don't do it,' you would just say, 'Aw, shut up!'" (Ross & Ross, 1988, p. 47).

The doctor as teacher is an essential role in pain management. Good explanations, accompanied by rough drawings or models of bones and muscles cannot be underestimated in terms of their positive influence in addressing children's concerns, pre-occupation, and beliefs about their pain. Well-done explanations have beneficial secondary effects on the convergence of pain processing within the child's neuromatrix and may influence recovery. The converse is also true. If children don't understand or don't have a satisfactory explanations of why they are in pain, they manufacture alternative explanations or blame themselves or others, which can interfere with recovery.

Diagrams, such as those supplied in Chapter 2, aid in imparting as clearly as possible what is causing or maintaining the pain. These consultations also require a somewhat longer appointment time, patience, and using appropriate phrases for a child's cognitive and emotional maturity; such as 'blue lines' for veins and 'little straw' for an IV (see Table 3.2). This educative process also can help close the gap between scientific research and practice, enabling children to understand and follow recommendations for their recovery. The more children and parents feel free to ask questions, voice concerns, check procedures, and request more information, knowing that they will be heard and respected, the healthier the doctor-patient partnership becomes. This cooperative partnership, between physician parent and an aware child, is needed most in times of pain or illness exacerbation and its associated stress, where the doctor as teacher informs sound clinical management. This reflects a change from traditional models of medicine that "emphasize the physician's role in prescribing treatment and the patient's role in following them, [to] newer models of care focused on child and parental communication with their providers (and visa versa) to set goals and share treatment decisions" (Drotar, 2009, p. 246). Here, physician behavior is an important but understudied influence on child and parental adherence to medical treatment.

The Examination of a Child in Pain

Examining a child requires a physician to become inventive and playful and, where possible, to give the child choices so that the examination is as non-distressing as possible (Kuttner, 1992). When the child is in pain, this process is even more challenging. Parents are a helpful resource in the process of working quickly and deftly, knowing that time is short with squirming, sore, fearful, or achy children. It is preferable for many toddlers or preschoolers to be examined on a parent's lap (Children's Hospital of Philadelphia, 2003; Sparks et al., 2007). This maintains a warm sense of security and allows the parent close contact to comfort and coach the child. This is also a good way to begin an examination – until a child is able to sit unaided on an examining table, which commonly occurs at about four years of age, depending on the child's level of independence.

Harnessing the Child's Imagination

Certain parts of the examination can be frightening to a child in pain. For example, holding still is upsetting and difficult to do for a toddler with an ear infection, whose orifices are being poked and prodded. Entering the child's world with imagination and a sense of play can stop the escalation of anxiety. On one occasion I heard a seasoned and playful pediatrician tell a squirming two-and-a-half-year-old with a possible otitis media (painful middle ear) infection:

> "Hold very, very still so that I can take a close look and find the bunny rabbit that jumped into your ear. That's great! Oh! I can see him; he's jumping over the fence. Hold still! Oh! He's gone across to the other ear. Quickly, let me look in the other ear. That's it! Ah, I've found him. Do you know what he's doing? He's wiggling his nose at me!"

The pediatrician rattled this off as he deftly completed his potentially painful examination. The child sat wide-eyed and remarkably still for the minute that was needed. Having something imaginative or playful to do with a child can take the monotony out of these routine procedures and harness the child's imagination adaptively to engage away from the pain. (Otitis media is associated with moderate or greater pain lasting for at least 48 hours [Hayden & Schwartz, 1985] which responds to ibuprofen and acetaminophen.)

Encouraging the Child's Self-Expression

Children need to be encouraged to speak for themselves with authority, relating specifically how their bodies feel, where they hurt, and providing the history and nature of their pain. However young, addressing the child in pain directly, sends an important message and establishes the child as capable of being this authority; competent and knowledgeable about his or her body. The earlier this process is established, the better it is for the child's developing sense of competency in dealing with pain, particularly if it's recurrent or ongoing. One of the measurement scales in Chapter 4 can be used to measure the different degrees of pain, along with asking the child some of the questions in Table 4.1.

Recognizing Fear and Anxiety

As explained previously, for children with persistent illness or medical problems, visiting the doctor conjures up memories of previous hospitalizations and painful treatments. These children are not novices; they're becoming experts on their conditions. Many have been sensitized by pain or have established anticipatory anxiety or catastrophic fears. One can recognize this by the child's watchful tense demeanor, white pallor, or anxious questions. Perhaps the doctor's visit was the prelude to intensive hospital treatments. A subsequent visit therefore evokes fears, including for some, the fear of death. These are children that require extra time in a busy practice to develop a rapport and working alliance. Approaches that involve physicians in active communication, support, and decision making with children and their parents are recommended (Drotar, 2009). These children have experience in identifying subtle and significant changes in their condition, responses to medications, and hunches about which analgesics offered the most benefit. They deserve to be consultants in their own treatment and will offer this information only if asked, as fear tends to inhibit children.

Avoiding Restraint

Children should not be restrained for a physical examination or a procedure. When children learn what they are expected to do when being examined, they become co-operative and the outcome is preferable. If restrained, toddlers and children remember and become fearful and panicky about future examinations. It is difficult subsequently to re-establish trust. Infants or toddlers, particularly if they are ill or in pain, have a difficult time settling, even on a parent's lap. A parent can be guided to firmly and calmly steady a child's hand, or support a wiggling head to assist a safe and thorough exam of the ears and throat. In these brief situations, delays by providing explanations and reassurance are of no benefit. They tend to promote the child's distress and resistance (Chambers, et al., 2002). When a child has 'lost it' it is hard to regain cooperation. Therefore stopping before that point is optimal, to minimize the child's distress and the consequent resistance that may occur.

Using a Parent's Containing Hug for an Injection

For a short examination, many family physicians prefer the child to be held by a parent. A parent's restraining hug for 15 seconds will not be traumatic for a young child. During an arm or leg injection, hugging containment takes this form: the child sits on the parent's lap facing the parent, with the parent's arms around the child, keeping one of the child's arms free for the injection (Penrose, 2006). For a leg injection, the child sits on the parent's lap with his or her back on the parent's chest. One leg, tucked in between the parent's knees, is held for the immunization and the other leg is free. Simultaneously the parent reads a pop-up book, blows bubbles, or holds a game-boy to focus the child's attention onto the more pleasant experience. This type of brief restraint is also useful for an ear, eye, or mouth examination, since the parent can subdue the child's flailing arms and stabilize the child's head. A parent's hugging containment is brief and prevents further escalation of distress.

The literature is consistent in recommending that it is not the parent's role to hold a child for longer than a brief examination or procedure. It is the health professionals' responsibility to position and help the child cope with distressing procedures. Parents are there to support, guide and be a safe haven. Biobehavioral coping techniques such as blowing bubbles, breathing techniques, imagery, distraction, and hypnosis can readily be used with children in an office practice (see Chapters 5 and 6). *Imaginative Medicine*, an informative DVD, shows how to use brain-body methods in a busy pediatric practice for examinations and routine immunizations (Sugarman, 2006). With these skills, restraint is not needed. Restraint is only an option in life-threatening and emergency situations.

Explaining While Doing a Painful Exam

At a doctor's office children in pain may feel protective and anxious, and will guard a tender stomach, broken bone or dislodged joint. Pediatric rheumatologist Pete Malleson talks about tracking a child's facial expression while palpating the child's body as a key aspect in diagnosing the child's pain (Kuttner, 1990). He eases a nine-year-old boy's fears by addressing the child directly. He talks warmly and calmly while he carefully examines the child's joints and tracks his facial expression to add to the physical evidence he collects while mobilizing each joint.

> When you start to examine the joint, the child will sometimes start to look anxious as you move the joint to the end of the range of movement that is pain free and it starts to become painful, then the child tenses up. It's no great skill if you keep watching the child's face... Doctors sometimes forget that what the child cares about is how sore it is, and we look to see if the swelling has gone down. I hope we're getting better at looking at the pain aspects as well. (Malleson, in Kuttner, 1990)

Children have complained that when they indicate an area is hurting, an inexperienced physician-in-training will poke around too much just to make sure he or she has got it, thereby causing even more pain and distrust. Fourteen-year-old Paul, who has Crohn's disease, said,

"When I tell some interns, they won't go near the pain. Some others poke around and I feel like hitting them!" (Kuttner, 1990).

Seeing Parents as Allies

Parents play a pivotal role in preparing and coaching their child through the physician's consultation. They are often attuned to the subtleties of their child's behavior and know how to interpret the child's unspoken reactions and facilitate discussion. For example, seven-year-old Jenny became visibly distressed when her doctor mentioned taking her blood pressure. Knowing her daughter's fear of needles, this mother realized that Jenny heard 'blood' and was heading for panic – so she immediately added, "Dr. Sandy is just measuring the pressure around your arm, Jenny. That tells your blood's pressure. It doesn't hurt. She's not going to take any blood." Parents can be invited to become allies by:

- Prompting the child to speak up for him or herself.

- Interpreting or clarifying the child's fears.

- Encouraging the child to settle, 'do a job to help,' and explain how to start coping.

- Distracting a distressed child with bubbles, a toy, or a favorite story.

Medical jargon easily leads to misunderstandings (refer to Table 3.2). It is always preferable to use words for bodily functions that children know, rather than polysyllabic medical words. Many families don't use words such as 'diarrhea' or 'constipation' with their children. While examining a child's abdomen, a physician may ask if a child is constipated, and wanting to be pleasing and cooperative, the five-year-old child may say 'yes' without understanding what 'being constipated' means. Simple words like 'pooing' and 'peeing', 'hurt' and 'owies' are easier for children to understand. Determine the family's words so that you can talk the same language.

Parents may fear their child's fear or their resistance. Because of this, some will avoid telling their child about the consultation and not adequately prepare the child. These parents need the nursing and office staff's coaching on how to prepare the child and provide coping skills, such as breathing away fears and bringing an iPod to distract and entertain. With information from parents about whether the child copes by seeking information or avoiding it (see Chapter 3), health care professionals will know how much information to share to elicit coping, yet not trigger fear and avoidance (Jaaniste, Hayes, & von Baeyer, 2007).

Encourage parents not to lie to or mislead their children. Let parents know that threats, or telling a child that the doctor is not going to hurt if pain will occur in the visit, will backfire and result in deep feelings of betrayal. We cause children more distress and anxiety when we try to spare them information they require to be prepared (more about this in Chapter 10). By avoiding the truth, we also deny children the opportunity to gather sufficient information through questions and discussion to mobilize their resources for the task. It is important not to lie to children. They remember!

Common Acute Painful Conditions

There are many ailments causing pain or discomfort that present in the pediatrician or general practitioner's office. These include teething, otitis media, fevers, pharyngitis, urinary tract infection – and all may be accompanied by pain. Many of these pains are short-lived and relatively easily treated with appropriate antibiotics for the infection and with mild analgesics for the pain itself (Schechter, 2008b). There are also a succession of injections, primarily immunizations, that children are required to undergo and incidental lacerations that the more boisterous or accident-prone children may incur.

There is little research on common pain problems in outpatient settings. They appear to lack the "urgency and poignancy that accompanies pain problems in the hospital" (Schechter, 2008b, p. 55). This is unfortunate, as it doesn't reflect the actual burden on children that these pain-related problems place. Regular immunizations and unexpected lacerations requiring sutures are common sources of acute pain that present in practice. In discussing these, I emphasize the importance of creating comfort, settling anxiety, using parents, and enabling the child to participate in the treatment process.

Immunizations

Immunizations for the common childhood infections of diphtheria, whooping cough, tetanus, polio, meningitis, measles, mumps, and rubella are one of the most frequent reasons for a consultation. For a healthy baby, it is also the first experience of the pain of an injection. Immunizations are given in the thigh muscle in babies and toddlers and in the arm in older children. These injections are given at least five or six times before the child starts kindergarten – sufficient exposures to develop fear and become sensitized to the needle! The immunizations are painful and unpleasant, and often leave local irritation or swelling that feels tender and sore for a few days. It's important to minimize this pain and to maximize the child's coping and parents' help in this process.

Prior to the injection, advise parents to:

- Use a locally available local anesthetic such as EMLA® on the leg or arm site 60 to 90 minutes before the immunization (see Chapter 7). It numbs the site and the child will not feel much pain when the skin is punctured. Give the recommended dose of acetaminophen half an hour before the immunization to minimize the pain and discomfort during and after the injection. Pediatricians recommend two subsequent follow-up doses, at 4 and 8 hours, and if needed every 4 hours up to 24 hours after the injection. Analgesics given around the clock will prevent the pain from recurring if the injection site is still red or painful a day or two following immunization.

Advise parents that when at home after the injection to:

- Use one of the cool aids, such as an Ouch Mouse, a cool cloth, or a frozen sponge, to reduce the inflammation at the site (see Chapter 6).

- Ensure that the child gets extra sleep.

When giving an injection:

- Give children a job to help themselves. For example, say to a child, "Let's work together to make sure that this injection doesn't bother you? OK. To do that, you have a job to do. Choose either this pinwheel or bubbles or this game-boy/pop-up book and blow/focus – that's it. Really blow/focus because that way the needle doesn't bother you? OK!"

- Prompt children to get into blowing *before* the injection is given. Don't show the needle; if children look for it, redirect them back to their job! (Sugarman, 2006). Don't count the injection down (as in "1, 2, 3!") as this heightens anxiety and distracts children from focusing on their job. Once the child is blowing give the injection. "Good job! You did well!" Team work like this creates an alliance between a clinician and child. Once established, it will be relied on for future injections, and may prevent a learned fear response.

- Harness the child's imagination by using hypnotic suggestions to reduce the perception of pain. This is useful for a series of immunization given at one time. Invite the child to imagine: "If you could be any place right now, where would you be, what is there, how does it look? What are you doing, seeing, wearing?"

- Tell older children riddles – a useful strategy. An eight-year-old girl reported that her penicillin injections took no more than a minute because her pediatrician always asks riddles when giving injections, and they only got through two on that injection! (Ross & Ross, 1988).

Immunizations do sting sharply. Even with a local topical anesthetic there may be some stinging. Alert the parent to increase the child's bubble blowing, or add another distraction such as a book, and provide immediate comfort after the procedure. Some medical offices have a treasure box from which the child can choose a little play toy or ball as a reward for helping. Particular care needs to be given to infants, who are at great risk for developing conditioned fear to needles, doctors, white coats, and the consultation room and office. (See Chapter 6 for methods of pain relief for newborns and infants during immunizations and other painful procedures.)

Lacerations

The pain with a cut or laceration is greatest at the time when the injury occurs. A young child is invariably startled and horrified seeing an open wound with flowing blood ensuing from his or her own body! After the injury and depending on the extent of the injury, the site usually remains very tender, throbbing, and sensitive. When the parent brings a child with a laceration into a physician's office, attempt to ensure that the child's natural anxiety not be magnified by the parent's anxiety. Parent's attitude is pivotal in how the child responds to this injury. Parents who calmly ask, "Do we need any stitches, or will a Band-aid do?" generally have children who cope equally well. If the parent is overwhelmed, it may be better for everyone, that the parent not be present for the laceration repair.

A child, when overwhelmed by fears, finds it hard to listen to staff, take in new information, or hold still for stitching. Once this anxiety takes over, it is very difficult for nursing and medical staff to rescue the situation and settle the child. Right from the very beginning, a very anxious child will benefit from calm, slow clear direction, explanation, direct eye-contact, a soothing touch, and suggestions about coping and healing (see Chapter 5), such as: "Your body knows exactly how to heal this perfectly."

Before suturing, a swab soaked with a topical spray of TAC (tetracaine, adrenaline, and cocaine), or an injectable local anesthetic of lidocaine or xylocaine, buffered to diminishes the sting, could be infused into the wound. Suturing should not start until the local anesthetic has had sufficient time to take effect – otherwise there is no purpose in providing it. Within two to five minutes the local anesthetic numbs the site, providing adequate pain relief for suturing. Meanwhile a story, riddle or imagery told with calm suggestions for comfort can transform the previous panic into a more manageable situation.

Recurrent and Persistent Pains

In general or pediatric practice the most common recurrent pain complaints are headaches and abdominal pain (Ghandour, Overpeck, Huang, et al., 2004; Perquin, Hazebroek-Kampschreur, Hunfeld, et al., 2000). The large majority may have no significant physical cause; however, they can be highly disruptive to the child and family's life, interfering with school and physical activities, and creating parent and sibling consternation (Fichtel & Larsson, 2002). Assessment and intervention requires a broad lens, starting with the pain itself and going wider to include psychosocial, emotional, and behavioral issues in the child's life (refer to Table 4.1 in Chapter 4).

Headaches

Tension headaches and migraines are common and disruptive to otherwise healthy children, and their prevalence increases with age. In one survey, headache was found to be the most prevalent (60%) pain complaint from school (Roth-Isigkeit, Thyen, et al., 2005). Headache is more common in pre-pubertal boys and in peri- and post-pubertal girls (Lewis, Ashwal, Dahl, et al., 2002). Recurrent headaches can be triggered by a combination of emotional and physiological stress, including irregular eating habits, insufficient sleep, sleep apnea, sinus congestion, referred pain from muscle tension in the back and neck (see Chapter 2), hormonal fluctuations, academic stressors, genetic factors, and psychosocial difficulties with peers and family. Ongoing headaches often limit school attendance and impact socialization, sleep, and quality of a child's life (Sethna & Lebel, 2008).

Most headaches are benign, but a neurological examination and pain history are required to exclude more serious pathology. The International Classification of Headache Disorders (ICHD) is a recently revised diagnostic resource, and includes criteria for children fifteen years and younger (ICHD-2, 2004). (See also an excellent resource, McGrath & Hillier, 2001: *The Child with Headache: Diagnosis and Treatment*.)

The ICHD-2 classifies children's headaches into four categories that often overlap and may form a continuum within the spectrum of these disorders: *migraine* (with or without aura); *childhood periodic syndromes* (a precursors of migraines that include abdominal migraines, cyclic vomiting syndrome); *tension-type headaches*, which has a prevalence of almost 10% among children from seven to fifteen years; and *new daily persistent headaches* that evolves from tension-type headaches and predominately affect girls in their mid-teens. Given the overlap of these, we'll consider the two more prevalent, migraines and tension-type headaches and their management in the sections below.

Migraine Headaches

Migraines with or without auras are common pain complaints in children and teens. Migraines with auras (that precede the headache within 60 minutes) present with fully reversible visual disturbances, sensory symptoms (often unilateral), speech disturbance, and motor weakness (hemiparesis). Migraines without auras have episodes that last 1–48 hours during which there is nausea, vomiting, photophobia, and phonophobia (very sensitive to bright light or loud noise).

Migraines with or without auras present with a unilateral (one-side of the head) location, a pulsating quality, and moderate to severe pain, and the headache is aggravated by physical exertion (ICHD-2, 2004). This pain can be severe. A seven-year-old boy described his migraine pain as being like a big monster that is growing like crazy, and there's no room. So it pulls the two sides of his head apart because the monster is getting so big! (Ross & Ross, 1988). In Figure 8.1 an artistically talented nine-year-old girl graphically depicts the restriction in her visual field when the aura first presents prior to the onset of her severe migraines.

Even very young children experience migraines. Children diagnosed with migraine at age seven or eight can sometimes trace their pain back to early childhood. Over 70 percent of children and teenagers with migraine headaches have close family members with similar headaches (McGrath & Hillier, 2001). The genetic influence is a predisposition to develop migraines, although stress triggers are usually required for a migraine episode. Hormonal factors play a role in the frequency of migraines, and contraceptive pills are considered a possible trigger for migraines. Weather shifts and changes in barometric pressure are commonly reported triggers. Teens who have insufficient sleep or disturbances in their sleep patterns appear to have an increased association with headaches (Gilman, Palermo, et al., 2007). When migraines persists despite medication use, medication rebound may be the culprit; that is that the medication may sustain rather than reduce pain. This includes anti-migraine medication and/or opioids that have been taken for ten days or longer, or other analgesics for longer than two weeks. When discontinued and the child improves, this confirms analgesic rebound (Sethna & Lebel, 2008).

Tension Headaches

Children often report that the pain from tension headaches feels like a tight band around both sides of their head, lasting from several minutes to days, or longer, and the presentation can be quite different from migraines, although the majority of headaches in children are not 'pure' and often have mixed features that don't fit cleanly into separate categories. In a recent descriptive study (Seshia, Phillips, & von Baeyer, 2008), 6% of patients had chronic migraine, 16% had chronic tension-type headaches, and 53% of patients had mixed or comorbid headaches with both tension and migraine features; 25% had other types, mostly concussion and medication overuse.

The pain of a tension headache can be mild or moderate and described as 'dull, diffuse and persistent' (McGrath & Hillier, 2001). The headache is in the front or spread over the head and on both sides. A seven-year-old girl explained her pain as : "When I get my headaches, my head feels hot and sore – it's like I'm wearing a tight swimming cap." This pain rarely wakes the child from sleep, and weather and food do not seem to precipitate episodes, unlike migraine headaches. Chronically blocked sinuses may cause the throbbing frontal sinus tension-type headache. As the study above noted, many or most headaches have mixed features.

The following variables can contribute to tension headaches:

• Tight and painful neck muscles.

• Poor posture or other sources of muscle strain, such as carrying a heavy book bag or holding a cellphone to an ear with a raised shoulder.

• Physiological stress, such as missing breakfast or over-exercising.

• Psychological stress such as exam anxiety, the pressures of a demanding schedule of extracurricular activities after a busy school day, homework burden, sleepless sleepovers at friends' houses, or unremitting anxiety. For teens, no breakfast or irregular eating (headaches can be triggered by hyperglycemia), irregular or very late sleep habits, or the overuse of over-the-counter medication.

Drs. McGrath and Hiller (2001) write that many of their patients with tension headaches "are overachievers, superior students who are active in extracurricular activities but despite doing well in school, they are not attending regularly" (p. 71). Disrupted school attendance is a compounding problem for these children. Returning to school (see further on in this chapter), initially part-time or in progressive steps returning to full-time, is an essential component of treatment.

Indication that a headache pain may be a 'red flag' – an indicator of more serious pathology and require a specialist referral, may include: sudden severe pain during vigorous exercise, a trauma to the head or neck, mental status changes during the headache, a history of cancer, HIV or recent infection or fever, or pain radiating to the child's back (posterior thorax) (Sethna, 2008).

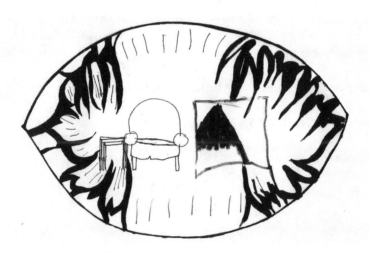

Figure 8.1: Migraine with Aura drawn by a 10-year-old girl

She explained, "Imagine I'm looking at a chair or out of the window - this is what I see. The black and white designs on the sides are usually a very bold colour at a time, say green, then it quickly changes to another colour, say red, I see every colour."

Management of Headaches

The starting point is the physician as educator. Often child and parent have fears that this pain may indicate more serious pathology such as a brain tumor. After a careful history and neurological examination, the physician can dispel the fears and provide an explanation of the prevalence and resolving nature of childhood-headache symptoms. Drawings and models can aid in this process.

In my office, I have a plastic brain that provokes fascination and an open discussion as the child holds and examines the brain. My goal is to convey how the brain perceives, makes sense of, and modulates the headache pain; we cover the full reversibility of the symptoms. Then we explore the critical need to modify stressors in the child's life, and the child learns self-regulation strategies to bring down the frequency and intensity of these headaches. Ultimately, the goal of headache management, whatever the type, is to control symptoms as early and as effectively as possible:

- *Prompt pharmacological treatment* is recommended as first line, initially using the mild analgesics, acetaminophen and ibuprofen, singly or in combination (Hämäläinen, Hoppu, et al., 1997). The triptans, though not yet FDA approved for use with children have been trialed and shown some efficacy and safety for children over twelve years old (Sethna & Lebel, 2008).

- *Physical intervention* for migraines includes lying down in a dark room, sleeping; and exploring food sensitivities such as cheese, chocolate or red wine for teenagers. Physical intervention for tension – type headache includes massage, postural shifts, stretching and outdoor exercise, warm shower and acupuncture (Diener, Kronfeld, et al., 2006; Hammill, Cook, & Rosecrance, 1996).

- *Psychological intervention* includes addressing how to minimize or eliminate the triggers, precipitating factors, such as peer and family stress, academic pressures, inadequate sleep hygiene, and developing coping strategies, such as hypnosis skills and relaxation training for pain and comfort management (McGrath & Hillier, 2001). A recent systemic review found that psychological treatments are effective in pain control for children with headaches and the benefits appear to be maintained (Eccleston, Palermo, Williams, et al., 2009).

Doing the detective work by keeping a pain diary (see Chapter 4) to identify the triggers of each episode, day and time of onset, what helps, and how long it takes for relief to be experienced, are useful variables in the creating a treatment plan. This process of 'being the detective' places the child in the driver's seat, promoting greater self-awareness and control, which may lead to better life-style choices.

Identifying Early Warning Signals

When children with migraines have auras, these are identified as a 'helper'. The aura, for example, light sensitivity, visual flickers or pain behind the eyes, serves as an alarm for the child to take action: promptly take the required medication, lie down in a dark room, and put on a relaxation or hypnosis CD and/or go to sleep. When nausea and vomiting accompany migraine pain, the gel form of acetaminophen and ibuprofen is recommended. If tolerated, rectal suppositories are extremely helpful to control pain. Medication should be taken early, well before the onset of nausea and vomiting, which disrupts analgesia absorption.

For children with tension-type headaches, the early warning signs may be the experience of throbbing in the right temple or pain intensification with head movement. Medication, rest, and the physical and psychological techniques discussed before and below are effective aids.

Controlling the Pain

With advances in technology, home treatments that are CD-ROM-or web-based have been created. These treatments have promising outcome data (Connelly, Rapoff, Thompson, et al., 2006; Hicks, von Baeyer, & McGrath, 2006). This self-management approach is an exciting development. It provides easier access for children and teens who are often comfortable with technology-based treatments. Here are some elements of treatment, as each child's headache has distinctive features:

• Learn not to fear the pain and instead to recognize and respond promptly to the early warning signals.

• Sleep may be one of the most effective interventions, particularly for full recovery from migraine pain.

• Regular and sufficient sleep helps prevent recurrence of migraine and tension headaches.

• With professional guidance, a child can take dietary supplements B 6 (riboflavin), magnesium, coenzyme Q10, and omega 3 fatty acids.

• Relaxation techniques may reduce and control tension headaches.

• Massage of the neck and trapezius muscles, and/or self-massage of tender points in the occiput or temples can reduce tension or pain build-up.

• Self-hypnosis or imagery practiced regularly may modulate pain intensity and reduce headache frequency.

• Taking a warm streaming shower or using a warm microwavable bag designed for placement on shoulders, or a cool cloth on the frontalis muscle may be beneficial.

Ten-year-old Matt, who regularly had tension headaches after school, liked to use the imagery experience from his favorite vacation, snorkeling in Hawaii. First he massaged a few key acupressure points in his temples, on his forehead and behind his ears where his glasses rested to get the pain release process underway. Then he took some deep breaths, closed his eyes, and traveled back to his snorkel experience, until he saw "a Moray eel that popped out to greet" him. Initially he needed 10 to 15 minutes to get his headache to diminish. After practicing his relaxation-imagery daily for ten days, he could ease the tension of school and reduce his headache from pain levels of 5 down to 0 within five minutes. He explained: "I'm so enjoying snorkeling again that my muscles relax and the pain just fades away because I'm doing something that I like!"

Even with a family history of headaches, coping techniques can help reduce the pain intensity, duration, and frequency of headaches. When children and their parents understand how a pain signal becomes a pain experience, they may be more open to treatment options that combine with medication for pain relief.

Abdominal Pain

Abdominal pains affect between 4–25% of school-age children in the United States (Mallaty, Abudayyeh, O'Malley, et al., 2005) and account for 2–4% of visits to a pediatrician per year (Starfield, Hoekelman, et al., 1984). It is one of the more troubling pains for clinicians in general practice as ruling out any organic disease is only the beginning of assessing and treating abdominal pains (Walker, 2004). Some complaints are one-time pain episodes, while others become recurrent or chronic. It is the latter that causes considerable parental worry, child distress, recurring consultations, and school absences that can lead to a disability.

In 1975 these pains were categorized as recurrent abdominal pain (RAP) by Apley (1975). To meet the criteria there needed to be three or more episodes of severe abdominal pain that interfere with normal daily activity, followed by pain-free periods over a period of three consecutive months. Girls appear to be affected slightly more than boys (12.3% girls and 9.5% boys). More recently there has been discussion that the diagnosis may be too vague and overlapping with the criteria for irritable bowel syndrome

(IBS) and functional dyspepsia – all part of a differential diagnosis of abdominal pain (Scharff, Leichtner, & Rappaport, 2003; von Baeyer & Walker 1999). In 2006, the Rome III criteria defined a broad scope of functional gastrointestinal disorders, that included IBS, functional dyspepsia, abdominal migraine, and functional abdominal pain (FAP), which was designed as a differential diagnostic guide rather Apley's descriptive criteria for RAP. It seems that these serve different purposes and Apley's criteria may be a good starting point in general practice. If the pain persists, FAP could be considered.

Functional Abdominal Pain

To diagnose FAP, Scharff & Simon (2008) provide a list of positive symptoms with the hope that this may reduce referrals to gastroenterologists. The symptom list requires all of the following:

- Episodic or continuous abdominal pain.

- Insufficient criteria for other functional gastrointestinal disorders, listed above.

- No evidence of inflammatory, anatomic metabolic, or neoplastic process that explains the patient's symptoms.

Functional abdominal pain usually has the following characteristics. The pain is usually periumbilical, and the child finds it hard to describe; it lasts less than an hour and no longer than three hours. Pain does not wake the child up at night and can be associated with autonomic symptoms, such as pallor, nausea, and sweating. There is rarely one intervention that reliably succeeds in reducing the pain (Scharff et al., 2003). A thorough examination is needed to rule out constipation, indigestion, Crohn's disease, ulcerative colitis, and other more serious pathology. Some 'red flag' indicators of an underlying pathology include weight loss, vomiting, ongoing diarrhea, bloody stools, pain that wakes the child up at night, abdominal pain that is not near the umbilicus, and any family history of inflammatory bowel disease (Scharff et al., 2003). However, when a child has persistent or recurrent abdominal pain, ongoing investigations to further rule out disease tend to heighten both the child and parents' anxiety. Laparoscopies and other invasive examinations are not usually warranted, as identifiable organic pathologies do not frequently occur, and optimal management "necessitates a clear marriage between the science and art of medicine" (Rappaport & Leichtner, 1993. p. 568). This requires recognizing the individual needs of the child and the family, and in a constructive discussion help them understand that the negative finding is the beginning of starting to cope and getting well.

Talking with the Child

A child and family frequently express distress and disappointment with the lack of an obvious organic cause for the persisting abdominal pain. It is estimated that one third of children with functional abdominal pain will continue to experience pain symptoms and some disability into adulthood (Jones & Walker, 2006). It is therefore important to clinically address these pain symptoms. With negative organic findings and persisting pain, an approach is required that begins by validating the child's pain, while simultaneously exploring and providing an explanation based on the confluence of physical, psychological, and/or social factors to sustaining this pain.

The notion of the 'brain-gut axis' – which has a bidirectional flow of information such that the perception of pain is modified by the brain and these brain centers may in turn affect gastrointestinal function – may open a discussion of how those factors operate in the child's daily life or are associated with a pain exacerbation. Gut-directed hypnotherapy (Vlieger et al., 2007) has been found effective as a treatment for abdominal pains. It takes the concept of brain-gut axis and develops a therapeutic process to repattern the pain pathways and with practice to provide relief (refer to Chapter 5, hypnosis for more details).

I recall a pediatric gastroenterology colleague, opening this exploration with a fifteen-year-old girl by saying words along these lines:

"The good news is that your endoscopy showed that your bowel is healthy and normal. Luckily you don't have any bowel disease. However, your pain is still there. I think the pain may be coming from higher nervous system factors. We know that the bowel and stomach, in fact the entire abdomen is richly supplied with nerves that are interconnected through the spinal cord and to brain and back again to the belly. So signals and stressors can be expressed in the abdomen. Have you noticed any link? (*pause for her response*) For example, when you are stressed does that worsen your abdominal pain? (*She nods*) There is a complex sophisticated interplay between brain and belly in abdominal pain. Do you think there may be some other factors that could trigger your abdominal pain? Or make it worse?"

It is rare for answers to come tumbling out after this opening. However, it reframes the problem. It allows the patient to consider other contributing factors and to know that a broader biopsychosocial approach is being taken in which other aspects of his life, such as his stressors, could possibly play a part in generating the pain.

Managing the Pain

Shifting the focus from attempts to find a cure, to determining how to cope with this distressing pain is fundamental for the child to recover. For some, exploring the child's daily stressors and achieving a consensus with the child and parent on the precipitating and or exacerbating factors can bring relief. Parents may need to be supported to move away from pain-focused conversations and onto encouraging a return to school, normal daily life, and home and academic responsibilities. A biopsychosocial approach to treatment once again is essential for optimal outcome (Weydert, Ball, & Davis, 2003):

- *Pharmacological treatment.* A Cochrane review has concluded that there is little evidence for the use of pharmacology in the treatment of FAP (Huertas-Cebbalos, Macarthur, & Logan, 2002). Of the range of pharmacological interventions to treat FAP, anti-depressants (a 12 week flexible dose of SSRIs) have emerged as potentially beneficial (Campo, Perel, Lucas, et al., 2004).

- *Physical treatment.* Mobilizing and increasing physical activity is a key part of recovery. Yoga has been found to hold promise for children with abdominal pain (Kuttner, Chambers, et al., 2006; Tsao, Meldrum & Zeltzer, 2009). Diet changes such as eliminating dairy if there is suspicious of lactose intolerance has been effective with a small proportion of children with FAP (Barr, Francoeur, et al., 1986).

- *Psychological Treatment.* The most commonly used intervention is cognitive behavior therapy focused on teaching coping, relaxation, and interpersonal strategies so that the child returns to attending school on a regular basis.

However, Abdominal pains (such as RAP/FAB, IBS) tend not to resolve quickly, and follow-up sessions continue to support the process of return to school and recovery. This counters feelings of being dismissed, when a clear organic cause hasn't been identified. Emphasizing the 'brain-gut' axis as a two-way process should be a central focus in these sessions. If there is no improvement, physicians should not delay or continue with further investigations so that disability sets in. A referral to a psychologist or other mental health professional with pain management expertise for biobehavioral treatment is strongly recommended, as psychological-based treatments show the most efficacy (Scharff & Simon 2008).

Returning to school

Providing reassurance, reframing of the pain and the impetus to return to school are pivotal in preventing further disability for children with chronic pain such as abdominal pains. These children can feel overwhelmed by how to manage this school return. Here are a few pointers and an excellent reference that provides guidelines by psychologist and researcher, Dr. Lynn Walker (2004). You can explore the psychosocial aspects of school questions, such as:

- How would it be for you *when* you go back to school? (Note: the use of 'when', not 'if'!)

- How will your friends be? What would you like to say to them about how you've been?

- How are your teachers this year? Has someone told them about your stomachache?

- What's happened about school work? Do you have much to makeup? How's that for you?

- What have you been doing during the day when you're home from school? (The answer to this question can reveal other home concerns, family issues, or academic boredom or overwhelm.)

Research has shown that mothers of approximately half of children with recurring abdominal pains, in an interview prior to a clinic visit, endorse that there were psychosocial triggers for their children's pain (Claar & Walker, 1999). Parents need to be part of the-return-to-school plan.

Schools are keen to accommodate children returning to school and in my experience welcome a letter from the child's physician or psychologist outlining special needs, such as bathroom breaks or permission to lie down in the nurses station if there is discomfort rather than returning home. Teachers value hearing from clinicians and are happy to discuss the best re-entry plan with a manageable work-load and to provide a supportive welcome back to the classroom. The school counselor is another useful resource for peer- or teacher-related obstacles.

Conclusion

Family physicians and pediatricians can help prevent and relieve children's pain. Given the many times children visit the doctor's office, the physician and nursing staff can have a significant impact on children's understanding of and experience with pain. Despite the acute pain of regular immunizations and other minor painful experiences, if pre-emptive pain measures, such as EMLA® and biobehavioral strategies, such as distraction, are systematically implemented in the office, children learn to cope and manage their fears, and the gap between research evidence and clinical practice is further closed. Allied with parents as interpreters and advocates, physicians help children when they experience themselves as heard and their pain concerns addressed.

A biopsychosocial approach using the 3Ps of treatment provides comprehensive and evidence-based pain treatment. The physician's role as educator using this approach within a collaborative relationship with the child and family, can positively change the course of recurring or chronic pain. Regular follow-up consultations, together with sleep and analgesic monitoring and a return-to-school plan, play a beneficial part in children's chronic pain management in pediatric practice. A positive experience in the doctor's office can generalize to the dental office, where regular visits are also a part of growing up, as we discuss in Chapter 9.

Chapter 9

Managing Pain and Anxiety in Dental Practice

"The dentist. I guess you could say that all children have a fear of them at one time or another. Who wouldn't? You're sitting in a chair, mouth wide open, and a person is sticking a drill in your mouth!"

Jeremy, age fourteen

Today the fear of pain and anxiety at the dentist's office is frequently more of a problem than the pain itself. We know that in the cascade of neural processes fear and anticipatory anxiety increases pain perception. Generally, dentists recognize that if children's fears are not adequately and effectively addressed they magnify discomfort and make good pain management difficult to achieve. Fear of going to the dentist is compounded by the physically vulnerable and awkward supine position required for dental work, as well as the complexity and shared nerve pathways of the structure of the head and face (Ferraro, 2003). Perhaps because of those factors, and unlike hospitals, today's many pediatric dental offices routinely address fears and general anxieties proactively, as they manage pain. But this may not be the case in non-pediatric dental offices. Many children don't have access to a pediatric dentist and are treated in a general dental practice, where there may or may not be the requisite skills to address children's fears and anxieties.

A retrospective uncontrolled study of returned questionnaires into the age of onset of dental anxiety indicated that 51% of adults reported the onset in childhood, 22% in adolescence and 27% in adulthood (Locker, Liddell, Dempster, & Shapiro,1999). These findings, which carry an inherent bias, suggest that almost three quarters of adults with dental anxieties and phobias acquired these fears early in their lives. A family history with a mother, father or sibling who was anxious about dental treatment was predictive of the onset of childhood dental anxiety, whereas the onset during adolescence occurred in subjects with higher trait or endogenous anxiety. There were different types of conditioning experiences in these two groups. Those subjects with child-onset dental anxiety were more fearful of the invasive procedures. In contrast, the adolescent onset group were more negative about the dentist's behaviour. The researchers also found that negative dental experiences were predictive of dental fear, regardless of age.

Pain prevention and control is a priority in dental procedures, since treatment can't be done without it. As a result dentists are specifically trained in pain management. Dental schools have included modules in management of pain and anxiety during third and fourth year as an essential part of their training curriculum, ahead of either nursing schools or medical schools. In fact, dentistry has been prominent in pioneering innovations in pain and anxiety management. To cite only some early achievements: In the 1840s, Horace Wells, a dentist, used nitrous oxide (see chapter 7), and in 1846, William Morton, a dentist and physician, first demonstrated the use of ether for a surgical procedure. Both Drs. Wells and Morton are considered founders in the field of general anesthesia.

The pain of toothache from a permanent tooth can be sharp and excruciating. It can radiate, for example, to the ear and to the jaw. Sometimes dental pain is easy to diagnose, such as a tooth with caries; other times it is complex and challenging, such as temporomandibular joint (TMJ) pain in children (Ferraro, 2003). Since dentists are trained to prevent pain and manage anxiety from the first encounter, the goal of this chapter will be to explore how this can be achieved developmentally with children, and with the involvement of parents. We'll cover how the planned prevention of pain helps control the child's natural anticipatory anxiety of "sitting in a chair on your back with your mouth wide open" (fourteen-year-old Jeremy); how dentists deal with pain using adept psychological, physical, and pharmacological techniques before, during, and after procedures; how the dental environment can attenuate dental anxieties and promote children's learning and adaptation to dental procedures; and how team-work between staff and with the child, supports the dental visit, especially when child-centered language is used. We'll also briefly discuss the use of general anesthesia, nitrous oxide, and evaluate a new injection technology, The Wand®.

The Pediatricians of Dentistry

Children's dental health requires a specialty because their physiology, anatomy, and psychological needs are different from those of adults (Moss, 2000). There is the recognition that dentists who treat young children need to be adequately trained in behavior management, since they may encounter anxious or uncooperative children, or those with special needs, who are unable to readily accept routine treatment (American Academy of Pediatric Dentistry, 2000).

A child needs only one negative experience, such as beginning to gag and the dentist becoming impatient, for them to develop anxiety and a strong desire to avoid further dental work. Special clinical skills, knowledge, and ability to relate sensitively to children are needed by pediatric dentists. They are taught to take active steps to prevent pain, rather than treating it after it arises and unsettles their patient.

Changes in Dental Practice

Over the last two or more decades, the training of dentists, and consequently the practice of dentistry in North America, has changed dramatically. Today the focus in dentistry is on preventing dental problems, and therefore preventing pain and dental fears. The recommendation of the American and Canadian Association of Pediatric Dentistry is that a child's first visit occurs within six months after the eruption of the first tooth to check development, provide oral hygiene and diet instructions, and establish good dental habits. Unfortunately, this doesn't always occur and the young children of new immigrants have a higher incidence of early childhood caries (Werneck, Lawrence, Kulkarni & Locker, 2008).

Ideally, dentists will see children before the age of one year, followed by regular six-month visits to monitor the eruption of the teeth and to identify cavities early. These visits can provide regular and pain-free opportunities for children to become familiar with the dentist, dental staff, the chair and procedures, and the practice environment. In the best of all possible worlds, the child's first exposure to the dental office is not a result of a dental trauma or a sleepless night from a toothache.

Not all children have the option to go to a pediatric dentist and may need to consult a general dentist. This may pose more challenges, as not all dentists enjoy working with children. Some dentists find it difficult when children are fearful and uncooperative, and some dental staff don't have the requisite psychological skills to reduce a child's anxiety. These are not ideal situations for children. Practices that welcome and accommodate children's unique needs, and those that are devoted to pediatric dentistry, tend to provide both a child-oriented environment and a child-centered staff. A pleasant environment with pictures on the walls, an opportunity to play in the waiting room, mobiles, and books is welcoming and reassuring for children, toddlers and their parents.

Some offices include video monitors so that the child can watch a video while sitting in the dental chair, or they have dress-up clothes, toys, and other child-oriented play experiences accessible in the waiting room. Many offices include a treasure box where the child can chose a reward at the end of the visit, to mitigate against any fear or avoidance the child may have about returning for another visit. The bonus of a reward may increase the likelihood that the child leaves the office with a sense of some success, however trying the session. Although children enjoy these 'extras', they aren't essential for a successful visit to the dentist. Many children can be successfully treated in general dental offices that have no special modifications, and where the dentist is perceived as caring and the staff responsive to the child. The impact of traumatic dental experiences depend on the interpersonal context in which they occur (Milgrom & Weinstein, 1993).

The Involvement of Parents

Most dental practices, pediatric or general, do not include parents in the procedure room with a child beyond the age of about three years. For children to be comfortable and develop trust, the dentist and dental staff need to create a highly supportive and a reliably comfortable environment with an open two-way relationship with the child, for the child to feel sufficiently safe to relinquish the security of his or her parent.

Some children of all ages may want their parents present for any potentially painful or anxiety-provoking experience, as we know that the parental presence is felt by children to be the most consoling of all interventions during procedures (Ross et al., 1988). Further research has indicated that if the parent can provide a comforting presence and encourage the child's coping, the parent should be allowed to be present and can be requested to sit and be a quiet supportive presence. If the parent isn't able to provide pain coping support and is fearful, threatens, or provides excessive reassurance, the parent's presence will not positively aid the completion of the procedure, and may not be advisable (Chambers, Craig, & Bennett, 2002).

It is a concern if the parent who accompanies a child has dental fears. Children of all ages readily hear and absorb their parents' fears and phobias. Information regarding past dental experience and dental attitude of parents can be gained from the first telephone call. It is known that parental anxieties affect how a child deals with a dental consultation (Locker et al., 1999). Statements such as "The dentist will try not to hurt you..." or "I am also very brave when I go to the dentist" tend to send the wrong message. Dental staff need to determine whether the accompanying parent can help the child in a positive, calm way, or not. Being aware and sensitive to this dynamic is an important part of preventing the fears of one generation from infecting the next.

In previous generations, dental practices were not as sensitive to children's anxieties or to the prevention of pain as they are today. This parallels medical practices. Historically, dentists believed that children's primary teeth were less sensitive than mature teeth and therefore they did not need to be anesthetized for dental work to be done. Topical anesthetics, which have revolutionized practice today by preventing or reducing the pain of dental anesthetic injections, were first available in the later half of the 19th Century. Yet it has taken nearly an entire century for effective and safe topical anesthetics to become readily available (Kundu & Achar, 2002).

Thus, some parents dental fears may be well-founded in negative dental experiences. For dental practitioners faced with a child with a puzzling and strongly persistent dental phobia, gaining a notion of the parents' attitude, history, or fears about dental work, can help gain a better understanding of the source of the problem. Addressing this empathically with the parent may begin to address or interrupt the intergenerational negative learned patterns. If not, it may require a referral to a psychologist or other mental health profession to treat a post-traumatic response. In all, it may be time well spent.

The Dental Examination

For the child's first number of dental examinations the American Academy on Pediatric Dentistry (2008–2009) has recommended that dental teams use a desensitization technique Tell Show Do (TSD). This technique helpfully explains the sounds and feel of instruments using age-appropriate language. Verbal explanations are given in developmentally appropriate language (Tell); the visual, auditory, tactile, olfactory aspects of the procedure are demonstrated in a non-threatening and carefully defined way (Show); then without any deviation from either the explanation or demonstration, the procedure is completed (Do). This is used to help the child become acquainted with the dentist and surroundings while sitting on the parent's lap, and eventually in the dental chair. This is a smart anxiety-prevention tool, which medical and nursing practice could do well to emulate.

Dental Terms Made Child-Friendly

Words that imply pain are naturally fear provoking for children, as well as for adults (Lang, 2005). Words such as *needles, shots, drills, pulling teeth,* and *blood* are emotive, negatively loaded, and provoke anxiety and the desire to escape. Since today, dental procedures can be virtually guaranteed to control or at least minimize any pain related to procedures (see below), the use of euphemistic and child-oriented terms is morally acceptable and helpful. Using such terms is not lying to or tricking children. It is not equivalent to administering an injection and saying – as has been heard – "This is just a little mosquito bite – it won't hurt!" Children don't easily forgive or forget such betrayals.

With Tell Show Do the child is introduced to each instrument. For example, the high power suction: "the suction makes a noise like a vacuum cleaner, but feels like little kisses on your hand." The child then witnesses a puddle of water suctioned from the dentist's hand and is invited to feel the little kisses on her or his own palm; the probe tickles the teeth and counts them, while the air syringe blows the teeth dry (J. Ronen, personal communication, 2009). Dental students are taught the importance of being truthful with children about a sensation they will experience but to avoid emotive and anxiety-provoking words. Pediatric dentists appear to have success in curtailing the child's fears, because they use everyday children's language while preventing or minimizing the occurrence of pain (see Table 9.1).

Table 9.1 Dental Terms made Child-friendly

- The explorer may be called a 'tooth counter, tooth tickler, or pointer'.

- The hand piece used for cleaning teeth is often called 'the electric toothbrush'.

- X-rays are usually called 'pictures of your teeth' or 'special pictures'.

- Local anesthetic is often called 'sleepy water, magic water, or sleepy medicine'.

- The injection of anesthetic may be referred to as 'sleepy-drops' and may be felt as a 'push, or pressure to put the tooth to sleep'.

- The feeling of numbness is described 'like a pillow' 'balloon' or 'pastry / dough'.

- The rubber dam may called a 'raincoat, rubber mask, or tooth raincoat'.

- The drill may be called 'Mr. Whistle, tooth washer, sugarbug chaser, or buzzer'.

- The suction may be called 'Mr. Thirsty'.

- Extracting a tooth is 'helping your tooth wiggle out.

Explanations in appropriate language about what will happen and what it will feel like ('cool' or 'a squirt of water', or 'wiggling your cheek as the sleepy medicine goes in') are given from the perspective of the child's sensory and procedural experience – and not from the clinician's perspective, another important principle for procedure management (Kuttner, 1988).

Dental Examining Techniques for Children of Different Ages and Abilities

Lying supine in a vulnerable position with mouth ajar and adults poised above with noisy instruments can be a frightening experience for adults, and more so for an inexperienced child. Remaining sensitive to this power differential, and the fears and helplessness that this supine position evokes is an important interpersonal and contextual factor. There are some useful developmental techniques to position and examine children to minimize any anxiety and enable learning and trust to develop.

Toddlers

Young children do not like being separated from their parents for dental exams. Children aged one to three are usually examined in the lap-to-lap technique, in which the parent sits knee-to-knee with the dentist. The parent holds the child on his or her lap, with the child's head on the dentist's knees. The dentist is able to carefully check the child's teeth and gums for signs of infection, the beginnings of decay, or evidence of injury. This takes only a few minutes, and the position also allows the parent a good view. Placing pictures or mobiles on the ceiling can stimulate a young child's curiosity to maintain lying in this position. Provided that nothing untoward is found in the examination, the dentist and parent usually discuss home care and preventive strategies. This again is a fine learning opportunity for young children to become familiar and develop some comfort and trust in the dentist and the environment.

Children Aged Three to Ten Years

Children aged three to ten years are usually able to sit by themselves in the dental chair, with or without their parent's help. Team-work can minimize the child's anxiety. In the best situation for this age-group, the dentist usually explains the set-up and instruments using the TSD method with child-friendly language, and repeats this on each subsequent visit. The session may start with the dentist asking the child to "Open your mouth wide so that I can have a 'look-see'. I want to see if there any tooth germs hiding on your teeth; if so, we'll wash them away", and "to count the teeth that have gone and the teeth that are coming."

The child is given a job in order to help, such as holding the suction ('Mr. Thirsty') to take the saliva away or watching carefully in the hand-held mirror. The dentist also explains how to use the 'stop' signal by raising the left hand, should anything not feel right, and the team will stop. This is practiced. In this way the child is incorporated into the team as a 'helper', and thanked for taking the task on. Children who have disabilities benefit significantly from the sensory experiences in the TSD method. Deaf children need to see the instruments being demonstrated on a hand or finger nail and feel their sensation. Children who are blind require a stronger auditory explanation of the sounds and what they mean, as well as the sensation experienced on their hand or finger nail (J. Ronen, personal communication, 2009).

Making the range of dental experiences normal for children in this age group happens in small and progressive steps and with regularly scheduled dental visits. Positive feedback to the child, referring to the specific help the child gave, is part of any successful visit. Comments such as, "Thank you, it helped us all that you sat so still", "You opened your mouth wide and that helped us to be quicker in mending your tooth – thank you!" or "Even though it wasn't easy holding your mouth open so wide, we sure got a good look at those molars coming in!" are a helpful guide to children. In the experience of regular (approximately every six months) preventive dental visits, children can develop positive dental attitudes. This positive learning process is aided when there no significant pain in these consultations – unlike the child's regular immunizations.

Using modeling for school-aged children

From a preschool or school-aged child's point of view, one of the easiest ways to learn about dentistry is to watch another child having his or her teeth checked, cleaned, and counted. Researchers found that children with no prior experience of dental treatment displayed heightened distress when shown a short video demonstration of the procedure, unless the demonstration used a peer model (Melamed, Yurcheson, Fleece, et al., 1978). Some pediatric dental practices are designed to promote positive modeling. They have an open plan seating with five or so dental chairs placed within the room and staff working side-by side, so that conversations can be overheard and there is a general, easy climate in the room. Witnessing another child coping, sitting in the chair, with an open mouth, relatively still, and comfortable is highly reassuring for an anxious child and an excellent anxiety-reduction strategy. However, learning by modeling can be for better or for worse. We know that observational learning via modeling is one of the three types of conditioning in the acquisition of fears (Rachman, 1977), and modeling can account for some dental fears in childhood (Locker et al., 1999).

Children learn very rapidly through observing, imitating, and modeling. Research (Melamed et al., 1978) suggests that children tend to trust to a greater extent that a situation is inherently safe when this information is obtained from another child, than when it is obtained from an adult. For modeling to be a positive learning experience, the model child needs to be around the same age and has agreed to be watched, and the procedure is known not to be complex. A positive and encouraging open atmosphere in the dental room needs to be consistently maintained for positive modeling to occur. This requires prompt, skilled, and calm intervention when a child in the open-plan practice becomes distressed – as it will be witnessed and absorbed by all the young observers. This requires full environmental management, which includes the front desk with scheduling instructions to pay attention to these factors. For example, a new patient should not follow an uncooperative patient in the open-plan office so to avoid hearing unpleasant sounds or seeing an unhappy face.

Pre-Teens and Teenagers

Generally by their teen years, adolescents will have had some dental experiences – for better or for worse – and will know what to expect. When a teen is feeling fearful, there may be a regression to behaviors typical of younger children, such as becoming restless in the chair, protesting or crying at the earliest sign of discomfort. This is when the skill of the team will be put to the test. Can they regain the teen's trust? Will they pause, and inquire about what triggered the fear, and give the teen more control in pacing the procedure? Will they offer options to regain comfort, repositioned with pillows, or propose a break for a discussion so that some confidence can be regained? And, will they do this in a respectful way so that the teen doesn't feel belittled? Can they transform this scary experience into an opportunity for the teen to learn, begin to cope, and feel good about the experience when it is over, rather than feeling ashamed and not wishing to return!

If a child or teen has had negative experiences with a previous dentist, it is important to review the situation to ascertain what went wrong from his or her perspective, and in this process, to re-define the situation, the working alliance, clarify procedures, and give the child or teen choices. Even when the procedure, such as in orthodontic work, is not pain-free, if the relationship with the dentist is essentially collaborative, then the teen will cooperate and feel respected, and trust will develop over time (Milgrom & Weinstein, 1993).

Children with Special Needs

The dentist and the dental team rely on the knowledge and skill of parents of children who are physically, intellectually, or emotionally challenged. When invited, these parents provide crucial guidance during dental treatment, particularly during the child's first dental visit to a new practice. The dentist should be well acquainted with the child's history, allow for extra time, and make accommodations to the child's physical limitations and level of tolerance in the dental chair (J. Ronen, personal communication,

2009). Since modeling has been shown to promote a child's learning, if the child is fearful and slow to 'warm up' to new situations, a useful anxiety control strategy is to invite the parent and child to sit on a bench in an open-plan pediatric dental office and watch the other children cope with the dental session. This provides an opportunity for the child to explore, play with toys, and assimilate the environment in an indirect and non-stressful way.

Many pediatric dental offices have a quiet room for children who are disruptive and noisy or who may upset other children in the office. The most common use of this room is for the examination of young children who commonly cry very noisily when having their teeth examined, even when being held by a parent. Being treated in the quiet room, however, may not always be in the best interests of the child.

Dr. Penny Leggott was treating Sam, a severely autistic eleven-year-old child, who tended to be very disruptive, noisy, and combative. He was generally seen for his recall examinations in the quiet room with both his mother and father present. On one occasion, the quiet room was in use, so Sam was seated in a chair in the open area, where he could see three other children seated around him. Much to everyone's surprise, particularly his mother's, instead of protesting, he was much more cooperative than usual and was relatively quiet. The dental staff and his parents realized that Sam was more sensitive to peer pressure than they had appreciated and changed their plans for future sessions.

Children are continually growing, changing individuals, and as pediatric health practitioners, we need to remain flexible and provide new opportunities for children to learn and develop competencies, whatever their temperament or limitations.

How Pain Is Controlled in Dental Procedures

Children in dental pain can present with swollen face, tender ulcerations (canker sores), abscesses, and impacted teeth (Ferraro, 2003). Let's explore how dental staff manage this pain. Pre-emptive and well-planned pain management practices have transformed dental experiences for children. Invasive procedures such as fillings and extractions need not be painful, when using topical and skillfully delivered local anesthesia (2% lidocaine with a vasoconstrictor, generally epinephrine). Local anesthetic is the cornerstone of modern dental treatment, and standard textbooks devote considerable space to the topic (Ferraro, 2003).

To prevent pain during invasive procedures, dentists commonly first use a topical anesthetic cream, which comes in a variety of child-friendly flavors, including bubble gum, banana, cherry, and mint. The cream takes approximately one minute to anesthetize the gum. The plan is explained to the child in age-appropriate language from the child's perspective, for example:

> "First I'm going to place cotton with tasty cream next to the tooth to make the gum go to sleep and then drip the sleepy drops to send the tooth to sleep. When the tooth germs and tooth are snoring, we can wash them away – this way you'll just feel water and hear this sound."

Then the local anesthetic is injected into the anesthetized gum to numb the tooth pulp, nerve, and surrounding tissue. It is important to describe the feeling to the child and show in the hand-held mirror that it is only a feeling and the nerves will wake up again: "This numbing will also make the side of your face go to sleep and feel a bit strange, but it'll all come back to normal in an hour or so." If there is lip numbness, it is important that the child not bite the lip. To help prevent this, petroleum jelly can be spread on the lip.

The pain caused by injecting a local anesthetic is controlled by using diversion and counter-irritant tactics with the following technique, which utilizes the concept of field anesthesia (Ferraro, 2003):

- *Inject the local very slowly* allowing for the infiltrate to anesthetize the tissue and create a small anesthetized field before repositioning the needle within that field and injecting further.

314

- *Simultaneously use the understanding of the 'gate control' to divert attention.* The large movement-detecting fibers that inhibit the smaller C fibers are stimulated to create deliberate sensory distracting movements, stretching and wiggling the cheek while talking to the child, and redefining uncomfortable sensations of the infiltrate into 'tingles'. The discomfort of the stretching and the cognitive distractions during positive chatter confuse the sensory uptake and absorb the child's attention, to minimize any discomfort.

- *Carefully monitor the facial expressions* of the child and adjust the technique accordingly; for example, wiggling more or pausing to minimize the pain.

This careful injection technique takes time and patience, but it pays dividends in the child's comfort (Ferraro, 2003). Proceeding through the anesthetized zone ensures that the child is largely unaware of pain as the local anesthetic infiltrates and all the teeth in a quadrant become anesthetized. During the three to five minutes that the local takes effect, dentists are trained to wait for the effect to be well-established. In this way local anesthesia in children is usually readily accomplished. If there is any anxiety, possibly from past experience about the anesthetic being effective enough, this needs to be tested by touching the tooth to be worked on with an ice stick. If no sensation of cold is felt, adequate anesthesia will have been attained (Dr. Bruce Marshall, personal communication, 2009).

The Wand® for Pain Relief?

New computerized devices for the delivery of local anesthetic have recently been developed for use in dentistry. One of these is The Wand®. The manufacturers maintain that the source of discomfort for most injections is not the needle, it is the flow of anesthetic into the tissue in the mouth. The Wand® which has a microprocessor, guides the anesthetic flow rate, and compensates for different tissue densities so that the anesthetic is delivered at a constant pressure and volume to reduce sensory perception. How effective is this device for reducing pain and anxiety in children?

There have been numerous studies across the world. A Mexican study (Martin-Lopez, Garrigos-Esparza, & Torre-Delgadillo, 2005) found that traditional syringe injections were more painful than the computerized injection device. In Israel (Ran & Peretz, 2003) with sedated children from two to four years, they found that the same efficacy of anesthesia was achieved with both techniques. While the children did not show signs of discomfort after treatment with The Wand®, they did while receiving conventional injections. In Turkey (Kuscu & Akyuz, 2007) they found no significant differences in injection pain scores with children aged nine to thirteen years. They did find that higher levels of pre-injection anxiety were related to more severe pain reports by the children. They concluded with the question whether it is the injection device or the anxiety that causes pain during dental local anesthesia. This was further explored in a study from The Netherlands (Versloot, Veerkamp, & Hoogstraten, 2008). They compared the behavioral reaction of children, from four to eleven years old, during, and the self-report after, the two types of injections. They found no difference between The Wand® nor the traditional injection. They did find that the child's level of anxiety was the important factor. Highly anxious children reported more pain, displayed more pain behavior and more distress than did the children with low anxiety. Children's anxiety plays a more important role in their pain reaction and pain perception than does the injection device. How then can anxiety be best managed?

Cognitive-Behavioral Principles Incorporated into Dental Practice

In addition to using local anesthetics, successful pediatric dental practices have effectively incorporated cognitive-behavioral principles of behavior management (see Chapter 5). A study with preschool children who were taught coping skills, such as relaxation, pleasant imagery, calming self-talk, and techniques that are similar to hypnosis, demonstrated significantly less distress in the dental office than the control group (Siegel & Peterson,1980). Attention to an external stimulus or an internal activity increases pain tolerance. Here is a report from an eleven-year-old on how she'd spontaneously developed her own effective distraction method.

> "Our dentist has this music, see, and I say to him turn it up real loud… Then I pretend that I have to really learn the music, like the tune, or something terrible will happen to me. And I keep telling myself to listen, listen, listen, and after a while sometimes I almost don't know I'm getting drilled." (Ross & Ross, 1988, p. 54)

In the following case, Dr. Jane Ronen (personal communication, 2009) explains how she used hypnosis to enable her patient Keren to overcome her anxiety about dental treatment:

Keren, aged 8, was one of twin sisters referred to me after seeing five different dentists, and five previous attempts to anesthetize a permanent molar. Keren had hypoplastic molars, an enamel defect which results in these teeth being hypersensitive. Keren's parents reported that in the past she had no problem with accepting dental treatment, however, now she had 'lost faith' that anyone could help her. She was very anxious. She was extremely frightened in spite of being assured that this visit was to be an examination only.

I asked Keren if she was prepared to try a new way of 'freezing her tooth' so that we could clean and cover it so that she would not have problems eating ice popsicles or ice cream, which she missed and wanted to be able to have again. As Keren lives in Israel, I asked her if she had ever seen and played in snow. She had, and told of her experience making snow balls.

I explained to Keren that the sensation she felt in her hands and fingers when holding the snowball she would feel on her face, jaw, and tooth when we numb her tooth. We also blew a few bubbles to help her to relax, and she decided she would like to have nitrous oxide as well when we do the treatment.

Keren asked if she was going to have "the painful injection". I explained to her about the Wand technique. Keren got up with a faint smile and

317

asked, "When could I come again?" The second visit went according to Keren's wish. While breathing nitrous oxide, I asked her to indicate with a raised finger when she was ready to set off for the trip to the snow with her family and best friends. She seemed to enjoy the outing, the special warm clothes, socks and shoes she had on. But, when it came to playing snow balls she had "no gloves" and as a result her fingers and hand started to tingle and feel frozen. Keren was asked to give a sign when she felt this sensation. She nodded to confirm. She was told in her own time to bring her frozen hand to her lower jaw and by stroking her jaw and face she will freeze her jaw and lower teeth. Within 3 minutes Keren said her jaw was stiff and numb, after which the Wand was used without difficulty to induce local anesthesia. The tooth was restored with a crown. Keren was asked by her father, "How did it go?" and she replied "Easy and good fun."

Common Dental Problems and Their Solutions

As explained earlier, when children have had a negative experience in the dental chair, they require skilled and sympathetic work by the dental team to mitigate the effects of this experience for subsequent visits. For other children, such as those with a sensitive temperament, one bad experience in the dental chair can be traumatic and destroy their trust and feeling of safety. The more sensitized the child, the harder it is to recover from the unexpected shock of pain in the dentist chair. This can be caused by inadequate preparation for a painful procedure, unexpected pain, an active gag reflex, a lengthy procedure with no relief, or the non-supportive manner of the dentist. If not therapeutically addressed, these fears can become phobias. We discuss below how to handle some of these problems.

Unexpected Pain

Occasionally local anesthesia is not sufficient or adequate. The child may perceive pain, or if the child is very anxious, may interpret pressure as pain. The dentist should immediately and carefully assess the situation, stop and explain what is happening, reassure the child, and re-anesthetize the child if appropriate. All these steps can help maintain or rebuild confidence.

Lack of Patience and Empathy for Children

Not all dentists are skilled in treating children. Given that one negative experience can have a very long-term impact on the child's attitude and willingness to have further dental work, the best solution is to refer the patient to a colleague who has the necessary experience and the staff to address the child's needs.

Excessive Fears

A few children develop excessive fears, becoming dental phobic over time, making it impossible for them to undergo routine dental care without help. A dentist who is skilled in communication and has an experienced staff may be able to manage these children with the help of nitrous oxide, local anesthesia, conscious sedation (such as midazolam), and a caring, empathetic manner. Some children, however, may need additional help, such as general anesthetic if the treatment is urgent, or psychotherapy to better manage anxiety. The following case illustrates how a procedure can go awry:

Six-year-old red-haired Theo had numerous cavities because his teeth had very thin enamel. After X-rays and a careful examination, his dentist said Theo would need to have four or perhaps five fillings done quite promptly. Theo, an intelligent and thoughtful boy, was overwhelmed by the news. The dental team began the procedure by giving Theo local anesthetic and then putting a rubber dam in his mouth. This new, uncomfortable experience unsettled Theo, who began whimpering and wriggling. The dentist said in a kindly way, "It is important that we carry on, because we will have at least another two or three more visits to get all your teeth fixed." This statement unsettled Theo even more. He tensed up and said, "I don't want that thing in my mouth!" The dentist then said he couldn't do this extensive work without the dam, and maybe they should consider doing the whole procedure under general anesthetic. Theo's mother went white. "No!" she said. "Please let's think about what else could help Theo. The dentist then suggested they look into some help for Theo and ended the session.

Less than happy, Theo's mother consulted me to enable him to cope with the dental procedures. It turned out that what troubled Theo the most was "having that thing across my throat". It became apparent that if the dam were eliminated Theo could handle the fillings using some coping methods. In the following two psychotherapy sessions, Theo learned and practiced relaxation and imagery methods which I digitally recorded. Lying on a reclining chair, relaxing his mouth wide open, he focused on his own iPod, newly acquired for the purpose. The audio experiences took him hang-gliding through the Grand Canyon, down through the different sedimentary levels so that he could study all the different ages embedded in the rocks. He gradually sailed down to the powerful Colorado River below, where he transferred onto a river raft. Theo's motivation was impressive. A consultation was then set up between me, his mother, and the dentist to determine if he were willing to do the procedures without a dam. The difference was that this time Theo was highly motivated, informed, prepared, co-operative and relaxed – and he would be hang-gliding in his mind. The answer was Yes, and to his mother's relief, Theo went on to complete all of his treatment with a feeling of accomplishment.

Gagging

Numerous children have an active gag reflex that gradually diminishes as the child grow older. When a child becomes anxious about gagging during dental work, it inevitably occurs more frequently. There are a number of techniques that the dental team can do to help diminish gagging:

- Allow the child to sit up partially, instead of fully reclining, in the dental chair.

- When they get the reflex, let the children bend their head forward with their chin towards their chest to prevent gagging.

- Administer nitrous oxide.

- Encourage the use of hypnosis and other coping, relaxation strategies.

- Spray topical anesthetic on the back of the tongue and palate.

- Take the procedures in small steps while building team work and the child's confidence.

I've quoted Jeremy before in this section, here is his story of dental fears and gagging:

Fourteen-year-old Jeremy had no awful dental experiences that he could recall, but the fear was always there. He said that it faded when he was nine years old, but an automatic gagging reflex remained whenever the dentist put an instrument into the back of his mouth or touched his sensitive tongue. This is what Jeremy wrote in a school essay on his experience:

"I did not want to gag. I tried really hard not to, but it was like a conditioned reflex. When I would gag it felt like I couldn't breathe. I would be out of breath and feel very nauseous. My eyes would water too. Even though the gag would only last a second, it seemed like a lot longer. It was very scary.

"I went to the dentist. I had eight teeth that needed to be sealed. All of them were at the back of my mouth. One is bad enough, and I could probably have handled it, but there were eight! My dentist was very supportive that I try hypnosis. So Dr. K. taught me breathing techniques and together we worked on a number of different strategies including hypnosis to overcome my problem. On the tapes were messages about how I could keep my mouth open without gagging. Night after night I would listen to these tapes as I fell asleep. My family was very supportive. I practiced seeing how many teaspoons I could get into my mouth.

I could get three pretty far back without gagging. There I was, walking around my house with my mouth wide open and spoons sticking out. It turned into a habit. Once I even walked in on my mom when she had a friend over, with my spoons sticking out of my mouth. The hypnosis was working.

"Dr. K spoke to my dentist on a number of occasions. He was very supportive. They went over the procedure; not all my teeth were going to be done at the same time. The job would be completed over a number of appointments. There were going to be no needles, and no pain. That was the relieving news, but I was still a little nervous." My first appointment was in September. I had major butterflies that day and the night before. I used one of the tapes. But to my surprise I did well. A lot better than I thought I'd do. There was almost no gagging, but I was still not satisfied. I wanted NO GAGGING! Call me stubborn, but if you're going to do something, do it right! I should mention this is no individual effort. We worked as a team, my dentist, Dr. K. and me. We took the problem, and if there were still some kinks, we improved on them. That's why we went through four tapes; we kept getting new ideas. Knowing all of that comforted me on my second visit. In a sense it was not just me in the chair but Dr. K. was there too. Not her, but her voice, which was coming out of my iPod.

"After my second appointment I was so happy. I had accomplished what I had set out to do. For over half an hour I sat in that chair, my mouth open while my dentist worked on me. And for over half an hour, there was no gagging whatsoever! The dentist also gave me breaks every little while; that helped a lot too. I was on top of the world. I did it! I conquered my problem. I was not the only one who was excited – my family, my dentist, the nurse, Dr. K. They were all proud of me. It felt good. There is probably no greater feeling than being proud of yourself. I was on cloud nine that whole day.

"What I'm trying to say is that no matter what, anything can be accomplished. I'm living proof. It's mind over matter. The mind has a lot of power. Being hypnotized was one of the most amazing experiences of my life. What's more amazing is what can be done with it. The mind is a terrible thing to waste!"

Orthodontics

Orthodontics is an area of dentistry for children that is not pain-free. Children report that orthodontic procedures are painful. The most painful procedures are the first fitting of the braces, the periodic adjustment to tighten them, and some discomfort between treatments. The discomfort from the pressure can be eased with acetaminophen or ibuprofen; the ulcers in the lips and cheeks can be helped by applying strips of soft wax supplied by the orthodontist. If children are well prepared for orthodontic procedures by the staff, shown photos and study models to demonstrate the plan, they are more likely to remain committed to their treatments and motivated to continue, however much discomfort.

Involving children in the initial decision to start treatment contributes to their capacity to tolerate the adjustments, endure the discomfort and pain, and follow through with the time-consuming oral hygiene procedures. There is significant reinforcement in the positive changes in personal appearance, and for many teens this is reward enough. Mild analgesics relieve orthodontic-related pain, which is also lessened when soft foods such as soup and ice cream are eaten.

Use of General Anesthesia and Sedation and Their Risks

General anesthesia should not be undertaken lightly as it carries risk. It does, however provide a means for taking care of extensive dental work for children under some circumstances. These include children under three years old who are too young to understand and cooperate in the dental office, but who have extensive decay resulting from the use of a night-time bottle of juice; medically compromised children who need the entire treatment undertaken within one session; older, mentally challenged children with numerous cavities; or children who have extensive dental needs and such extreme anxiety that psychotherapy and behavioral strategies will not have sufficient impact.

There is the notion that sedation has less serious consequences than anesthesia, but this is not necessarily so. Sedation techniques for young children are generally less reliable than for adults: children can become over-excited instead of sedated. The dosage levels often tend to be low to ensure the safety of the child, but this in turn reduces the sedative effect. Medications can elicit unpredictable and different responses in different children. The younger the child, the more unpredictable is the medication's effect. A certain dosage may make a child quite sleepy and sedated, while the exact same dose will not have much effect on the next child. Sedation for children appears to carry significant potential for adverse outcomes such that the American Academy of Pediatric Dentistry has drawn up guidelines (2006). In addition, some dentists have commented that many children have negative feelings about dentistry after a series of visits using sedation perhaps due to its confusing or amnestic effects (P. Leggott, personal communication, 1996). If other methods of intervention are not effective, general anesthesia may be a better option for extensive work than the use of sedation. For young or challenged children with extensive dental needs, treatment under general anesthesia is a justified and humane option.

Conclusion

In this chapter, we discussed that children's fear of dental pain and their anxiety may be even more of a problem than the occurrence of pain itself during dental procedures. Given that children may be reluctant to talk, let alone reveal these fears, the burden is on the dental professional to be vigilant and to address these in a constructive and compassionate manner. Teaching children how to help in the procedure, employing reinforcing cognitive-behavioral techniques and rewards, using child-centered language within a child-friendly environment is the optimal process for successive good dental experiences. This promotes children's competence and reduces their fear. Flexibility and attentiveness to the developmental and individual needs of each child remains fundamental. Generally, pain in pediatric dentistry is preventable; and if pain does occur, it can quickly be well-controlled. In many respects, the management of pain in dentistry is a model for other areas of health care, such as in hospitals, which we take up in Chapter 10.

Chapter 10

Managing Pain and Anxiety in the Hospital

"I didn't fear sickness, I was afraid of pain
and I was afraid of strange people coming into my room
to give me pain and why are they?"

*Lesley, a ninteen-year-old leukemia survivor, recalling her experience
in the hospital thirteen years earlier (Kuttner, 1998)*

Many hospitals now consider pain the fifth vital sign. However, for children in pain, it is number one! Our increasing appreciation of the plasticity and complexity of children's pain has profound implications for how procedures are approached and managed in hospital, and the long-term consequences of this treatment, as highlighted in Lesley's comment thirteen years after she had been discharged from hospital. How confused and frightened she must have been, lying in her bed fearing when the next stranger would pop in to prick her finger, prod her body, put in another IV line, or perform another nasty surprise. Children's memories of painful experiences can have long-term consequences for their reaction to later pain experiences as well as their acceptance of future health care (von Baeyer, Marche, Rocha & Salmon, 2004).

The seven teenagers and young adults in the documentary *No Fears No Tears – 13 Years Later* (Kuttner, 1998) talk about their recall of their hospital experiences, when they were young children, being treated for cancer. Their memories are vivid. Courageously they have moved on, grateful to be alive, but unanimously they say that the invasive treatments and regular procedures were the hardest part to deal with. Kelsey recalls being very angry early in her diagnosis at three years old: "I was lashing out at people. I didn't know what was happening to me!" Her mother felt that if she accompanied Kelsey into her painful treatments she would become "the bad guy" because she was unable to protect her daughter (Kuttner, 1986). Twelve-year-old Brian, brought up on a farm, said, "As a child you always say, what am I doing wrong? Why am I sick? Then you realize there are some things that just come your way and you just have to deal with it. Now when I look back I wonder how I was such a tough little kid." Adam at sixteen years recalls, when he was barely three years old, feeling fear "like I was a fragile little egg that could be easily broken." He would complete his play with his doctor's kit with his nurse's words, "That's all for today!" – comforting himself with the reminder that there would be no more painful experience that day in the hospital (Kuttner, 1998).

In a busy complex hospital environment where there are a lot of players in the system, not one discipline owns pain, and as a result all of us need to. Everyone within the hospital, parent and child included, needs to assume a part in providing pain and anxiety management. Let's briefly review why:

As explained in Chapter 2, the gate control theory informs us that a child's pain is not entirely determined by the degree of tissue damage caused by a procedure. This means we cannot completely control the child's pain by controlling the physical tissue damage. We also know there are other key factors that influence pain perception. The neuromatrix (refer to Figure 2.8), proposed by Dr. Melzack (1999), helps us to appreciate that the multi-dimensional ongoing input into the child's neural network pathways influence the outer expression of pain. The input includes cognitive-related brain areas, emotion-related brain areas, and sensory signaling systems. This includes the child's previous hospital pain history; the meaning of the current pain; the child's beliefs and fears about the anticipated medical intervention; the child's disease state, fatigue level; the degree of trust in the nursing and medical staff; and the presence or absence of the child's parent in the hospital.

These interacting variables create a dynamic neuronal network within the child's body-brain system and is expressed by the child when engaging within the hospital. The convergence and processing of this information happens very rapidly – particularly if the child is uncertain or fearful, and the environment unfamiliar (see Figure 10.1). Children learn and become sensitized very quickly in a hospital environment with its strange smells, strange people, upsetting sounds, and the possibility of pain. Therefore, it is everyone's responsibility to attend to how best to minimize children's anxiety and pain.

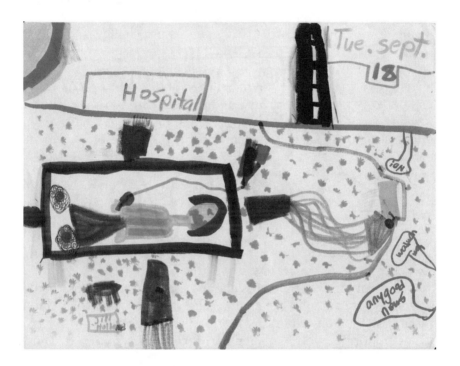

Figure 10.1. Hospital

Child's drawing of her hospital experience in which she remembers the cries ("wa, wa") of other children, someone asking if there was "Any good news" and the reply coming "No!"

In this chapter I first want to share a highly instructive story of one U.S. hospital that wanted to establish uniform practice for children's pain-relief and realized they needed to change the institution's culture of care. We'll learn about their experience at system change and the critical elements that emerged of leadership, education, parent empowerment, and the impact of the physical environment – all of which has significant implications for other hospitals seeking to undertake these necessary changes.

Next we will turn to the legal and practical requirements in hospitals of providing information to children of different ages as a cornerstone of good pain and anxiety management. We also address the concerns of children who are hospital inpatients. The chapter will close with what we can learn from the a case of a resilient teenager who is an out-patient, living with a complex life-long painful condition.

Making a Hospital Stay Less Painful

Here is a story in two parts. It's about a group of committed pediatric professionals who decided to take steps to make their community hospital an environment in which children's pain would be systematically well-managed and their anxiety reduced. They wanted to address the discrepancy between what we know and what we do (Schechter, 2008a).

Part One: The Ouchless Place

In 1997 Dr. Neil Schechter and his colleagues developed a program, which they called "The Ouchless Place" (Schecter, Blankson, Pachter, Sullivan, & Costa, 1997). Their goal was to overcome the impediments to adequate pain management on their pediatric inpatient unit. They recognized that hospital care placed a significant and added burden on children that went beyond their illness or medical condition. The pediatric professionals attempted to systematically reduce pain associated with hospitalization by doing the following:

- *Developing protocols* for post-operative pain management, sedation for painful procedures and sickle cell vaso-occlusive pain, using patient-controlled analgesia (PCAs). This they hoped would develop a uniformity in pain management practice, and reduce the wide variability of practice that was evident in the hospital (for example, giving a child the more painful intramuscular injection, when less painful alternatives are available and known). Nurses were to act as patient advocates and were empowered to question the resident physician if the protocol was not followed. If the resident was unable to justify the change in procedure, the nurse could contact a more senior staff member. "Most of the time, house officers and attendings [physicians] were happy to have these protocols and be spared the humiliation of not knowing appropriate doses or approaches to children" (Schechter et al., 1997, p. 891).

- *Using standardized pain assessment techniques* and pain relief protocols. They compiled the protocols into a book, and displayed them prominently on the floor so that they were easily available to all staff. The nurses reviewed and selected child self-report measures, since self-report is the most appropriate starting point in pain assessment. The visual analogue scale was selected for use with children aged eight years and older, and for children from three to seven years, the Wong-Baker FACES Pain Rating Scale was selected. Nurses also redesigned the vital sign flow sheets to include a prominent column for pain, as the fifth vital sign. This allowed the nurses to do ongoing assessments of the child's pain, which would then inform subsequent interventions. With this change, "the nurses took some pride in their ability to influence children's comfort in the hospital" (p. 892).

- *Decreasing needle pain.* Since it is possible for needle procedures to be essentially painless when topical local anesthetic is used (Clark & Radford, 1986) they created a standing order for EMLA® (see Chapter 7) on all patients on the inpatient unit who required scheduled blood work. This included children who would have blood drawn early in the morning. For these children, the night staff were required to apply EMLA® onto two sites. They reported that although the children displayed some anxiety on seeing the needle and anticipating pain, "in general, this approach dramatically reduces the pain associated with needle sticks" (Schechter et al., 1997, p. 892). As part of the plan to decrease needle pain, the resident physicians were encouraged to order blood work only when they had a good reason to do so, particularly for a child who already had a recent blood draw.

- *Empowering the parents.* Parents were invited to participate in all aspects of their child's care. They were given a pamphlet requesting their help to develop a suitable program for their child because they knew their child's unique needs. Signage placed in the hospital stated this commitment. Parents were also permitted to be present if they so chose, at all procedures and to participate in making decisions. This empowered parents to play an active role in their children's care, to express their concerns, and to be assured that these concerns would be taken seriously. The group considered this to be their most important change.

One of the lessons learned when they reviewed their program and ventured into institutional change, was the extreme difficulty they encountered in controlling the hospital environment. They noted that deviations from the best-practice protocols happened on numerous occasions. Unevenness of pain control for children continued. Children did not always receive the applications of EMLA® for procedures, despite the standing order. Laboratory technicians, for example, would come to draw children's blood without using EMLA®, or not draw from the site on which EMLA® had been applied! Because of the transdisciplinary nature of the hospital, there were many difficulties in maintaining an adherence to the basic concepts of pain management. Continued vigilance and obtaining administrative leadership was critical.

Part Two: Comfort Central

Ten years later in 2008, with the formation of a new children's hospital, Dr. Schechter and his colleagues reviewed what they had learned from their previous experience and developed a new initiative (Schechter, 2008a). They moved from creating The Ouchless Place to Comfort Central. Dr. Schechter writes that they found the concept of The Ouchless Place helpful, but with the constant changes within a busy hospital environment, its efficacy eroded over time. Importantly he added: "It was clear that, despite our best efforts, pain could never be entirely eliminated in the hospital or in outpatient facilities. Our pledge had to be to provide the most comfort we could, while not implying an unrealistic 'ouchless' experience" (p. S157).

Spurred on by the development of a new hospital, these pediatric clinicians planned their new Comfort Central as a stable and enduring program to create a culture of comfort and to reduce pain for all children in the complex hospital system. With a more seasoned vision, Schechter and his colleagues had learned more about how to institute change within the ever changing multi-disciplinary domain of a children's hospital. With Comfort Central their approach this time was broader, more systemically inclusive, and also more detail specific. This is what they did:

1. *Established institutional leadership* with the administrative authority to mandate change. They convinced the hospital administration that establishing a systemic approach to pain management should be a philosophical cornerstone of the hospital. A Pain Steering Committee was formed with the hospital vice-president as the chair to create the needed institutional change to establish pain management throughout the hospital.

2. *Recognized that pain management belongs to no one discipline* because of the complex nature of pain. In fact, every discipline – pediatrics, pharmacy, child life, nursing, psychology, anesthesia, and more – contributes an aspect to the whole care of children's pain. The Steering Committee realized that their next essential task should be directed toward

collaboration on pain management between disciplines, as all were affected and each could be effective in this shared task.

3. *Fostered collaboration across disciplines and services,* leading to a fundamental organizational change in the hospital, establishing a *decentralized model of hospital pain management.* The pain service that previously was responsible for attending to pain now served as a catalyst and resource for other services wanting to provide children with pain relief, such as the palliative care service and the orthopedic department.

4. *Created a child-centered environment*: They recognized the therapeutic value in pain management of absorbing and distracting a child's attention. Art work was put up on walls throughout the hospital, particularly in procedure rooms. The hospital auxiliary supported the purchase of passive and active distraction tools so that children, parents, and staff could use these therapeutically in the blood collection labs and treatment rooms. They also included complementary medicine intervention in their hospital care.

5. *Extended their influence* into the community pediatric offices, outpatient clinics, and external labs by developing an educational program for all staff on anxiety and pain management practices. They prepared teaching materials and adopted active learning approaches for their educational initiatives using case-based small seminars and group and ward discussions.

6. *Promoted a more realistic parental attitude.* Experience had taught the group that they needed to reduce parents' expectations that all medical encounters would be pain-free. As a result, parents continued to be empowered to play a more active role as a team member, and were encouraged to advocate for their child with staff members who were resistant to now-established hospital protocol and policy regarding pain management.

Why Is This Story Important?

This account of Comfort Central mirrors the efforts and struggle that many other children's hospitals across the world are currently engaged in: how to think systemically and act collaboratively to change entrenched systems that don't consistently address or prevent children's anxiety and pain, despite the very best of intentions. Entrenched habits and the chaos factor in hospitals are hard to control and change. For hundreds of years, children didn't have rights. Their fears were dismissed, their pain undertreated or not treated at all. Health professional of all stripes were entitled to carry out painful interventions, and their task took precedence over children's preparedness. Children's pain or fear really didn't matter: "They'd get over it!" We've shown with research and evidence collected in the last thirty years from all parts of the world that children's pain and fear does matter (Finley, Franck, Grunau, & von Baeyer, 2005). It has significant psychological and physiological impact, with short-term and long-term consequences.

The story of Comfort Central serves as a call to other children's hospitals to develop a cohesive system-wide approach to pain-reduction for children. Changing hospital practice, systemically and consistently, is one of the remaining barriers to effective pediatric pain management. Schechter and his colleagues realized in 2008 that their struggle to bring about an Ouchless Place and then Comfort Central to their hospital mirrored the national trends in the United States. In fact, it also mirrors international trends. Across the world there now is a greater recognition and knowledge of pain management for children, even though significant gaps and uneven and unpredictable services remain. In the electronic age with resources such as the internet, there is a dramatic increase in knowledge exchange and information on how to provide state of the art management of pain and fear in hospitals. However, for children in the hospital, their pain experiences and sense of safety and comfort remain hit or miss – and this is neither acceptable or humane!

Providing Information to Children

At the chapter opening, Lesley questions why these strangers were coming into her room to give her pain. She wanted to know what was going on! This raises the ethical and legal issues of informed consent for children, and our clinical responsibility to provide children with information sensitively, therapeutically, and in a timely fashion. How best to do this? What choices do children have?

Legal and Ethical Issues

It is a legal requirement to provide detailed medical information to both parent and child, and to obtain consent from a parent prior to any medical or surgical intervention. The process of obtaining informed consent is more than a legality for health care professionals – it is a moral and ethical responsibility. Based in the legal recognition of dignity, individual autonomy, and the capacity for self-determination, consent is not a single event or episode, but a complex process that occurs within the therapeutic alliance between physician and patient (Krener & Mancina, 1994). The power to make a decision is shared by physicians and patients as partners. Both have roles and responsibilities in the consent process (American Academy of Pediatrics Committee on Bioethics, 1995; American Medical Association, 1992).

According to the law, consent is only required from parents if the child is still a minor. Yet in practice, there is a general consensus that children too need to be accurately informed about what the procedure entails and their assent obtained. Assent is an important concept when working with children who have not reached legal majority. Here is part of a statement from a European pediatric working group on ethics:

> *Informed assent* means a child's agreement to medical procedures in circumstances where he or she is not legally authorized or lacks sufficient understanding for giving consent competently. Doctors should carefully listen to the opinion and wishes of children who

are not able to give full consent and should strive to obtain their assent. Doctors have the responsibility to determine the ability and competence of the child for giving his or her consent or assent. All children, even those not judged as competent, have a right to receive information given in a way that they can understand and give their assent or dissent. This consent/assent process must promote and protect the dignity, privacy and confidentiality of the child and his or her family. Consent or assent is required for all aspects of medical care, for preventive, diagnostic or therapeutic measures and research. Children may effectively refuse treatment or procedures which are not necessary to save their lives or prevent serious harm. Where treatment is necessary to save a life or prevent serious harm, the doctor has the duty to act in the best interest of the child. (De Lourdes Levy, Larcher, Victor, Kurz, et al., 2003, p. 629)

In Canada, according to the Family Law Reform Act of 1969 (section 8), a person aged 16 may give consent to treatment in the same way as an adult. The Act provides guidance that "it is good practice to involve the child's family in the decision-making process unless the child specifically requests that this should not happen." Furthermore,

a child under 16 years who is mentally disordered may have sufficient competency and intelligence to enable him or her to understand fully what is proposed... There is no specific age at which a child becomes competent to consent... This depends on the particular child and on the seriousness and complexity of whatever treatment or procedure is proposed (EIDO Healthcare, 2004).

In the United States, state legislation requires parental consent for medical treatment for minors, those eighteen years and under. In law, minors are considered incapable of understanding and making decisions about medical treatment, and their parents are permitted to make decision on behalf of their child. However, in practice most states allow minors aged thirteen through eighteen to provide consent for some medical care, such as contraception. In these States they are considered 'mature minors' and considered able to understand the nature and consequences of their medical treatment, and to consent to or to refuse treatment (AMA, 1992).

How to Implement a Legal Process Therapeutically

Obtaining informed consent and assent requires providing information, and in a hospital this legal process needs to be therapeutic in its intent and outcome. It is a key aspect of cognitive and emotional preparation, which if sensitively done could support coping and minimize anxiety or avoidance. How should this be done? What should be covered? By whom and when? And does this change with children of different ages? What about children's different coping styles and temperament differences – does this determine how information should be provided? There is a strong body of research evidence in this area to guide us in answering many of these questions, though some still remain unanswered.

Benefits for Children and Parents

There is a consensus of evidence that providing information that is developmentally appropriate in a time-sensitive fashion has many potential benefits, not only for the child and parents, but also for the health care professionals (Jaaniste et al., 2007). Children who are better informed about an upcoming procedure generally have better outcomes, as measured by lower distress and better adjustment during and after the procedure (Claar & Walker, 1999; Margolis et al., 1998; Schmidt, 1990). Researchers in Los Angeles found that when a child can accurately recall positive aspects of a medical procedure, this minimizes the child's anticipatory anxiety for future procedures (Chen et al., 1999). This is an encouraging finding. Added to that is the evidence that accurate information seems to assist a child in regulating their expectation and separating fantasy from reality (Mahajan et al., 1998). Thus, we can proceed knowing that accurate information is helpful in a number of ways for children. What about parents?

Parents' level of satisfaction with their child's medical care is closely associated with whether or not they perceive that the information that they have received is adequate (Magaret, Clark, Warden, et al., 2002). Parents also report that their own stress levels could have been reduced if, prior to their child's elective surgery, they had received more information from the health care professionals (Shirley, Thompson, et al., 1998). Further support for the benefit of providing information to parents in timely fashion comes from Canadian researchers Rugg & von Baeyer, (2000). They found that parents, who received a mailed package of information that was suited to the age of their child to read with their child prior to their tonsillectomy, were less likely to search for information from the Internet and friends – less reliable sources – than did parents who did not receive this information.

Form of Delivery

The Interaction. Providing information about an anticipated medical procedure requires a discussion and should not be a one-way delivery. "Once the child learns something about a forthcoming procedure, a communication process starts whereby the child may avoid or seek further information via asking questions or being vigilant" (Jaaniste et al., 2007). The amount of information that the health care professional then provides is signaled by both the child's non-verbal behavior and questions. Responses of curiosity, anxiety, or avoidance will result in quite different discussions and amounts of shared information. Creating an environment in which children feel comfortable to discuss their concerns and questions is a key to the success of this process.

What About Timing? When to tell a child about a procedure is largely determined by the child's age as well as the significance of the procedure. Most of the evidence comes from research on providing information prior to surgery. Younger children seem to need less time than older children. Children who were given information 5 to 7 days prior to a surgery were less anxious than those told within 24 hours of their surgery (Kain, Mayes, & Caramico, 1996). Some researchers recommend that the child should be informed of the procedure when it is scheduled, as most of the relevant information can be provided at the time, and definitely not just before or during the procedure (Blount, Piira & Cohen, 2003). This allows the child time to do the 'work of worry' (Janis,

1958), a form of getting ready, becoming used to, and rehearsing what may occur.

What to Cover. Words of explanation need to be elaborated in a child-centered manner by using rough sketches, charts, displays, instructional videos, and modeling (as described in Chapter 9); medical play; interactive computer programs; or a tour of the site (commonly used for day surgery preparation).

Younger children respond spontaneously to playing out hospital procedures, for example, using a child's version of a doctor's kit to become accustomed to the medical equipment of stethoscope, tourniquet, injections, bandages, and Band-aids. These pre-school-aged children develop their coping skills, procedural language, and sensory markers to work through their fears with repetitive play of what happened. They sometimes adopt different roles simultaneously as the nurse or the doctor.

Children seven to twelve years, in contrast, process information internally, yet require information in clear simple language that is concrete, retaining the primacy of their sensory experience: "You may feel it as cool, maybe tingly as the freezing goes in, or some 'pressure', you'll let me know." It isn't optimal to providing a sensory analogy – 'like a bite' or 'like a pinch' – as that often carries a negative connotation. Make the language playful; for example, "If you stay tense like this, guarding the pain, it won't be able to leave – and we want it to go away!"

Teenagers benefit from a more complex, physiological explanation. Given their capacity for abstract thought, they need more time for questions and to understand the implication of the intervention for their treatment. Unlike younger children, school-aged children and teens engage in fantasies and images on their own to prepare for procedures. Seeing a model of the brain or other part of the body can fill in the gaps.

We know little from the literature about who best should give this information – parents or healthcare professionals, or a combination of the two, at different time periods. Yet in hospital it is common practice that children will hear about a planned procedure a number of different times from different adults. We know little about the impact of this on the child and on developing readiness. We do know as a start that the information needs to be consistent.

Providing information should never be separated from its therapeutic intent to *empower the child* to deal as well as possible with the often taxing experience. Although this has been mentioned before, it is so central to sound clinical practice that it bears repeating. We need to explore with the child what to do to cope and feel better and how to retain or regain feelings of self-control while the procedure progresses. We need to ask questions such as, "What helped you the most when you had this last?" "Do you remember how to help yourself get rid of scary feelings?" or "Do you know how to drain the pain away? What would you like to use this time? Would you like to practice or rehearse it with me?"

We've know for over thirty years from research evidence (Melamed, Meyer, Gee & Soule, 1976) that for children who have had prior negative medical experiences, giving them information about the impending procedure tended to make them more sensitized. However, if information about the procedure is coupled with advice on strategies of how to cope with the procedure, this reduces the child's level of distress and sense of helplessness (Melamed & Ridley-Johnson, 1988). This is one of the main themes of this book: Simply telling a child about a painful procedure is insufficient preparation. The child needs to be guided as to how best to help him or herself through the taxing experience, what other aid (analgesics, hypnosis) or support (parent) is available, and how to use it most effectively (Refer to Chapter 9 where Dentists do this well with their Tell Show Do).

Children who have had many medical procedures or those with chronic illnesses develop an expertise over time with an elaborate cognitive grasp and a sophisticated understanding of their condition (Crisp, Ungerer, & Goodnow, 1996). These children will often counter with specific fears, preferences, or provisos about who should be present or what equipment or procedure helps their pain to go. Part of the responsibility of the health care professional in preparing the child is to relay this information on to the team, to advocate and co-ordinate to ensure that the child's reasonable requests are incorporate into the scheduled procedure. This is part of the process of collaborative team work, in which the child becomes a more active player in his or her own treatment.

A Mandate for More Than Information

The discussion above provides a clear rationale for the role of Child Life Specialists and Pediatric Psychologists in hospitals. Trained to provide play therapy for medical preparation and psychotherapy, respectively, in a child-centered and therapeutic context, these health professionals treat children who have become traumatized, or who are depressed, angry, confused, or fearful. Unless these children are given psychological treatment, they can develop further complications and also may become a significant stressor and management concern for the medical and nursing team.

Psychologist Anne Kazak and colleagues (2006) looked at the accumulated psychological and physiological responses of pain, injury, serious illness, medical procedures, and invasive or frightening treatment experiences on children, in research into a concept related to post-traumatic stress response (PTSD), called 'pediatric medical traumatic stress'. They found that traumatic stress could unfold at various points in the course of the child's illness and treatment, such as at a recurrence or deterioration. It would present with symptoms of intrusive thoughts, hyper-arousal, and avoidance in both the child and, of note, in other members of the family. When traumatic stress responses such as a high arousal, re-experiencing negative aspects, and avoidance occurred, daily lives were disrupted. The child's pain and frightening, negative experiences then have an impact beyond the child and onto siblings and parents, changing the quality of the family's life, well beyond the days or months spent in hospital.

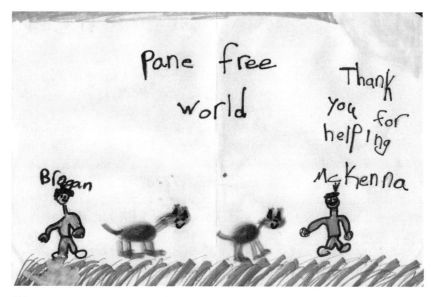

Figure 10.2a A younger sibling of a child in pain drew this, and reveals his wish that the world was pain-free and that his sister was no longer suffering.

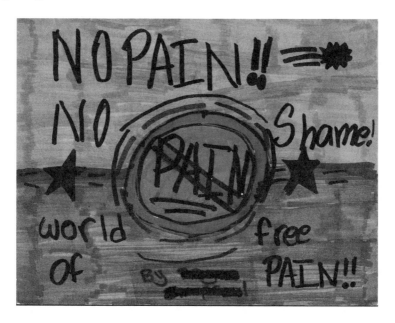

Figure 10.2b An older sibling spontaneously drew this as a statement in support of his sister's struggle with pain and moving on with her life.

In Summary

Some health care professionals fear that imparting information about an unpleasant upcoming procedure will upset a child. If the professional decides to underplay or minimize the pain of the impending procedure to 'spare the child', this is likely to compound the child's distrust. We also know that under-predicting pain tends to increase children's fear and their physiological responses (von Baeyer, Carlson, & Webb, 1997). A health care professional need not undertake this process alone. Allied with the parent, the two can come to a judgment as to when, what, and how to give information, so that a sensitive 'fit' is achieved, considering the child's temperament, history, and condition at the time. It is important to stay attuned in the discussion and the transactional process to determine when to stop, that is when it is enough and not too much for this particular child, such that the information overwhelms the child creating a sense of helplessness and doom. This is where individual differences and issues of temperament and coping come into play.

Addressing the Pain Concerns of Hospitalized Children

If a painful procedure has to be done, where is the best place – in a child's bed or the treatment room? Can the child have a choice to make bed a safe place? What about a training hospital's obligation to train new staff; and what limits need to be in place to reduce the risk of further trauma being inflicted on a child?

Should a Child's Bed Be a 'Safe Place'?

The issue emerged in hospitals as to whether to make the child's bed a 'safe-zone'. Clinicians recognized that we need to create environments for children that minimize their anxiety and accumulated trauma, and established more predictability and comfort during hospitalization. This meant that the child's bed became a non-treatment area and all invasive painful treatments would occur in a specially designated treatment room, supplied with distraction items such as bubble-blowing equipment, pop-up books, and DVDs. For children like Lesley, with a leukemic condition that required many needle sticks, knowing that her bed was a 'no-poke' zone would have diminished her fears. She may then have been more comfortable when staff entered her room, knowing that 'owies' only occurred in the treatment room.

This is not straightforward. For other children, this would magnify their fears. The accumulated painful treatments in one location creates a dread for that room. The treatment room becomes a place of fear and they protest when taken there. Parents need to be consulted by staff as to what is optimum for the child, so that together they can reach the best decision. Little Megan's Mom (in Chapter 3) knew that she would straddle the treatment table to position and hold her daughter for the IV access and that despite her daughter's whimpering, the procedure would be done more quickly and safely than in Megan's bed. For some children, however, the bother of having to leave their bed, wheel their attached equipment (IV, PCA, or other devices) along into the treatment room, takes too much energy and creates too much discomfort. They prefer to opt for procedures in their own bed. Having choice and predictability in the fast changing and often unpredictable hospital environment have far-reaching impacts on minimizing the traumatic effects of hospital experiences on children.

Responsibility to "Do No Harm"

In a fine book on procedure-related cancer pain in children, psychologist Christina Liossi (2002) draws attention to the impact of the environment, advising that eliminating loud noises, cold examining tables, and beepers that suddenly go off loudly in a treatment room, creates a less threatening environment. She raises a troubling aspect of many modern hospitals, which also serve as training hospitals. Often "the least experienced person is assigned the task of performing a painful procedure." This is not an uncommon practice, and another institutional barrier to ensuring the consistency of comfort for children in hospital. Dr. Liossi continues, "Every attempt should be made to ensure that the person who performs the procedure has proficient technical skill" (p. 106). With this concern some hospitals have developed protocols that limit procedure access attempts to two per trainee before a more senior colleague is called. For routine invasive procedures, such as lumbar punctures, other centers have selected either a dedicated nurse practitioner, or a dedicated physician to perform all such procedures. These are humane hospital decisions to reduce the burden of suffering on ill children.

Despite the very best of intentions, hospital practices may still be a source of immediate and long-term suffering for children and their families. As health care practitioners, we have an ethical, moral, and professional responsibility to "do no harm." Dr. Gary Walco (2008), Director of Pain Medicine, Seattle Children's Hospital, summarized this ethical challenge by saying:

> A fundamental principle of responsible medical care is not "do not hurt" but "do no harm." Harm occurs when the amount of hurt or suffering is greater than necessary to achieve the intended benefit. Since pain is harmful to patients, and caregivers are categorically committed to preventing harm to their patients, not using all the available means of relieving pain must be justified. (p. 5)

Collaboration Across Disciplines

There is considerable accumulated knowledge and skill within our modern day hospitals. Collaboration across disciplines, services and education in an active engaged fashion emerged as an important factor in the project to develop Comfort Central. "Using all available means" includes hospital-wide, discipline-inclusive efforts that are ongoing. It also requires the leadership and financial support of medical, nursing, and administrative personnel. "Unless people in each field recognize the importance of pain control, assume ownership of the problem and sit together and focus their collective energy and experience, any clinical approach [to pain and anxiety management] is potentially incomplete" (Schechter, 2008a).

Successful collaboration requires a sharing of skills and 'cross-pollination' between the different disciplines, regular rounds, inservice sessions (a Joint Commission requirement), and efforts to disseminate research from scholarly journals more broadly (such as the online *Pediatric Pain Letter*, www.childpain.org/ ppl/). As mentioned before, communication is the most common procedure in hospitals. Developing a common effective language across disciplines in a hospital to impart information, jointly solve problems, deliver bad news, and create smoother team work is a worthy goal. Learning from one another is particularly relevant to treating complex and ongoing pain where we don't know all the answers. Openly sharing across disciplines our concerns, our specific knowledge of the impact of the analgesics, the child and family's psychological dynamics, the disease or illness vulnerabilities specific to the child's disease, prognosis, and physical assessment, as well as our limitations and risks can only enhance the outcome for a child and family.

Helen's story: Living with Pain

I have spoken throughout the book about reducing, relieving, and preventing pain. However, there are some children who, despite our very best efforts, live a life in which pain is a frequent, familiar, and unwelcome visitor. In this last section I'll share the experience of Helen, now a teenager, who was born at our hospital with a congenital condition, which would become more painful as she developed and grew into adulthood. Managing pain would be a consistent part of her life. Over the years she would come to know the hospital well as an outpatient, and develop relationships with the pain service, her subspecialists, her physiotherapist and psychologist. Ultimately she would become an authority on her own condition, on optimal pain management and treatment. Until that time, all of us, Helen, her parents and the professionals involved would be learning, humbled by our limitations and the power of pain. As Albert Schweitzer (1931) said, "Pain is a more terrible lord of mankind than even death itself" (p. 62).

History

Helen's rare disorder, Klippel-Trenaunay Syndrome (KTS), consists of capillary vascular malformations, venous malformations that often develop into varicose veins, and hypertrophy (overgrowth and enlargement) of soft tissue and bone. With vascular, soft tissue, and bone malformations, she experiences different types of pain at unpredictable times, in different areas in her body, most commonly in her legs, her back and her stomach. Pain is a debilitating problem for Helen, something she always has to manage during the day and at night, although its intensity varies and there are days she feels fine. These are the days she'll happily go to school, then head for her part-time job at the bakery or home where she can play with her dog, involve herself in her creative crafts and hang out with her friends and family.

Reason for referral. I met Helen when she was eight, referred by a pediatric neurologist for headaches and dizzy episodes. The neurologist mentioned that even at that young age Helen was "an excellent historian" and able to accurately chronicle her condition. Her headaches were resolved quite quickly by addressing sleep patterns and giving her skills in self-hypnosis and breathing.

During those treatment sessions, social issues emerged of feeling different from other children. She hated going to Children's Hospital and being examined. Coming to terms with her different, changing, and painful body wove its way through many of our sessions in the early years. She was resourceful and a key resource was swimming. She was good at it and felt accepted by her team. She was and is still a strong-willed 'gutsy' girl, who loves her independence and wants to boldly engage with life.

Over the years Helen has developed the vascular malformations characteristic of this syndrome. She developed swellings, bruises, and bleeds in her arms, knees, legs, and abdomen; thrombosis in her varicose veins (she finds wearing the compression stockings hot and painful). As she has grown into her teens, subcutaneous tissue in her upper body has increased, and she has developed hypertrophy and asymmetry in her arms, legs, and hands.

In this condition pain can be severe and debilitating (Lee, Driscoll, Gloviczki, Clay, Shaughnessy, & Stans, 2005), and it comes from many different sources: (1) chronic venous insufficiency; 2) cellulites; (3) superficial thrombophlebitis; (4) deep vein thrombosis; (5) calcification of vascular malformations; (6) growing pains; (7) intraosseous vascular malformation; (8) arthritis and (9) neuropathic pain (Lee et al, 2005). Helen has five of these pain sources. Managing her pain depends on understanding its cause and determining the best treatment, while supporting her through it.

Biopsychosocial Analysis

Working with Helen, we have struggled to better understand her multiple sources of pain and find therapies to alleviate these pains. These have steadily and significantly increased over the last five years. There have been consultations with pain colleagues across the country to determine other analgesic options and she and her parents have consulted with leaders in KTS. She has taught us as much as we have taught her! As the closing case in this book let's use Figure 3.1, the Biopsychosocial Model of Pain, and do a functional analysis to better understand the sources of her pain.

Psychological Factors

Helen has grown up with KTS and the different types of pain. Her pain reports are reliable though she tend to minimize her distress and pain level. She is stoic and remarkably resilient. As soon as an episode of pain is over, it becomes history. She has well-developed coping skills, no evident anxiety, and likes to be independent. She is forthright, optimistic, social, intelligent, and courageous. She is determined to be 'in her life' and persevere through more painful episodes. But when these painful episodes persist beyond three or four days, she tires, feels despondent, and retreats to bed. She rests, elevates her legs, and sleeps a lot, and talks with her Mom.

Academic achievement is a high priority for her. (I am raising academic aspects here rather than under Social, as it applies to her sense of self.) Helen is suitably ambitious and plans to go on to higher education. She is committed to attending and doing well at school, but often misses a day or two per week. She can become very fatigued and despondent. In earlier years, anti-depressants were helpful, but she has not needed them since turning sixteen years of age. She has good support from her teachers to make-up work. Since her sixteenth birthday we have noticed her growing sense of confidence and self-assertion. Helen knows better than ever what is going on and expresses it even more succinctly, so that we 'get it!'

Social Factors

Family. She has a close, committed, loving family. Her pain is independent of any family issues. She attends to her physical discomfort and pain at home. Even though she'll incur the wrath of her siblings for not doing her chores, she takes her analgesics, lies down on the couch, props her stocking legs up, and calls to her Mom to resolve any tension or conflict with her siblings. Her siblings report feeling conflicted. They have their own struggles coming to terms with their sister's suffering. Her brother openly says that he worries about her when she's lying on the couch in pain. Yet he adds, within a heart beat, that he gets furiously mad with her for not unloading the dishwasher. It's a simple chore – and now it falls to him and he has to do it: "I wish she were healthier and didn't have pain."

Friends. Helen would much prefer to go to the mall and hang out with her friends, but "I'm making the best of it" she said on a day when we spoke and she was too fatigued to leave the house. She has developed and maintained good friendships. Her irregular social life does not seem to feed her pain, though it is a source of frustration for her. She is candid about it when she cannot join a social event, or fatigues too early. This may factor into her 'slump episodes' when she reports feeling despondent. She seems to be coming to terms with some of her losses.

Biological Factors

The major following sources of her pain derive from her KTS disorder:

1. *Chronic venous insufficiency.* She has dull achy sensations in her legs from the pooling of venous blood and varicose veins. After years of struggle coming to terms with the heat and discomfort of pressure stockings, she now accepts this key treatment as a standard part of her life. She also now routinely elevates her legs, including during her sessions with me. This reduces her leg pain significantly. She finds daily Celebrex and acetaminophen helpful and is taking them more reliably.

2. *Cellulitis.* It is not clear whether as a result of venous stasis, thrombosis, or localized lymph accumulation, but Helen developed chronic lymphedema. This has changed her body, and she's struggled in her earlier years to come to terms with these physical changes.

3. *Thrombophlebitis.* Helen has some inflammation of her superficial veins that respond to the analgesics.

4. *Deep vein thrombosis.* She recently had spontaneous painful bleeds in her knees. This was very troubling, and her physician has ordered a Venogram to better understand what is occurring.

5. *Growing pains.* Helen had considerable growing pain during puberty, which has now stabilized. Her muscles were more affected than her joints. She reported back and leg pains, and

found her mother's gentle massage and soaks in a warm bath gave some relief.

Additionally: Fatigue is significant factor. She tires more easily than her peers as a result of the KTS and the continual pain. Yet she experiences periods of difficulty falling asleep, and during more painful episodes, her sleep is unsettled. Amitriptyline has recently been helpful in re-establishing more settled sleeps.

Her health care team consists of many disciplines in the hospital and community. All these professionals value the importance of pain control as a key part of the management of her condition. We've had many discussions, and pooled our collective experience and knowledge to find the best treatment at different times during her taxing pain-filled growing years. Given that she will be living with this syndrome for the rest of her life, any complications that can be prevented now will increase her function and quality of life in the future. Helen's drive, creativity, and determination help many of us when faced with the limitations of our capacity to remove her pain and suffering.

What Helen Has to Say to Us

As an authority on living with pain, I asked her about what she would like health professionals to know. Here is what she had to say:

Helen: "It's hugely important for me to have the support group of key people who are easily accessible to see and help me: Dr. B, my pediatrician; you; my family doctor, Dr. L; Dr. C, my plastic surgeon; and the complex pain clinic. Knowing that you guys are there and will help me makes it easier for me to go on.

Dr. K: What has helped you recently?

Helen: Going back to the complex pain clinic helped. I'm now on 10 mg amitriptylene every night, because sleeping became harder for me. It's helping me sleep a lot better. Also, I enjoyed my summer. It was a big improvement on the previous summer, when we thought I had a DVT [deep vein thrombosis] and couldn't do much. This time I could hang out with friends, go to a friend's cabin, and make the most of this summer. But I overdid it! So I've had to be in bed the last 10 days resting and sleeping in late. But it was worth it – I have no regrets.

Dr. K: What physical treatments do you find helpful?

Helen : I enjoy swimming, my best way to exercise. Sometimes it can aggravate the pain, but I do it anyway because I find it beneficial and relaxing because of the stretching. I'm now wearing the compression stockings daily because the pain in my legs is getting worse, so I've moved up to 50-60 mmHg pressure. This weekend I also wore knee tensors to give extra pressure when I was out and walking around – it helps. I wear them under my jeans so no one will notice. I also like walking, but I get tired quickly so I need to pace myself. My family bought me my dream pink, cute, small electric scooter to get to school and home. When I get home, I lie down with my legs elevated. I also sleep with my bed elevated. I use a heating pad in bed, under or on top of my knees – wherever it's aching. I find heat helps me more than cold.

Dr. K: What would you like health professionals to know about pain?

Helen: Everyone is different! It's taken me seventeen years to figure out what is best. It's taken so long to get to where I am. Today I'm on Celebrex 400 mg per day; acetaminophen up to six a day, this definitely helps with the pain. My family doctor wants me off the acetaminophen and gave me some alternatives to try. But they didn't agree with me. If I forget to take my meds, I feel a big difference within the hour, and I'm hurting a lot more. I must remember to take them with me in a little bag. What else? Hypnosis helped in the beginning. It got me to know how to focus and use my imagination and brain to bring comfort into my body. I don't use it any longer because I've got it, and I just love the breathing to calm myself – it definitely helps with the pain. Having someone to talk through things in my life – you, my mom, my family, and my friends – is the best. At the Mayo I met a group at the KT conference. Talking with them I realized how important it was to wear stockings. Great to learn more from people who know!"

Pain is a singular experience. While it may to some extent be known medically, it is as personal and unique as pleasure. The framework may be 'generic' but the experience is anything but – as in Helen's case.

Conclusion

Beyond a psychological, physical, or pharmacological focus for pain management, the adoption of a child-centered approach makes children's experience of pain the number one vital sign. This requires collaboration of health care professionals across all disciplines who hold the value that pain deserves the best of our skill, talent, and efforts. Pain belongs to all disciplines, as we all have something to contribute to reduce children's suffering. This dedicated collaboration is essential in a children's hospital, where pain accompanies many conditions and illnesses. It is also caused during diagnosis and treatment, where it is our duty to act to prevent pain and anxiety. Thought and planning for pain relief is a central part of delivering humane clinical care.

There is now international interest and momentum to integrate pain management across all services in hospitals and in education and training. To do this consistently and create uniformity, state of the art pain practices must be embedded within hospital policy and protocols, adhered to by all professionals, and be led and supported by administration. These protocols address children's fears, anxiety, and concerns with respect. Children then become active, vocal, and valued members of the team in managing their pain relief – this is a worthy and humane goal for any hospital.

Afterword

Knowing is Not Enough:
Strategies to Improve Pain Management
in Healthcare Institutions

"Knowing is not enough, we must apply; willing is not enough,
we must do."

Goethe

This volume is testimony to the enormous growth over the past few decades in our understanding of children's pain and in our strategies to treat it. It is probably unimaginable to younger colleagues that a scant 25 years ago (the wink of an eye for some of us), highly painful procedures such as bone marrow aspirations were performed on infants and children with essentially no sedation, that postoperative pain was ignored or addressed with intramuscular analgesics, and that even the possibility of pain in infants was viewed with a jaundiced eye (no pun intended). This sorry state of affairs stemmed not from malevolence but from the lack of a research base from which to derive informed decisions regarding pain management. We had only a cursory understanding of the developmental neurobiology of nociception, few standardized assessment tools with which to measure pain and gauge response to treatment, and limited research on what strategies (pharmacologic, physical, or psychologic) actually worked to alleviate it. There was no recognition of the short and long term consequences of inadequately treated pain which might provide the urgency to drive research forward. As a result, there were essentially no books on pediatric pain, no review articles, no national guidelines, and few research articles in peer reviewed publications to inform attitudes or practice.

As is evident from this volume, however, much has changed. New knowledge has accrued at a rapid rate and has been translated for use at the bedside. As a result, clinical practice has clearly changed. When compared to studies done 25 years ago, postoperative pain, cancer pain, procedure pain, and infant pain are much more likely to be addressed with the result being that average pain scores in hospital have plummeted. Despite this improvement, however, in study after study, a significant number of children (up to 25% in most studies), regardless of their medical problem or the hospital in which they are being treated, continue to experience severe pain during their medical treatment. In a study by Ammendorp, (2005), families were asked to list their most important goals for the hospitalization of their child as well as to report their level of satisfaction with meeting those goals. The area of pain management had the greatest disparity between the importance of the goal to families (second after accurately diagnosing the problem) and their satisfaction with how successfully it was accomplished. There also continues to be vast inter- and intra-hospital variations. For example, in one study, one hospital used twenty eight times more morphine in their neonatal intensive care unit than another hospital with a similar sized unit.

What accounts for the persistence of significant numbers of children in pain even in our most sophisticated hospitals? I would assert that the lack of research is no longer the main impediment. Although there certainly remain gaps in our understanding of pain in children, the main culprit appears to be the lack of uniform application of what we already know. This problem is not new and clearly not confined to the area of pediatric pain management. As early as 1990, one of the pioneers of pain medicine, John J. Bonica (Bonica, 1990) said of adult postoperative pain control:

> I have studied the reasons for inadequate management of postoperative pain, and they remain the same...inadequate or improper application of available information and therapies is certainly the most important reason for inadequate postoperative pain relief.

How then are we to assure that all children benefit from the advances that have occurred in the area of pain management? Many strategies have been employed to attempt to address this deficiency. These include increasing the education of healthcare providers, development of guidelines to promote ideal practice, and use of audits to document that such practices are occurring. Unfortunately however, these strategies often have limited impact on practice patterns. In the remainder of this afterword, I hope to review what we presently know about how to change the behavior of practicing physicians and offer some suggestions about what seems to work and what doesn't. The goal of course, is to put into place many of the ideas about pediatric pain that have been so elegantly elucidated by Dr. Kuttner throughout this book.

Education

There are many forms of and venues for continuing medical education. What we do know is that the traditional model, a single lecture about a topic in a large auditorium, is often ineffective. Study after study demonstrates that sleepy practitioners, overwhelmed by the ever-increasing demands of modern medicine, often do not incorporate what they hear in such a passive environment into what they subsequently do in practice. The literature suggests that information shared at the site of care (on rounds, in the office) and in small groups using case based examples is far more likely to have an impact. This explains the relative success of pharmaceutical representatives who tend to meet practitioners in their offices who can address the specific barriers or concerns that exist within that setting. Another important characteristic of any educational effort is that it needs to be repeated frequently so that questions that arise when the information provided is used can be addressed. Educational initiatives therefore need to be active, occur at the site of care in small groups and be repeated frequently. Another important educational strategy that is effective at changing practice is the education of consumers. When parents are made aware that there may be techniques available to reduce their child's suffering, they will often aggressively advocate for those approaches and spur on health care providers to consider pain management as an essential element of their care.

Guidelines

The new information that has emerged regarding pediatric pain has been organized into guidelines by many professional organizations and NGOs such as the World Health Organization. These guidelines theoretically offer 'best practices' to providers based on rating the quality of the available evidence. One would think that guidelines would immediately become the standard of care once they are produced, but despite their availability, they often have very limited impact on practice. A number of reasons for this have been offered – practitioners may not know that they exist or may not agree with them; they may be perceived as hard to implement or lacking in relevance to the local community; and finally, a variety of non-clinical factors such as limited logistical or financial support may impede their integration into practice. Studies suggest that if a local team examines national guidelines and modifies them to address local concerns and practice patterns they are more likely to be used.

Audit

Audits with feedback are often considered to be the cornerstone of creating change in healthcare settings. The notion is that if individuals are given information about how their practices or patient outcomes compare with some internal or external standard, they will modify their practice accordingly. Audits are moderately successful at producing some change in specific behaviors but are not nearly as successful as one might hope. There appear to be a few reasons for this. One problem is in the selection of indicators to monitor practice. One commonly used indicator is patient satisfaction, but unfortunately this does not provide an accurate reflection of the individual's pain experience. Many studies have shown that patients will report that they are satisfied with the pain control they had during a hospital stay despite the fact that, when their charts are examined, high levels of unrelieved pain were frequently documented. Specific 'indicators' have been developed by professional societies such as the American Pain Society to help develop an appropriate quality improvement program for pain management. There are other problems with audits as well. Frequently, the review occurs long after the event that is being audited. This lack of immediate feedback tends to diminish its impact. Additionally, there are often no consequences for not responding to the findings of the audit. Audits therefore as education and guidelines are valuable as part of an overall approach to pain control but should not be used in isolation.

Institutionalizing Pain Management

How then can we change practice if each of these seemingly powerful tools are minimally effective at doing so? One of the answers that seems obvious to me, is not to focus on individual behavior change but rather to institutionalize the importance of pain management. Although individual initiatives are valuable, they are more beneficial and sustainable if they are part of an overall institutional plan. In that way, appropriate pain management does not rely on the memory or good graces of any one practitioner but instead becomes part of the fabric and culture of care, similar to issues of safety and confidentiality. For this to occur, all of the measures previously mentioned (education, guidelines, audit) need to be put in place in a coordinated way with full administrative support. Inadequate pain management should be seen as everyone's responsibility to remedy.

The key components to creating an institutional approach to pain management have been discussed in Chapter 10. Briefly, they consist of: Creating an interdisciplinary work group with administrative authority to mandate change; An initial self study to identify the current status of pain management within the institution; Development of explicit policies and protocols which are evidence informed but developed locally with buy-in from relevant stakeholders; Informing families of the importance of pain management and soliciting their active involvement in the process; An ongoing education and audit process.

While it is easy to identify these principles, there are often numerous roadblocks to their implementation and these are described somewhat in Chapter 10 and in more detail in our article (2008a). At present, our attempt to provide a systematic, institution-wide uniform approach to pain management, has three main elements: clinical, educational, and advocacy. From the clinical side, we have a Pain Steering Committee with broad representation and administrative and moral authority to make change. We have protocols that are accessible and continuously reinforced and updated for all major pain problems. Pain discussion is emphasized on rounds and at the nursing interview at admission. We have frequent quality audits to identify infractions. From the educational side, we have yearly pain lectures for the practicing medical community, an ongoing educational series for trainees, a pain handbook, and brochures and signage for families emphasizing the importance of pain management and urging their involvement in the process. Finally, in the area of advocacy, we have buttons, tee shirts, awards for those who do an especially good job, and a newsletter to highlight pain relief activities. Although we feel we have had a significant impact on the quality of pain control within our institution, continuous vigilance is necessary to maintain those changes. While this model is what has evolved in our hospital, each institution will find different ways to implement these basic principles depending on local factors.

International Accreditation

Although an institution-wide commitment to pain relief seems to hold promise as a strategy to assure the uniform application of new knowledge about pain, few institutions are able to put in place such an approach. Lack of a local champion, inadequate resources, issues of territoriality and personality, and a host of other factors may provide impediments to the implementation of such an approach. However, many of these barriers could be overcome if there was enough motivation for an institution to do so and if there was a mechanism through which international expertise and experience could be imported and adapted. The Child-Kind initiative, a project emerging from the Special Interest Group on Pain in Children of the International Association for the Study of Pain, is one strategy to provide the motivation to institutions to overcome the barriers that prevent the available knowledge in pediatric pain from being applied to the every child.

ChildKind is modeled on the Baby Friendly Hospital Program, a highly successful joint effort of WHO and UNICEF to encourage breast-feeding in hospitals. In this model, if institutions meet a list of specific criteria, they are awarded the prestigious Baby Friendly Hospital designation. Desire to gain this international accreditation and recognition is a driving force for many institutions to overcome internal barriers to breast-feeding. There are presently 15,000 Baby Friendly hospitals so one can only imagine how powerful the impact of this technique has been on the nutrition of the world's children.

The ChildKind initiative will encompass a similar model applied to pediatric pain prevention and relief. If institutions can demonstrate that they have incorporated the five key principles of Child-Kind into the care they provide, they will receive this international award. Those principles are: the presence of a facility-wide, evidence-informed, written policy on pain assessment, prevention, and management; comprehensive and on-going pain education and awareness programs for all staff, students/trainees, patients, and caregivers; routine pain assessment using an evidence-informed, developmentally-appropriate process, and recorded in the patient record; use of specific, evidence-informed protocols for pain prevention and management, including pharmacological, psychological, and physical methods; and, a regular institutional self-monitoring program of the above criteria. If institutions can document that they are adhering to these principles, they will be granted the international recognition that ChildKind certification offers. Although ChildKind is in the early phases of development, it is hoped that when it is fully formed and operational, it will have as powerful an impact on pain reduction as Baby Friendly has had on increasing breast-feeding

Rights-based approaches

Creation of an institution-wide systematic approach to pain requires significant effort. The motivation to offer such effort may stem from the passion and commitment of staff members or from the recognition that may accrue either locally or internationally once this has been accomplished.

There certainly will be situations in which this 'carrot approach' is inadequate to produce change. Another approach to improving pain management is the 'stick approach' where inadequate pain relief is considered malpractice or even 'illegal.' There are many examples of this strategy and many more are emerging. In the United States, there have been lawsuits that have asserted that failure to provide pain relief has caused irreparable harm to the patient and damages have been awarded to patients in response to those claims. In Australia, the Medical Treatment Act of the Australian Capital Territory states explicitly that individuals have the "right to receive relief from pain and suffering to the maximum extent possible." There are three specific statutes in California law that mandate attention to pain. One insists on yearly physician education in pain; one states that physicians who are not comfortable with prescribing opioids must refer patients to physicians who are comfortable; and finally, one provides a mechanism to follow up complaints of inadequate pain treatment. It is unfortunate that legal remedies are sometimes necessary to bring about change.

There is one 'legal' strategy that specifically applies to children. The UN Convention on the Rights of the Child (1989) has 194 signatories and asserts that children have the same inherent value as adults and the same human rights. Specific articles of the Convention (article 2 on non-discrimination, article 3 on 'best interests,' article 6 on the right to survival and development, and article 12 on the right to be listened to) have been offered to support the contention that pediatric pain relief is a human right and that failure to provide it should be considered a violation of the convention. Although such arguments may seem extreme, they offer insight into the depth of concern that many have when children's healthcare facilities fail to offer the compassionate care that should be their hallmark.

Summary

In this outstanding volume, Dr. Kuttner has presented an overview of our present understanding of children's pain. New research has helped to unravel some of its complexity. We now know that unrelieved pain can have significant long and short-term consequences on the developing child. We also know that there are clearly techniques that we have available to us that can reduce the pain that children experience during medical illness or its treatment. These strategies are effective, however, only if they are used. In this afterword, I have tried to suggest some approaches that can be put in place to assure that most children, in whatever setting they find themselves, have access to the comfort that the application of these techniques can offer. If we, as health professionals and advocates for children, do not lead the way, who will?

"Although the world is full of suffering,
it is also full of the overcoming of it. "

Helen Keller

Neil L. Schechter, MD
Professor and Head, Division of Pain Medicine
Department of Pediatrics, Connecticut Children's Medical Center
University of Connecticut School of Medicine
Hartford, CT, USA

References

Core references are marked with a *

Abu-Saad, H. (1984a). Cultural components of pain: The Asian-American child. *Children's Health Care, 13,* 11-14.

Abu-Saad, H. (1984b). Cultural components of pain: The Arab-American child. *Issues in Comprehensive Pediatric Nursing, 7,* 91-99.

Abu-Saad, H. (1984c). Cultural group indicators of pain in children. *Maternal-Child Nursing Journal, 13,* 187-196.

Achterberg, J. (1985). *Imagery in healing.* Boston: New Science Library.

American Academy of Pediatric Dentistry. (2000). *American Academy of Pediatric Dentistry reference manual.* Chicago.

American Academy of Pediatric Dentistry. (2006). Guidelines for monitoring and management of pediatric patients during and after sedation for diagnostic and therapeutic procedures. *American Academy of Pediatric Dentistry reference manual, 31,* 6, 09/10 152-168. Retrieved 1 November 2009 from: http://www.aapd.org/media/Policies_Guidelines/G_Sedation.pdf

*American Academy on Pediatric Dentistry Clinical Affairs Committee, Behavior Management Subcommittee and American Academy on Pediatric Dentistry Council on Clinical Affairs. (2008-2009). Guideline on behavior guidance for the pediatric dental patient. *Pediatric Dentistry, 30* (Suppl. 7), 125-133.

American Academy of Pediatrics Committee on Bioethics. (1995). Informed consent, parental permission, and assent in pediatric practice. *Pediatrics, 95,* 314-317.

American Academy of Pediatrics Committee on Bioethics and Committee on Hospital Care. (2000). Palliative care for children. *Pediatrics, 106,* 351-357.

American Academy of Pediatrics Subcommittee on Abdominal Pain in Children. (2005). Chronic abdominal pain in children. *Pediatrics, 115,* 812-815.

American Medical Association. (1992). *Confidential care for minors.* Retrieved August 3, 2008, from: http://www.ama-assn.org/ama1/pub/upload/mm/369/40b.pdf

American Pain Society. (2001). *The Assessment and Management of Acute Pain in Infants, Children, and Adolescents: A Position Statement from the American Pain Society.* Retrieved October 21, 2009 from: http://www.ampainsoc.org/advocacy/pediatric2.htm

American Pain Society. (2005) *Pediatric Chronic Pain: A Position Statement from the American Pain Society.* Retrieved October 21, 2009 from: http://www.ampainsoc.org/advocacy/pediatric.htm

Ammentorp, J., Mainz, J., & Sabroe, S. (2005). Parents' Priorities and Satisfaction with Acute Pediatric Care. *Archives of Pediatric Adolescent Medicine. 159(2),* 127-131.

Anand, K.J.S., & Aynsley-Green, A. (1988). Measuring the effects of surgical stress on newborn infants. *Journal of Pediatric Surgery, 23,* 297-305.

Anand, K.J., & Hickey, P.R. (1987). Pain and its effects in the human neonate and fetus. *New England Journal of Medicine, 317(21)*, 1321-1329.

*Anand, K. J. S. and the International Evidence-Based Group for Neonatal Pain. (2001). Consensus statement for the prevention and management of pain in the newborn. *Archives of Pediatric & Adolescent Medicine, 155*, 173-180.

Anand, K. J. S., Sippell, W. G., & Aynsley-Green, A. (1987). Randomized trial of fentanyl anesthesia in preterm babies undergoing surgery: Effects of stress response. *The Lancet, 8524*, 62-67.

*Annequin, D., Carbajal, R., Chauvin, P., Gall, O., Tourniaire, B., & Murat, I. (2000). Fixed 50% nitrous oxide mixture for painful procedures: A French survey. *Pediatrics, 105*, E47.

Apley, J. (1975). *The child with abdominal pains*. Oxford, United Kingdom: Blackwell Scientific.

Asmundson, G.J.G., Vlaeyen, J.W.S., & Crombez, G. (Eds.). (2004). *Understanding and treating fear of pain*. New York: Oxford University Press.

Asprey, J.R. (1994). Postoperative analgesic prescription and administration in a pediatric population. *Journal of Pediatric Nursing, 9*, 150-157.

Bamigbade, T.A., & Langford, R.M. (1998). The clinical use of tramadol hydrochloride. *Pain Reviews, 5*, 155-182.

*Bandstra, N.F., Skinner, L., Leblanc, C., Chambers, C.T., Hollon, E.C., Brennan, D., et al. (2008). The role of child life in pediatric pain management: A survey of child life specialists. *Journal of Pain, 9*, 320-329.

*Barber, J. (1989). Suffering children hurt us. *Pediatrician, 16*, 119-123.

Barber, J. (2004). Hypnotic analgesia: Mechanisms of action and clinical approaches. In: D.D. Price & C. Bushnell (Eds.), *Psychological methods of pain control: Basic science and clinical approach. Progress in pain and research management: Vol. 29*. (pp. 269-300). Seattle, WA: IASP Press.

*Barber, J., & Adrian, C. (Eds.) (1982). *Psychological approaches to the management of pain*. New York. Brunner/Mazel.

Barber, J., & Mayer, D. (1977). Evaluation of the efficacy and neural mechanism of a hypnotic analgesia procedure in experimental and clinical dental pain. *Pain, 4*, 41-48.

Barr, R., Francoeur, T.E., Westwood, M., & Walsh, S. (1986). Recurrent abdominal pain due to lactose intolerance revisited. *American Journal of Diseases of Childhood, 140*, 302.

Bédard, G.B.V., Reid, G.J., McGrath, P.J., & Chambers, C.T. (1997). Coping and self-medication in a community sample of junior high school students. *Pain Research & Management, 2*, 151-156.

*Beecher, H.K. (1956). Relationship of significance of wound to pain experienced. *Journal of the American Medical Association, 161*, 1609-1613.

*Beider, S., Mahrer, N. E., & Gold, J. I. (2007). Pediatric massage therapy: An overview for clinicians. *Pediatric Clinics of North America, 54*, 1025-1041.

Beider, S., O'Callaghan, E.T., & Gold, J.I. (2009). A pediatric perspective on massage. In: T. Culbert & K. Olness (Eds.), *Integrative pediatrics* (pp. 248-266). New York: Oxford University Press.

*Berde, C.B., Lebel, A.A., & Olson, G. (2003). Neuropathic pain in children. In: N. Schechter, C.B. Berde, & M. Yaster (Eds.), *Pain in infants, children* *and adolescents* (2nd ed., pp. 620-641). Philadelphia: Lippincott, Williams & Wilkins.

*Berde, C.B. (2008). Foreword. In: G.A. Walco, & K.R. Goldschneider (Eds.), *Pain in children. A practical guide for primary care* (pp. vii-x). New Jersey: Humana Press.

Bieri, D., Reeve, R.A., Champion, G.D., Addicoat, L., & Ziegler, J.B. (1990). The Faces Pain Scale for the self-assessment of the severity of pain experienced by children: Development, initial validation, and preliminary investigation for ratio scale properties. *Pain, 41,* 139-150.

Blount, R.L, Piira, T., & Cohen, L.L. (2003). Management of pediatric pain and distress due to medical procedures In: M.C. Roberts (ed.), *Handbook of pediatric psychology* (pp. 216-233). New York: Guilford Press.

*Blount, R.L., Zempsky, W.T., Jaaniste, T., Evans, S., Cohen, L.L., Devine, K.A., et al. (2009). Management of pain and distress due to medical procedures. In M.C. Roberts & R. Steele (Eds.), *Handbook of pediatric psychology* (4th ed., pp. 171-188). New York: Guilford Press.

Bonica, J.J., *The Management of Pain, 2nd Ed.* Phililedphia, PA: Lea & Febiger.

Bozkurt, P. (2005). Use of tramadol in children. *Pediatric Anesthesia, 15,* 1041-1047.

Bradley, D. (1991). *Hyperventilation syndrome: A handbook for people with disordered breathing.* Auckland, New Zealand: Tandem Press.

Breau, L., McGrath, P., Finley, A., & Camfield, C. (2004). *Non-communicating Children's Pain Checklist – Postoperative Version* (NCCPC-PV). Retrieved October 10, 2009, from http://www.aboutkidshealth.ca/Shared/PDFs/AKH_Breau_post-op.pdf

Breau, L., McGrath, P., Finley, A., & Camfield, C. (2004). *Non-communicating Children's Pain Checklist – Revised* (NCCPC-R). Retrieved October 10, 2009 from http://www.aboutkidshealth.ca/Shared/PDFs/AKH_Breau_everyday.pdf

Brent, M., Lobato, D., & LeLeiko, N. (2009). Psychological treatments for pediatric functional gastrointestinal disorders. *Journal of Pediatric Gastroenterology and Nutrition, 48,* 13-21.

Brett, D. (1988). *Annie's stories: A special kind of story telling.* New York: Workman.

Broome, M.E., & Stieglitz, K.A. (1992). The consent process and children. *Research in Nursing and Health, 15,* 147-152.

Bruce E., & Franck, L. (2000). Self-administered nitrous oxide (ENTONOX) for the management of procedural pain. *Paediatric Nursing, 12,* 15-19.

Bursch, B., Walco, G., & Zeltzer, L. (1998). Clinical assessment and management of chronic pain and pain-associated disability syndrome (PADS). *Journal of Development & Behavioral Pediatrics, 19,* 44-52.

Campo, J.V., Di Lorenzo, C., Bridge, J., Chiappetta, L., Colborn, D.K., Gartner, J.C., Gaffney, P., Kocoshis, S., & Brent, D. (1999). *Adult outcomes of recurrent abdominal pain: Preliminary results.* Orlando, FL: American Gastroenterological Association, Orlando, Fl. May 16, 1999.

Campo, J.V., Perel, J., Lucas, A., Bridge, J., Ehmann, M., Kalas, C., et al. (2004). Citalopram treatment of pediatric recurrent abdominal pain and comorbid internalizing disorders: An exploratory study. *Journal of the American Academy of Child and Adolescent Psychiatry, 43,* 1234-1242.

Cervero, F. & Laird, J. (1991). One pain or many pains? A new look at pain mechanisms. *News in Physiological Sciences, 6*, 268-273.

Chambers, C.T., Craig, K.D., & Bennett, S. M. (2002). The impact of maternal behavior on children's pain experiences: An experimental analysis. *Journal of Pediatric Psychology, 27*, 293-301.

Chen, E., Zeltzer, L.K., Craske, M.G., & Katz, E.R. (1999). Alteration of memory in the reduction of children's distress during repeated aversive medical procedures. *Journal of Consulting and Clinical Psychology, 67*, 481-490.

*The Children's Hospital of Philadelphia. (2003). *Positioning for comfort.* Retrieved October 1, 2009, from http://www.chop.edu/consumer/jsp/division/generic.jsp?id=82113

Ciszkowski, C., Madadi, P., Phillips, M.S., Lauwers, A.E., & Koren, G. (2009). Codeine, ultrarapid-metabolism genotype, and postoperative death. *New England Journal of Medicine, 361*, 827-828.

Claar, R.L., & Walker, L.S. (1999). Maternal attributions for the causes and remedies of their children's abdominal pain. *Journal of Pediatric Psychology, 24*, 345-354.

Clark, S., Radford, M. (1986). Topical anesthesia for venipuncture. *Archives of Diseases in Childhood 16*, 1132–1134

Cohen, L.L., Blount, R.L., & Panopoulos, G. (1997). Nurse coaching and cartoon distraction: An effective and practical intervention to reduce child, parent, and nurse distress during immunizations. *Journal of Pediatric Psychology, 22*, 355-370.

Cohen, L.L., McLaren, J.E., DeMore, M., Fortson, B., Friedman, A., Lim, C.S., et al. (2009). A randomized controlled trial of vapocoolant for pediatric immunization distress relief. *The Clinical Journal of Pain, 25*, 490-494.

*Compas, B.E., & Boyer, M.C. (2001) Coping and attention: Implications for child health and pediatric conditions. *Journal of Developmental & Behavioral Pediatrics, 22*, 323-333.

Compas, B.E., Connor-Smith, J.K., Saltzman, H., Thomsen, A.H., & Wadsworth, M.E. (2001). Coping with stress during childhood and adolescence: problems, progress, and potential in theory and research. *Psychological Bulletin, 127*, 87-127.

Connelly, M., Rapoff, M.A., Thompson, N., & Connelly, W. (2006). Headstrong: A pilot study of a CD-ROM intervention for recurrent pediatric headache. *Journal of Pediatric Psychology, 31*, 737-747.

Coté, C.J., Karl, H.W., Notterman, D.A., Weinberg, J.A., & McCloskey, C. (2000). Adverse sedation events in pediatrics: Analysis of medications used for sedation. *Pediatrics, 106*, 633-644.

Coté, C.J., Notterman, D.A., Karl, H.W., Weinberg, J.A., & McCloskey, C. (2000). Adverse sedation events in pediatrics: A critical incident analysis of contributory factors. *Pediatrics, 105*, 805-814.

*Coté, C.J., Wilson, S., & American Academy of Pediatrics and American Academy of Pediatric Dentistry Work Group on Sedation. (2006). Guidelines for monitoring and management of pediatric patients during and after sedation for diagnostic and therapeutic procedures: An update. *Pediatrics, 118*, 2587-2602.

*Crisp, J., Ungerer, J.A., & Goodnow, J.J. (1996). The impact of experience on children's understanding of illness. *Journal of Pediatric Psychology, 21,* 57-72.

Crombez, G., Bijttebier, P., Eccleston, C., Mascagni, T., Mertens, G., Goubert, L., et al. (2003). The Child version of the Pain Catastrophizing Scale (PCS-C): A preliminary validation. *Pain, 104,* 639-646.

Culbert, T.P., & Olness, K. (Eds.), (2009). *Integrative pediatrics.* New York: Oxford University Press.

Curtis, C.P. (1999). *Bud, not Buddy.* New York: Delacorte Press.

Dampier, C., & Shapiro, B.S. (2003). Management of pain in sickle cell disease. In: N. Schechter, C.B. Berde, & M. Yaster (Eds.), *Pain in infants, children and adolescents* (2nd ed., pp. 489-516). Philadelphia: Lippincott, Williams & Wilkins.

De Lourdes Levy, M., Larcher, V., Kurz, R., & Ethics Working Group of the Confederation of European Specialists in Paediatrics (CESP) (2003). Informed consent/assent in children. Statement of the Ethics Working Group of the Confederation of European Specialists in Paediatrics (CESP). *European Journal of Pediatrics, 162,* 629-633.

Department of Pediatrics, University of Saskatchewan (n.d.). Retrieved October 2, 2009, from http://ww.usask.ca/pediatrics/services/pain

Diener, H.C., Kronfeld, K., Boewing, G., Lungenhausen, M., Maier, C., Molsberger, A., et al. (2006). Efficacy of acupuncture for the prophylaxis of migraine: A multicentre randomised controlled clinical trial. *The Lancet Neurology, 5,* 310-316.

Drotar, D. (2009). Physician Behavior in the Care of Pediatric Chronic Illness: Association With Health Outcomes and Treatment Adherence. *Journal of Developmental & Behavioral Pediatrics, 30,* 246-254.

Ebner, C.A. (1996). Cold therapy and its effects on procedural pain in children. *Issues in Comprehensive Pediatric Nursing, 19,* 197-208.

*Eccleston, C., Crombez, G., Scotford, A., Clinch, J., & Connell, H. (2004). Adolescent chronic pain: Patterns and predictors of emotional distress in adolescents with chronic pain and their parents. *Pain, 108,* 221-229.

Eccleston, C., Morley, S., Williams, A., Yorke, L., & Mastroyannopoulou, K. (2002). Systematic review of randomized controlled trials of psychological therapy for chronic pain in children and adolescents, with a subset meta-analysis of pain relief. *Pain, 99,* 157-165.

*Eccleston, C., Palermo T.M., Williams A.C., Lewandowski A., & Morley S. (2009). Psychological therapies for the management of chronic and recurrent pain in children and adolescents. *Cochrane Database of Systematic Reviews,* CD 003968.

Eccleston, C., Yorke, L., Morley, S., Williams, A., & Mastroyannopoulou, K. (2003). Psychological therapies for the management of chronic and recurrent pain in children and adolescents. *Cochrane Database of Systematic Reviews,* CD 003968.

EIDO Healthcare (2004). Consent – be informed: Module two. Treatment of people under the age of 16 years. Retrieved October 14, 2009, from http://www.eidohealthcare.com/consent/module2/section3.html

Eland, J.M. (1974). *Children's communication of pain.* Unpublished masters thesis, University of Iowa, Iowa City, Iowa.

*Epstein, G. (1989). *Healing visualizations: Creating health through imagery*. New York: Bantam Books.

Erickson, M., Rossi, E., & Rossi, S.I. (1976). *Hypnotic realities. The induction of clinical hypnosis and forms of indirect suggestion*. New York: Irvington.

Evans, S., Tsao, J., & Zeltzer, L. (2009). Iyengar yoga for pediatric chronic pain. *Pediatric Pain Letter, 11*, 12-16.

Fearon, I., Kisilevsky, B.S., Hains, S.M., Muir, D.W., & Tammer, J. (1997). Swaddling after heel lance: Age specific effects on behavioural recovery in preterm infants. *Journal of Developmental & Behavioral Pediatrics, 18*, 222-232.

Fearon, I., McGrath, P.J., & Achat, H. (1996). 'Booboos': The study of everyday pain among young children. *Pain, 68*, 55-63.

*Ferraro, N.F. (2003). Facial pain in children and adolescents. In: N. Schechter, C.B. Berde, & M. Yaster (Eds.), *Pain in infants, children and adolescents* (2nd ed., pp. 765-806). Philadelphia: Lippincott, Williams & Wilkins.

Fichtel, A., & Larsson, B. (2002). Psychosocial impact of headache and comorbidity with other pains among Swedish school adolescents. *Headache, 42*, 766-775.

Field, T., Hernandez-Reif, M., Seligman, S., Krusnegor, J., Sunshine, W., Rivas-Chacon, R., et al. (1997). Juvenile Rheumatoid Arthritis: Benefits from massage therapy. *Journal of Pediatric Psychology, 22*, 607-617.

*Finley, G.A., Franck, L.S., Grunau, R.E., & von Baeyer, C.L. (2005). Why children's pain matters. *Pain: Clinical Updates, XIII(4)*, 1-6.

Finley, G.A., McGrath, P.J., Forward, S.P., McNeill, G., & Fitzgerald, P. (1996). Parents' management of children's pain following 'minor' surgery. *Pain, 64*, 83-88.

Finley, G.A., & Schechter, N.L. (2003). Sedation. In: N. Schechter, C. B. Berde, & M. Yaster (Eds.), *Pain in infants, children and adolescents* (2nd ed., pp. 563-577). Philadelphia: Lippincott, Williams & Wilkins.

Finnerup, N.B., Otto, M., McQuay, H.J., Jensen, T.S., & Sindrup, S.H. (2005). Algorithm for neuropathic pain treatment: An evidence based proposal. *Pain, 118*, 289-305.

*Fitzgerald, M., & Howard, R.F. (2003). The neurobiologic basis of pediatric pain. In: N. Schechter, C.B. Berde, & M. Yaster (Eds.), *Pain in infants, children and adolescents* (2nd ed., pp. 19-42). Philadelphia: Lippincott, Williams & Wilkins.

Fitzgerald, M., & Walker, S.M. (2009). Infant pain management: A developmental neurobiological approach. *Nature Clinical Practice Neurology, 5*, 35-50.

French, S.D., Cameron, M., Walker, B.F., Reggars, J.W. & Esterman, A.J. (2006). Superficial heat or cold for low back pain. *Cochrane Database of Systematic Reviews*, CD 004750.

Friedrichsdorf, S.J. (2008). Pain management in pediatric palliative care. *ChiPPS Pediatric Palliative Care Newsletter, 13*, 5-21.

Friedrichsdorf, S.J. (2008). Unpublished data on Opioid Use.

Friedrichsdorf, S.J., & Kang, T.I. (2007). The management of pain in children with life limiting illnesses. *Pediatric Clinics of North America, 54*, 645-672.

Gall, O., Annequin, D., Benoit, G., Glabeke, E., Vrancea, F., & Murat, I. (2001). Adverse events of premixed nitrous oxide and oxygen for procedural sedation in children. *The Lancet, 358*, 1514-1515.

*Gertz, D.S., & Culbert, T. (2009). Pediatric self-regulation. In: W.B. Carey, A.C. Crocker, E.R. Elias, H.M. Feldman, & W.L. Coleman (Eds.), *Developmental-Behavioral Pediatrics* (4th ed., pp. 911-922). Philadelphia: W B Saunders.

Ghandour, R.M., Overpeck, M.D., Huang, Z.J., Kogan, M.D., & Scheidt, P.C. (2004). Headache, stomachache, backache, and morning fatigue among adolescent girls in the United States: Associations with behavioral, sociodemographic, and environmental factors. *Archives of Pediatrics & Adolescent Medicine, 158*, 797-803.

Gilman, D.K., Palermo, T.M., Kabbouche, M.A., Hershey, A.D., & Powers, S.W. (2007). Primary headache and sleep disturbances in adolescents. *Headache, 47*, 1189-1194.

Goldstein, A., & Hilgard, E. (1975). Lack of influence of the morphine antagonist naloxone on hypnotic analgesia. *Proceedings of the National Academy of Sciences, 72*, 2041-2043.

Gonzalez, J.C., Routh, D.K., Saab, P.G., Armstrong, F.D., Shifman, L., Guerra, E., et al. (1989). Effects of parent presence on children's reactions to injections: behavioral, physiological, and subjective aspects. *Journal of Pediatric Psychology, 14*, 449-462.

Goodman, J.E., & McGrath, P.J. (1991). The epidemiology of pain in children and adolescents: A review. *Pain, 46*, 247–264.

Gradin, M., Ericksson, M., Holmqvuist, G., Holstein, A., & Schollin, J. (2002). Pain reduction at venepuncture in newborns: Oral glucose compared with local anesthetic cream. *Pediatrics, 110*, 1053-1057.

*Grunau, R.V.E., & Craig, K.D. (1987). Pain expression in neonates: Facial action and cry. *Pain, 28*, 395-410.

Hadjistavropoulos, H.D., Craig, K.D., Grunau, R.V., & Johnston, C.C. (1994). Judging pain in newborns: Facial and cry determinants. *Journal of Pediatric Psychology, 19*, 485-491.

*Hämäläinen, M.L., Hoppu, K., Valkeila, E., & Santavuori, P. (1997). Ibuprofen or acetaminophen for the acute treatment of migraine in children: A double-blind, randomized, placebo-controlled, crossover study. *Neurology, 48*, 103-107.

*Hammill, J.M., Cook, T.M., & Rosecrance, J.C. (1996). Effectiveness of a physical therapy regimen in the treatment of tension-type headaches. *Headache, 36*, 149-153.

Hayden, G.F., & Schwartz, R.H. (1985). Characteristics of earache among chldren with otitis media. *American Journal of Diseases of Children, 139*, 721-723.

Headache Classification Subcommittee of the International Headache Society. (2004). The International Classification of Headache Disorders, 2nd edition. *Cephalalgia, 24 (Suppl. 1)*, 9-160.

Hermann, C., & Blanchard, E.B. (2002). Biofeedback in the treatment of headache and other childhood pain. *Applied Psychophysiology and Biofeedback, 27*, 143-162.

Hernandez-Reif, M., Field, T., Largie S, Hart, S., Redzepi, M., Nierenberg, B., et al. (2001). Children's distress during burn treatment is reduced by massage therapy. *Journal of Burn Care & Rehabilitation, 22,* 191-195.

Hester, N.O. (1975). *Poker Chip Tool instruction sheet.* Retrieved October 10, 2009, from http://painresearch.utah.edu/cancerpain/attachb7.html

Hester, N. (1979). The preoperational child's reaction to immunization. *Nursing Research, 28,* 250-255.

Hicks, C.L., von Baeyer, C.L., & McGrath, P.J. (2006). Online psychological treatment for pediatric recurrent pain: a randomized evaluation. *Journal of Pediatric Psychology, 31,* 724-36.

Hicks, C.L., von Baeyer, C.L., Spafford, P.A., van Korlaar, I., & Goodenough, B. (2001). The Faces Pain Scale – Revised: Toward a common metric in pediatric pain measurement. *Pain, 93,* 173-183.

Hilgard, E.R. (1977). *Divided consciousness: Multiple controls in human thought and action.* New York: Wiley.

Hilgard, E.R., & Hilgard, J.R. (1994). *Hypnosis in the relief of pain* (Rev. ed.). New York: Brunner/Mazel.

Hilgard, E.R., Morgan, A.H., & Macdonald, H. (1975). Pain and dissociation in the cold pressor test: A study of hypnotic analgesia with "hidden reports" through automatic key pressing and automatic talking. *Journal of Abnormal Psychology, 84,* 280-289.

Holden, E.W., Deichmann, M.M., & Levy, J.D. (1999). Empirically supported treatments in pediatric psychology: Recurrent pediatric headache. *Journal of Pediatric Psychology, 24,* 91-109.

Huertas-Ceballos, A., Macarthur, C., & Logan, S. (2002). Pharmacological interventions for recurrent abdominal pain (RAP) in childhood. *Cochrane Database Systematic Reviews,* CD 003017.

Hunt, A., Wisbeach, A., Seers, K., Goldman, A., Crichton, N., Perry, L. & Mastroyannopoulou, K. (2007). Development of the Paediatric Pain Profile: Role of video analysis and saliva cortisol in validating a tool to assess pain in children with severe neurological disability. *Journal of Pain and Symptom Management, 33,* 276-289.

International Association for the Study of Pain (1979). Pain terms: A list with definitions and notes on usage. *Pain, 6,* 249-252.

*International Association for the Study of Pain (2004). Pain Relief as a Human Right. *Pain Clinical Updates, September, XII, 5,* 1-4.

Ireland, M., & Olson, M. (2000). Massage and therapeutic touch in children: State of the science. *Alternate Therapies in Health and Medicine, 6,* 54-63.

Ireland, M. (1998). Therapeutic touch with HIV-infected children: A pilot study. *Journal of the Association of Nurses in AIDS Care, 9,* 68-77.

*Jaaniste, T., Hayes, B., & von Baeyer, C.L. (2007). Providing information to children about forthcoming medical procedures: A review and synthesis. *Clinical Psychology: Science and Practice, 14,* 124-143.

Janis, I.L. (1958). *Psychological stress.* New York: Wiley.

*Jay, S.M., Ozolins, M., Elliott, C.H., & Caldwell, S. (1983). Assessment of children's distress during painful medical procedures. *Health Psychology, 2,* 133-147.

Johnston, C.C., Stevens, B.J., Franck, L.S., Jack, A., Stremler, R., & Platt, R. (1999). Factors explaining lack of response to heel stick in preterm infants. *Obstetric, Gynecologic & Neonatal Nursing, 28,* 587-594.

*Johnston, C.C., Stevens, B., Pinelli, J., Gibbons, S., Filion, F., Jack, A., et al. (2003). Kangaroo care is effective in diminishing pain response to heelstick in preterm neonates. *Archives of Pediatrics & Adolescent Medicine, 157,* 1084-1088.

*Johnston, C.C., Stremler, R.L., Stevens, B.J., & Horton, L.J. (1997). Effectiveness of oral sucrose and simulated rocking on pain response in preterm neonates. *Pain, 72,* 193-199.

Jones, D.S., & Walker, L.S. (2006). Recurrent abdominal pain in children. In R.F. Schmidt & W.D. Willis (Eds.), *Encyclopedia of pain.* New York: Springer-Verlag.

Kain, Z.N., Mayes, L.C., & Caramico, L.A. (1996). Pre-operative preparation in children: A cross-sectional study. *Journal of Clinical Anesthesia, 8,* 508-514.

Kalso, E. (2007). How different is oxycodone from morphine? *Pain, 132,* 227-228.

Karl A., Mühlnickel, W., Kurth, R. & Flor, H. (2004). Neuroelectric source imaging of steady-state movement-related cortical potentials in human upper extremity amputees with and without phantom limb pain. *Pain, 110,*1, 90-102.

Karl, H.W., Rosenberger, J.L., Larach, M.G., & Ruffle, J.M. (1993). Transmucosal administration of midazolam for premedication of pediatric patients: Comparison of the nasal and sublingual routes. *Anesthesiology, 78,* 885-891.

Kaur, G., Gupta, P., & Kumar, A. (2003). A randomized trial of eutectic mixture of local anesthetics during lumbar puncture in newborns. *Archives of Pediatrics & Adolescent Medicine, 157,* 1065-1070.

*Kazak, A.E., Kassam-Adams, N., Schneider, S., Zelikovsky, N., Alderfer, M.A., & Rourke, M. (2006). An integrative model of pediatric medical traumatic stress. *Journal of Pediatric Psychology, 31,* 343-355.

Kemper, K.J., & Gardiner, P. (2003). Complementary and alternative medical therapies in pediatric pain treatment. In: N. Schechter, C.B. Berde, & M. Yaster (Eds.), *Pain in infants, children and adolescents* (2nd ed., pp. 449-461). Philadelphia: Lippincott, Williams & Wilkins.

*Kennedy, R.M., Luhmann, J., & Zempsky, W.T. (2008). Clinical implications of unmanaged needle-insertion pain and distress in children. *Pediatrics, 122 (Suppl. 3),* S130-S133.

*King, N.M.P., & Cross, A.W. (1989). Children as decision makers: Guidelines for pediatricians. *Journal of Pediatrics, 115,* 10-16.

*Klassen, J.A., Liang, Y., Tjosvold, L., Klassen, T.P., & Hartling, L. (2008). Music for pain and anxiety in children undergoing medical procedures: A systematic review of randomized controlled trials. *Ambulatory Pediatrics, 8,* 117-128.

Klenerman, L., Slade, P.D., Stanley, I.M., Pennie, B., Reilly, J.P., Atchison, L.E., et al. (1995). The prediction of chronicity in patients with an acute attach of low back pain in a general practice setting. *Spine, 20,* 478-484.

Kline, R.M., Kline, J.J., Di Palma, J., & Barbero, G.J. (2001). Enteric-coated, pH-dependent peppermint oil capsules for the treatment of irritable bowel syndrome in children. *Journal of Pediatrics, 138*, 125-128.

Koh, J.L., Harrison, D., Myers, R., Dembinski, R., Turner, H., & McGraw, T. (2004). A randomized, double-blind comparison study of EMLA® and ELA-Max for topical anesthesia in children undergoing intravenous insertion. *Paediatric Anaesthesia, 14*, 977-982.

*Koren, K. (2009). Codeine, Ultrarapid-Metabolism Genotype, and Postoperative Death. *NEJM, 8(361)*, 827-828.

Krane, E., & Mitchell, D. (2005). *Relieve your child's chronic pain: A doctor's program for easing headaches, abdominal pain, fibromyalgia, Juvenile Rheumatoid Arthritis, and more.* New York: Fireside.

Krener, P.K., & Mancina, R.A. (1994). Informed consent or informed coercion? Decision-making in pediatric psychopharmacology. *Journal of Child and Adolescent Psychopharmacology, 4*, 183-200.

*Kundu, A., & Berman, B. (2007). Acupuncture for pediatric pain and symptom management. *Pediatric Clinics of North America, 54*, 885-899.

Kundu, S., & Achar, S. (2002). Principles of office anesthesia: part II. Topical anesthesia. *American Family Physician, 66*, 99-102.

Kuscu, O.O., & Akyuz, S., (2007). Is it the injection device or the anxiety experienced that causes pain during dental local anesthesia? *International Journal of Paediatric Dentistry 18, 2*, 139-145. Published Online: 20 Nov 2007 Retrieved 21 October 2009. From: http://www3.interscience.wiley.com/journal/119410838/abstract

Kuther, T.L. (1997). Ethical issues in longitudinal research with at-risk children and adolescents. In B. Schrag (Ed.), *Research ethics: Fifteen cases commentaries* (pp. 89-100). Bloomington, IN: Association for Practical and Professional Ethics.

Kuttner, L. (Director/Producer) (1986). *No fears, no tears: Children with cancer coping with pain* [DVD]. (Available from BC Children's Hospital, http://bookstore.cw.bc.ca or 1-800-331-1533 x 3)

Kuttner, L. (1988). Favourite stories: A hypnotic pain reduction technique for children in acute pain. *American Journal of Clinical Hypnosis, 30*, 289-295.

Kuttner, L., (Director/Producer) (1990). *Children in Pain: An Overview* [documentary video]. Oakville, Canada: Magic Lantern Communications.

Kuttner, L. (1992). Managing children's pain: "Hello, I'm Dr. Seuss". *Contemporary Pediatrics*, Nov/Dec. 14-21.

Kuttner, L. (Producer) (1998). *No fears, no tears...13 years later* [DVD]. (Available from BC Children's Hospital, http://bookstore.cw.bc.ca or 1-800-331-1533 x 3)

Kuttner, L., Bowman, M., & Teasdale, M. (1988). Psychological treatment of distress, pain and anxiety for young children with cancer. *Journal of Developmental and Behavioral Pediatrics, 9*, 374-381.

Kuttner, L., Chambers, C.T., Hardial, J., Israel, D.M., Jacobsen, K., & Evans, K. (2006). A randomized trial of yoga for adolescents with irritable bowel syndrome. *Pain Research & Management, 11*, 217-223.

Kuttner, L., & Kohen, D.P. (1996). The language that helps pain go. In: L. Kuttner, *A child in pain: How to help, what to do* (pp. 93-98). Vancouver, Canada: Hartley & Marks.

Kuttner, L. (1996) *A child in pain: How to help, what to do*. Vancouver, Canada: Hartley & Marks. Available through www.crownhousepublishing.com

*Kuttner, L., & Solomon, R. (2003). Hypnotherapy and imagery for managing children's pain. In: N. Schechter, C.B. Berde, & M. Yaster (Eds.), *Pain in infants, children and adolescents* (2nd ed., pp. 317-328). Philadelphia: Lippincott, Williams & Wilkins.

Lander J., & Fowler-Kerry, S. (1993). TENS for children's procedural pain. *Pain, 52*, (2): 209-16.

*Lang, E.V., Hatsiopoulou, O., Koch, T., Berbaum, K., Lutgendorf, S., Kettenmann, E., et al. (2005). Can words hurt? Patient-provider interactions during invasive procedures. *Pain, 114*, 303-309.

*Larsson, B. S. (1991). Somatic complaints and their relationship to depressive symptoms in Swedish adolescents. *Journal of Child Psychology and Psychiatry, and Allied Disciplines, 32*, 821-832.

*Lavelle, E.D., Lavelle, W., & Smith, H.S. (2007). Myofascial trigger points. *Anesthesiology Clinics, 25*, 841-851.

Lawler, K. (1995). Entonox: Too useful to be limited to childbirth? *Professional Care of Mother and Child, 5*, 19-21.

Lee, A., Driscoll, D., Gloviczki, P., Clay, R., Shaughnessy, W., & Stans, A. (2005). Evaluation and Management of pain in patients with Klippel-Trenaunay Syndrome: A review. *Pediatrics, 45*, 3 March, 744-749.

Lee, B.H. (2000). Lobbying for pain control. *Journal of the American Veterinary Medical Association, 221*, 233-237.

*Lewis, D.W., Ashwal, S., Dahl, G., Dorbad, D., Hirtz, D., Prensky, A., et al. (2002). Practice parameter: Evaluation of children and adolescents with recurrent headaches: Report of the Quality Standards Subcommittee of the American Academy of Neurology and the Practice Committee of the Child Neurology Society. *Neurology, 59*, 490-498.

Li, B., & Balint, J.P. (2000). Cyclic vomiting syndrome: The evolution of understanding of a brain-gut disorder. *Advances in Pediatrics, 47*, 117-160.

*Lin, Y. (2003). Acupuncture. In: N. Schechter, C.B. Berde, & M. Yaster (Eds.), *Pain in infants, children and adolescents* (2nd ed., pp. 462-470). Philadelphia: Lippincott, Williams & Wilkins.

Linton, S.J., Buer, N., Vlaeyen, J.W.S., & Hellsing, A. (2000). Are fear-avoidance beliefs related to the inception of an episode of back pain? A prospective study. *Psychology and Health, 14*, 1051-1059.

*Liossi, C. (2002). The psychological management of paediatric procedure-related cancer pain. In: C. Liossi, *Procedure-related cancer pain in children* (pp. 141-172). Oxford, United Kingdom: Radcliffe Medical Press.

Liossi, C., White, P., & Hatira, P. (2009). A randomized clinical trial of a brief hypnosis intervention to control venepuncture-related pain of paediatric cancer patients. *Pain, 142*, 255-263.

Locker, D., Liddell, A., Dempster, L., & Shapiro, D. (1999). Age of onset of dental anxiety. Journal of Dental Research, 78,790. Retrieved on November 1, 2009 from http://jdr.sagepubp.com/cgi/content/abstract/78/3/790

Luhmann, J.D., Schootman, M., Luhmann, S.J., & Kennedy R.M. (2006). A Randomized Comparison of Nitrous Oxide Plus Hematoma Block

Versus Ketamine Plus Midazolam for Emergency Department Forearm Fracture Reduction in Children. *Pediatrics, 118(4):* e1078-1086.

*MacLaren, J., & Kain, Z. (2008). Research to practice in pediatric pain: What are we missing? *Pediatrics, 122,* 443-444.

Magaret, N.D., Clark, T.A., Warden, C.R., Magnusson, A.R., & Hedges, J.R. (2002). Patient satisfaction in the emergency department – a survey of pediatric patients and their parents. *Academic Emergency Medicine, 9,* 1379-1388.

Mahajan, L., Wyllie, R., Steffen, R., Kay, M., Kitaoka, G., Dettorre, J., et al. (1998). The effects of a psychological preparation program on anxiety in children and adolescents undergoing gastrointestinal endoscopy. *Journal of Pediatric Gastroenterology & Nutrition, 27,* 161-165.

Mallaty, H.M., Abudayyeh, S., O'Malley K.J., et al., (2005). Development of a multidimensional measure for recurrent abdominal pain in children: Population-based studies in three settings. *Pediatrics 115,* e210-215.

*Malnory, M., Johnson, T.S., & Kirby, R.S. (2003). Newborn behavioral and physiological responses to circumcision. *MCN: The American Journal of Maternal Child Nursing, 28,* 313-317.

*Malone, A. B. (1996). The effects of live music on the distress of pediatric patients receiving intravenous starts, venipuncures, injections and heel sticks. *Journal of Music Therapy, 33,* 19-33.

Margolis, J.O., Ginsberg, B., Dear G.D., Ross, A.K., Goral J.E., & Bailey A.G. (1998). Paediatric preoperative teaching: Effects at induction and postoperatively. *Paediatric Anaesthesia, 8,* 17-23.

Marquardt, K.A., Alsop, J.A., & Albertson, T.E. (2005). Tramadol exposures reported to statewide poison control system. *Annals of Pharmacotherapy, 39,* 1039-1044.

Martin-Lopez, A.M., Garrigos-Esparza, L.D., & Torre-Delgadillo, G., et al., (2005). Clinical comparison of pain perception rates between computerized local anesthesia and conventional syringe in pediatric patients Journal of Clinical Pediatric Dentistry pp. 239-243 Retrieved October 21 2009 from: http://pediatricdentistry.metapress.com/content/kt048u24x774/?sortorder=asc&p_o=10

Mawhorter, S., Daugherty, L., Ford, A., Hughes, R., Metzger, D., & Easley, K. (2004). Topical vapocoolant quickly and effectively reduces vaccine-associated pain: Results of a randomized single-blinded placebo-controlled study. *Journal of Travel Medicine, 11,* 267-272.

*McCaffery, M. (1972). *Nursing management of the patient in pain.* Philadelphia: Lippincott.

McCaffery, M., & Pasero, C. (1999). Practical non-drug approaches to pain. In: M. McCaffery, & C. Pasero (Eds.), *Pain: Clinical manual* (2nd Ed.). St. Louis, MO: Mosby.

*McCarthy, C.F., Shea, A.M., & Sullivan, P. (2003). Physical therapy management of pain in children. In: N. Schechter, C.B. Berde, & M. Yaster (Eds.), *Pain in infants, children and adolescents* (2nd ed., pp. 434-448). Philadelphia: Lippincott, Williams & Wilkins.

McCracken, L.M., & Eccleston, C. (2003). Coping or acceptance: What to do about chronic pain? *Pain, 105,* 197-204.

*McGrath, P.A., & Hillier, L.M. (Eds.) (2001). *The child with headache: Diagnosis and treatment. Progress in pain and research management: Vol. 19.* Seattle, WA: IASP Press.

McGrath, P.A., Seifert, C.E., Speechley, K.N., Booth, J.C., Stitt, L., & Gibson, M.C. (1996). A new analogue scale for assessing children's pain: An initial validation study. *Pain, 64,* 435-43.

McGrath, P.J., Cunningham, S.J., Lascelles, M.J., & Humphreys, P. (Eds.). (1990). *Help yourself: A program for treating migraine headaches. Patient manual and tape.* Ottawa, Canada: University of Ottawa Press.

McGrath, P.J., Cunningham, S.J., Lascelles, M.J., & Humphreys, P. (Eds.). (1990). *Help yourself: A program for treating migraine headaches. Professional handbook.* Ottawa, Canada: University of Ottawa Press.

*McGrath, P.J., Finley, G.A., & Ritchie, J. (1994). *Pain, pain go away.* Washington, DC: Association for the Care of Children's Health. (Also published in Dutch and Canadian editions.)

*McGrath, P.J., Finley G.A., & Turner C.J. (1992). *Making cancer less painful: A handbook for parents.* Halifax, Canada: IWK Children's Hospital. (Also available in American, Italian, French, Swedish, and Norwegian.)

*Melamed, B.G., Meyer, R., Gee C., & Soule, L. (1976). The influence of time and type of preparation on children's adjustment to hospital. *Journal of Pediatric Psychology. 1,* 31-37.

*Melamed, B.G., & Ridley-Johnson, R. (1988). Psychological preparation of families for hospitalization. *Journal of Developmental and Behavioral Pediatrics. 9,* 96-102.

Melamed, B.G., Yurcheson, R., Fleece, E.L., Hutcherson, S., & Hawes, R. (1978). Effects of film modeling on the reduction of anxiety related behaviours in individuals varying in levels of previous experience in the stress situation. *Journal of Consulting and Clinical Psychology, 46,* 1357-1367.

Melzack, R. (1973). *The puzzle of pain.* New York: Basic Books.

*Melzack, R. (1999). From the gate to the neuromatrix. *Pain, Suppl. 6,* S121-126.

Melzack, R. (2005). Evolution of the Neuromatrix Theory of Pain. The Prithvi Raj Lecture: Presented at the Third World Congress of World Institute of Pain, Barcelona 2004. *Pain Practice, 5,* 85-94.

*Melzack, R. Introduction: The challenge of pain in the twenty-first century In: R. Melzack & P.D. Wall. (2008). *The challenge of pain* (2nd ed.) (pp. ix-xvi). New York: Penguin Books.

Melzack, R., & Wall, P.D. (2008). *The challenge of pain* (2nd ed.) New York: Penguin Books.

*Miaskowski, C., Bair, M., Chou, R., D'Arcy, Y., Hartwick, C., Huffman, L., et al. (2008). *Principles of analgesic use in the treatment of acute pain and cancer pain* (6th ed.). Glenview, IL: American Pain Society.

*Milgrom, P., Weinstein, P. (1993). Dental fears in general practice: new guidelines for assessment and treatment. *International Dental Journal 43,* 288-293.

Moore, A., Collins, S., Carroll, D., & McQuay, H. (1997). Paracetamol with and without codeine in acute pain: A quantitative systematic review. *Pain, 70,* 193-201.

Moore, M., & Russ, S.W. (2006). Pretend play as a resource for children: Implications for pediatricians and health professionals. *Journal of Developmental and Behavioral Pediatrics, 27*, 237-248.

Morris, D.B. (1991). *The Culture of Pain.* Berkeley: University of California Press.

Moss, S.J. (2000). Children's dental health: The past is the present and the gateway to the future. *Alpha Omegan, 93*, 31-39.

Murdock, M. (1987). *Spinning inwards.* Boston: Shambhala.

Nagasako, E.M., Oaklander, A.L., & Dworkin, R.H. (2003). Congenital insensitivity to pain: An update. *Pain, 101*, 213-219.

*Neugebauer, V., Galhardo, V., Maione, S., & Mackey, S.C. (2009). Forebrain pain mechanisms. *Brain Research Reviews, 60*, 226-242.

*Oberlander, T.F., & Symons, F.J. (Eds.). (2006). *Pain in children and adults with developmental disabilities.* Baltimore: Paul H. Brookes.

*Olness, K., & Kohen, D.P. (1996). *Hypnosis and hypnotherapy with children* (3rd ed.). New York: Guilford.

Olness, K., & MacDonald, J. (1981). Self-hypnosis and biofeedback in the management of juvenile migraine. *Journal of Developmental and Behavioral Pediatrics, 2*, 168-170.

Olness, K.N., & MacDonald, J.T. (1987). Recurrent headaches in children: Diagnosis and treatment. *Pediatric Reviews, 8*, 307-311.

*Palermo, T. (2000). Impact of recurrent and chronic pain in child and daily functioning. A critical review of the literature. *Journal of Developmental and Behavioral Pediatrics, 21*, 58-69.

Penrose, S. (2006). *Positioning for comfort* [DVD]. (Available from Educational Resources Royal Children's Hospital, Melbourne Australia.)

*Perquin, C.W., Hazebroek-Kampschreur, A.A.J.M., Hunfeld, J.A.M., van Suijlekom-Smit, L.W.A., Passchier, J., & van der Wouden, J.C. (2000). Chronic pain among children and adolescents: Physician consultation and medication use. *Clinical Journal of Pain, 16*, 229-235.

Petersen, S., Brulin, C., & Bergström, E. (2006). Recurrent pain symptoms in young schoolchildren are often multiple. *Pain, 121*, 145-150.

Pickup, S., & Goddard, J. (1996). *Entonox protocol.* Retrieved September 27, 2009, from the Pediatric Pain Sourcebook: http://pediatric-pain.ca/files/pps24b.pdf

*Piira, T., Sugiura, T., Champion, G.D., Donnelly, N., & Cole, A.S. (2005). The role of parental presence in the context of children's medical procedures: A systematic review. *Child: Care Health and Development, 31*, 233-243.

Piira, T., Taplin, J.E., Goodenough, B., & von Baeyer, C.L. (2002). Cognitive-behavioural predictors of children's tolerance of laboratory-induced pain: Implications for clinical assessment and future directions. *Behaviour Research and Therapy, 40*, 571–584.

*Power, N., Liossi, C., & Franck, L. (2007). Helping parents to help their child with procedural and everyday pain: Practical, evidence-based advice. *Journal for Specialists in Pediatric Nursing, 12*, 203-209.

Powers, S.W. (1999). Empirically supported treatments in pediatric psychology: Procedure-related pain. *Journal of Pediatric Psychology, 24*, 131-145.

Rachman S. (1977). *Contributions to medical psychology, Vol. 1.* Oxford: Pergamon Press.

*Rainville, P., Hofbauer, R.K., Bushnell, M.C., Duncan, G.H., & Price, D.D. (2002). Hypnosis modulates activity in brain structures involved in the regulation of consciousness. *Journal of Cognitive Neuroscience, 14*, 887-901.

Rainville, P., Hofbauer, R.K., Paus, T., Duncan, G.H., Bushnell, M.C., & Price, D.D. (1999). Cerebral mechanisms of hypnotic induction and suggestion. *Journal of Cognitive Neuroscience, 11*, 110-125.

*Ramachandran V.S. & Hirstein, W. (1998). The perception of phantom limbs: The D.O. Hebb Lecture. *Brain, 9*, 121, 1603-1630.

Ramachandran, V. S. & S. Blakeslee (1998), *Phantoms in the brain: Probing the mysteries of the human mind.*, New York, William Morrow & Company.

Ran, D., & Peretz, B. (2003). Assessing the pain reaction of children receiving periodontal ligament anesthesia using a computerized device (Wand). *Journal of Clinical Pediatric Dentistry. 27(3)* 247-50. Retrieved 21 October, 2009 from: http://www.ncbi.nlm.nih.gov/pubmed/12739685

Rappaport, L.A., & Leichtner, A.M. (1993). Recurrent abdominal pain. In: N. Schechter, C.B. Berde, & M. Yaster (Eds.), *Pain in infants, children and adolescents* (1st ed., pp. 561-569).Baltimore: Williams & Wilkins.

Rasquin, A., Di Lorenzo, C., Forbes, D., Guiraldes, E., Hyams, J.S., Staiano, A., et al. (2006). Childhood functional gastrointestinal disorders: Child/adolescent. *Gastroenterology, 130*, 1527-1537.

Rey, M. (1995). *Curious George Goes to Hospital*, Boston: Houghton Mifflin.

*Rey, R. (1995). *The history of pain*. Cambridge, MA: Harvard University Press.

*Robinson, P., Wicksell, R.K., & Olsson, G.L. (2004). ACT with chronic pain patients. In: S.C. Hayes, & K.D. Srosahl (Eds.), *A practical guide to acceptance and commitment therapy* (pp. 315-345). New York: Springer.

Robb, S.L., & Carpenter, J.S. (2009). A Review of Music-based Intervention Reporting in Pediatrics. *Journal of Health Psychology, 14, 4*, 490-501.

Rose, J.B., Finkel, J.C., Arquedas-Mohs, A., Himelstein, B.P., Schreiner, M., & Medve, R.A. (2003). Oral tramadol for the treatment of pain of 7-30 days' duration in children. *Anesthesia and Analgesia, 96*, 78-81.

Ross, D.M. (1984). Thought-stopping: A coping strategy for impending feared events. *Issues in Comprehensive Pediatric Nursing, 7*, 83-89.

Ross, D.M., & Ross, S.A. (1984a). The importance of type of question, psychological climate and subject set in interviewing children about pain. *Pain, 19*, 71-79.

Ross, D.M., & Ross, S.A. (1984b). Childhood pain: The school-aged child's viewpoint. *Pain, 20*, 179-191.

*Ross, D.M., & Ross, S.A. (1988). *Childhood pain: Current issues, Research and Management.* Baltimore: Urban and Schwarzenberg.

Roth-Isigkeit, A., Thyen U., Stöven, H., Schwarzenberger, J., & Schmucker, P. (2005). Pain among children and adolescents: Restrictions in daily living and triggering factors. *Pediatrics, 115*, e152-e162.

Rugg, L., & von Baeyer, C.L. (2000). Preoperative information about pain management for children undergoing tonsillectomy: A randomized trial. *International Journal of Behavioral Medicine, 7 (Supp. 1)*, 131.

Savedra, M., Gibbons, P., Tesler, M., Ward, J., & Wegner, C. (1982). How do children describe pain? A tentative assessment. *Pain, 14*, 95-104.

Scharff, L., Leichtner, A.M., & Rappaport, L.A. (2003). Recurrent abdominal pain. In: N. Schechter, C.B. Berde, & M. Yaster (Eds.), Pain in infants, children and adolescents (2nd ed., pp. 719-730). Philadelphia: Lippincott, Williams & Wilkins.

*Scharff, L., & Simons, L.E. (2008). Functional Abdominal Pain. In: G.A. Walco, & K.R. Goldschneider (Eds.), *Pain in children: A practical guide for primary care* (pp. 163-171). Totowa, NJ: Humana Press.

*Schechter, N.L. (2008a). From the ouchless place to comfort central: The evolution of a concept. *Pediatrics, 122 (Suppl. 3)*, S153-S160.

*Schechter, N.L. (2008b). Pain management in the primary care office. General considerations and specific approaches. In: G.A. Walco, & K.R. Goldschneider (Eds.), *Pain in children: A practical guide for primary care* (pp. 55-64). Totowa, NJ: Humana Press.

*Schechter, N.L., Blankson, V., Pachter, L.M., Sullivan, C.M., & Costa, L. (1997). The ouchless place: No pain, children's gain. *Pediatrics, 99*, 890-894.

Schmidt, C.K., (1990). Preoperative preparation: Effects on immediate pre-operative behavior, post-operative behavior and recovery in children having same-day surgery. *Maternal-Child Nursing Journal, 19*, 321-330.

Schowalter, J.E. (1994). Fears and phobias. *Pediatric Reviews, 15*, 384-388.

Schwartzman, R.J., Grothusen, J., Kiefer, T.R., & Rohr, P. (2001). Neuropathic central pain: Epidemiology, etiology, and treatment options. *Archives of Neurology, 58*, 1547-1550.

Schweitzer A. (1931). *On the Edge of the Primeval Forest*. New York: Macmillan. p. 62.

*Selye, H. (1956).*The stress of life*. New York: McGraw-Hill.

Seshia, S.S., Phillips, D.F., & von Baeyer, C.L. (2008). Childhood chronic daily headache: A biopsychosocial perspective. *Developmental Medicine and Child Neurology, 50*, 541-545.

Sethna, N.F., & Lebel, A.A. (2008). Headaches. In: G.A. Walco, & K.R. Goldschneider (Eds.), *Pain in children: A practical guide for primary care* (pp. 173-184). Totowa, NJ: Humana Press.

*Shah, V., Taddio, A., Rieder, M.J., HELPinKIDS Team. (2009). Effectiveness and tolerability of pharmacologic and combined interventions for reducing injection pain during routine childhood immunizations: Systematic review and meta-analyses. *Clinical Therapeutics, 31 (Suppl 2)*, S104-S151.

Shirley, P.J., Thompson, N., Kenward, M., & Johnston, G. (1998). Parental anxiety before elective surgery in children: A British perspective. *Anaesthesia, 53*, 956-959.

*Siegel, D. (1999). *The developing mind: Toward a neurobiology of interpersonal experience*. New York: Guilford.

Siegel, L.J., & Peterson, L. (1980). Stress reduction in young dental patients through coping skills and sensory information. *Journal of Consulting and Clinical Psychology, 48*, 785-787.

Smith, J.L., & Madsen, J.R. (2003). Neurosurgical procedures for the treament of pediatric pain. In: N. Schechter, C.B. Berde, & M. Yaster (Eds.), *Pain in infants, children and adolescents* (2nd ed., pp. 329-338). Philadelphia: Lippincott, Williams & Wilkins.

Snow, C.E. (1999). Social perspectives on the emergence of language. In B. MacWhinney (Ed.), *Emergence of language* (pp. 257-276). Hillsdale, NJ: Lawrence Erlbaum.

Solomon, S. (2002). A review of mechanisms of response to pain therapy: Why voodoo works. *Headache, 42*, 656-662.

*Song, S., & Carr, D.B. (1999). Pain and memory. *Pain: Clinical Updates, VII(1)*, 1-7.

*Sparks, L., Setlik, J., & Luhman J. (2007). Parental Holding and Positioning to Decrease IV Distress in Young Children: A Randomized Controlled Trial. *Journal of Pediatric Nursing, 22, 6*, 440-447.

*Stanford, E.A., Chambers, C.T., & Craig, K.D. (2005). A normative analysis of the development of pain-related vocabulary in children. *Pain, 114*, 278-284.

Starfield, B., Hoekelman, R.A., McCormick, M., Benson, P., Mendenhall, R.C., Moynihan, C., et al. (1984). Who provides health care to children and adolescents in the United States? *Pediatrics, 74*, 991-997.

Stein, C. (1995). The control of pain in peripheral tissue by opioids. *New England Journal of Medicine, 25*, 1685-1690.

Stevens, B.J., Johnston, C.C., Franck, L., Petryshen, P., Jack, A., & Foster, G. (1999). The efficacy of developmentally sensitive interventions and sucrose for relieving procedural pain in very low birth weight neonates. *Nursing Research, 48*, 35-43.

*Stevens, B.J., Yamada, J., & Ohlsson, A. (1998). Sucrose for analgesia in newborn infants undergoing painful procedures. *Cochrane Database of Systematic Reviews*, CD 001069.

*Stinson, J., Yamada, J., Kavanagh, T., Gill, N., & Stevens, B. (2006). Systematic review of the psychometric properties and feasibility of self-report measures for use in clinical trials in children and adolescents. *Pain, 125*, 143-157.

Sugarman, L.I. (Director/Producer) (2006). *Hypnosis in pediatric practice: Imaginative medicine in action* [Book and DVD]. Carmarthen, United Kingdom: Crown House Publishing.

Swami Rama, Ballentine, R., & Hymes, A. (1979). *The science of breath: A practical guide*. Honesdale, PA: Himalayan Institute Press.

*Taddio, A., Katz, J., Ilersich, A.L., & Koren, G. (1997). Effect of neonatal circumcision on pain response during subsequent routine vaccination. *The Lancet, 349*, 599-603.

Thomson, L. (2005). *Harry the hypno-potamus: Metaphorical tales for the treatment of children*. Carmarthen, United Kingdom: Crown House Publishing.

Thomson, L. (2009). *Harry the hypno-potamus: More metaphorical tales for the treatment of children, volume 2*. Carmarthen, United Kingdom: Crown House Publishing.

Taddio, A., Ohlsson, A., Einarson, T.R., Stevens, B., & Koren, G. (1998). A systematic review of lidocaine-prilocaine cream (EMLA®) in the treatment of acute pain in neonates. *Pediatrics, 101*, E1.

Thorek, M. (1938). *Modern surgical technique: Vol. III*. Montreal, Canada: Lippincott.

*Tsao, J.C.I., Meldrum, M., & Zeltzer, L.K. (2006). Efficacy of complementary and alternative medicine approaches for pediatric pain: State of the science. In: G.A. Finley, P.J. McGrath, & C.T. Chambers (Eds.), *Bringing pain relief to children: Treatment approaches* (pp. 131-158). Totowa, NJ: Humana Press.

*Tsapakis, E.M., Soldani, F., Tondo, L., & Baldessarini, R.J. (2008). Efficacy of antidepressants in juvenile depression: Meta-analysis. *British Journal of Psychiatry, 193*, 10-17.

Turner, J.G., Clark, A.J., Gauthier, D.K., & Williams, M. (1998). The effect of therapeutic touch on pain and anxiety in burns patients. *Journal of Advanced Nursing, 28*, 10-20.

* Twycross, A., Dowden, S.J., & Bruce, E. (Eds.) (2009). *Managing pain in children: A clinical guide*. Oxford, United Kingdom: Wiley-Blackwell.

*Uman, L.S., Chambers, C.T., McGrath, P.J., & Kisely, S. (2008). A systematic review of randomized controlled trials examining psychological interventions for needle-related procedural pain and distress in children and adolescents: An abbreviated cochrane review. *Journal of Pediatric Psychology, 33*, 842-854.

University College, London/Institute of Child Health and Royal College of Nursing Institute (2003). *Paediatric Pain Profile*. Retrieved October 3, 2009 from http://www.pppprofile.org.uk/PDF/PPPp1-16.pdf

Upledger, J.E., & Vredevoogd, J.D. (1983). *Craniosacral therapy*. Seattle, WA: Eastland Press.

van Tilberg, M.A.L., Chitkara, D.K., Palsson, O.S., Turner, M., Blois-Martin, N., Ulshen, M. & Whitehead, W.E. (2009) Audio-Recorded Guided Imagery Treatment Reduces Functional Abdominal Pain in Children: A Pilot Study. *Journal of Pediatrics, 124*, 5, 890-897.

Versloot, J., Veerkamp, J.S.J., Hoogstraten, J. (2008). Pain behaviour and distress in children during sequential dental visits:comparing a computerized anaesthesia delivery system and a traditional syringe. *British Dental Journal 12*: 205, 1, 30-31.

*Vervoort, T., Goubert, L., Eccleston, C., Bijttebier, P., & Crombez, G. (2006). Catastrophic thinking about pain is independently associated with pain severity, disability, and somatic complaints in school children and children with chronic pain. *Journal of Pediatric Psychology, 31*, 674-683.

Vetter, T.R., & Heiner, E.J. (1994). Intravenous ketorolac as an adjuvant to pediatric patient-controlled analgesia with morphine. *Journal of Clinical Anesthesia, 6*, 110-113.

*Vlieger, A.M., Menko-Frankenhuis, C., & Wolfkamp, S.C.S. (2007). Hypnotherapy for children with functional abdominal pain or Irritable Bowel Syndrome: A randomized controlled trial. *Gastroenterology, 133*, 1430-1436.

*von Baeyer, C.L. (2007). Understanding and managing children's recurrent pain in primary care: A biopsychosocial perspective. *Paediatrics and Child Health, 12*, 121-125.

von Baeyer, C.L. (2009). Children's self-report of pain intensity: What we know, where we are headed. *Pain Research & Management, 14*, 39-45.

von Baeyer, C.L., Carlson, G., & Webb, L. (1997). Underprediction of pain in children undergoing ear-piercing. *Behaviour Research & Therapy, 35,* 399-404.

*von Baeyer, C.L., Marche, T., Rocha, E. & Salmon, K. (2004). Children's memory for pain: Overview and implications for practice. *Journal of Pain, 5,* 241-249.

von Baeyer, C.L., & Spagrud, L.J. (2003). Social development of pain in children. In: P. J. McGrath, & G.A. Finley (Eds.), *The context of pediatric pain: Biology, family, culture. Progress in Pain Research and Management: Vol. 26* (pp. 81-97). Seattle, WA: IASP Press.

*von Baeyer, C.L., & Spagrud, L.J. (2007). Systematic review of observational (behavioral) measures of pain for children and adolescents aged 3 to 18 years. *Pain 127,* 140-150.

von Baeyer, C.L., Spagrud, L.J., McCormick, J.C., Choo, E., Neville, K., & Connelly, M.A. (2009). Three new datasets supporting use of the Numerical Rating Scale (NRS-11) for children's self-reports of pain intensity. *Pain, 143,* 223-227.

von Baeyer, C.L., & Walker, L.S. (1999). Children with recurrent abdominal pain: Issues in the selection and description of research participation. *Journal of Developmental and Behavioral Pediatrics, 20,* 307-312.

Walco, G.A. (2008). Needle pain in children: Contextual factors. *Pediatrics, 122 (Suppl. 3),* S125-S129.

*Walco, G.A., Cassidy, R.C., & Schechter, N.L. (1994). Pain, hurt and harm. The ethical issue of pediatric pain control. *New England Journal of Medicine, 331,* 541-544.

Walco, G.A. (2008). Pain and the pediatric primary practitioner. In: G.A. Walco, & K.R. Goldschneider, (Eds.) (2008). *Pain in children. A practical guide for primary care.* (pp.3-8) Totowa, NJ: Humana Press.

*Walco, G.A., & Goldschneider, K.R., (Eds.) (2008). *Pain in children. A practical guide for primary care.* Totowa, NJ: Humana Press.

*Walker, L.S., Garber, J., Van Slyke, D.A., & Greene, J.W. (1995). Long-term health outcomes in patients with recurrent abdominal pain. *Journal of Pediatric Psychology, 20,* 233–245.

*Walker, L.S. (2004). Helping the child with recurrent abdominal pain return to school. *Pediatric Annals, 33,* 128-136.

Walsh, M.T. (1996). Hydrotherapy: The use of water as a therapeutic agent. In: S.L. Michlovitz (Eds.), *Thermal agents in rehabilitation: Vol 3* (pp. 139-168). Philadelphia: FA Davis.

*Weisman, S.J., Bernstein, B., & Schechter, N.L. (1998). Consequences of inadequate analgesia during painful procedures in children. *Archives of Pediatrics and Adolescent Medicine, 152,* 147-149.

Werneck, R.I., Lawrence H.P., Kulkarni G.V., & Locker, D. (2008). Early childhood caries and access to dental care among children of Portuguese immigrants in the city of Toronto. *Journal of the Canadian Dental Association. 74, 9;* 805.

Wester, W., & Sugarman, L.I. (Eds.). (2007). *Therapeutic hypnosis with children and adolescents.* Carmarthen, United Kingdom: Crown House Publishing.

Weydert, J.A., Ball, T.M., & Davis, M.F. (2003). Systematic review of treatments for recurrent abdominal pain. *Pediatrics, 111,* e1-e11.

Wicksell, R.K. (2007). Values-based exposure and acceptance in the treatment of pediatric chronic pain: From symptom reduction to valued living. *Pediatric Pain Letter, 9,* 17-24.

*Wicksell, R.K., Melin, L., Lekander, M., & Olsson, G.L. (2009). Evaluating the effectivness of exposure and acceptance strategies to improve functioning and quality of life in longstanding pediatric pain – a randomized controlled trial. *Pain, 141,* 248-257.

Wilkins, K.L., McGrath, P.J., Finley, G.A., & Katz, J. (1998). Phantom limb sensations and phantom limb pain in child and adolescent amputees. *Pain, 78,* 7-12.

Williams, D.G., Patel, A., & Howard, R.F. (2002). Pharmacogenetics of codeine metabolism of children in an urban environment and its implication for analgesic reliability. *British Journal of Anesthesia, 89,* 839-845.

Wood, C., & Bioy, A. (2008). Hypnosis and pain in children. *Journal of Pain and Symptom Management, 35,* 437-446.

*Yamada, J., Stinson, J., Lamba, J., Dickson, A., McGrath, P.J., & Stevens, B. (2008). A review of systematic reviews on pain interventions in hospitalized infants. *Pain Research & Management, 13,* 413-420.

Yaster, M., Kost-Byerly, S., & Maxwell, L.G. (2003). Opioid agonists and antagonists. In: N. Schechter, C.B. Berde, & M. Yaster (Eds.), *Pain in infants, children and adolescents* (2nd ed., pp. 181-224). Philadelphia: Lippincott, Williams & Wilkins.

*Zeltzer, L.K., Bush, J.P., Chen, P., & Riveral, A. (1997). A psychobiologic approach to pediatric pain: Part 1. History physiology and assessment strategies. *Current Problem in Pediatrics, 27,* 225-253.

*Zeltzer, L.K., Dolgin, M.J., LeBaron, S., & LeBaron, C. (1991). A randomized controlled study of behavioral intervention for chemotherapy distress in children with cancer. *Pediatrics, 88,* 34-42.

Zeltzer, L.K., & LeBaron, S. (1982). Hypnosis and nonhypnotic techniques for reduction of pain and anxiety during painful procedures in children and adolescents with cancer. *Journal of Pediatrics, 101,* 1032-1035.

*Zeltzer, L.K., & Schlank, C.B. (2005). *Conquering your child's chronic pain: A pediatrician's guide for reclaiming a normal childhood.* New York: Harper Collins.

* Zeltzer, L.K., Tsao, J.C.I., Stelling, C., Powers, M., Levy, S., & Waterhouse, M. (2002). A phase 1 study on the feasibility of an acupuncture/hypnotherapy intervention for chronic pediatric pain. *Journal of Pain and Symptom Management, 24,* 437-446.

Zhao, H., & Chen, A.N.C. (2009). Both happy and sad melodies modulate tonic human heat pain. *Journal of Pain, 10,* 953-960.

Zier, J.L., Drake, G., McCormick, P.C., Clinch, K.M., & Cornfield, D.N. (2007). Case-series of nurse-administered nitrous oxide for urinary catheterization in children. *Anesthesia & Analgesia, 104,* 876-879.

Index

Immunization, 283-85
Infants, 216-220
    Assessing pain, 115-16
    Pain relief, 216-20
Inflammatory bowel disease, 295
Information provided to children
    See also Explanation of Pain
    under Pain), 334-44
Injections, 30, 31, 57, 98, 99, 187,
    188, 196, 206, 243, 250, 282-85,
    306, 315, 316, 338, 369, 374
International Association for the
    Study of Pain, 3, 11, 36, 37, 359,
    370
Intravenous line (IV), 82, 188, 235,
    247, 372, 374
Irritable bowel syndrome, 16, 89,
    161, 210, 231, 294, 371, 372, 380

Journal,
    Kept by child, 108, 177
    Kept by parent, 108-110
Juvenile Idiopathic Arthritis, 30,
    175, 197

Kohen, D., vii, 54, 148, 151, 152,
158, 159, 372, 376

Lacerations, 73, 149, 273, 283, 285
Language, xiv, 20, 32, 76, 78, 88,
    99, 148, 150, 152, 338, 372,
    378At dentist's office, 307-08
Lawson, J., 35
Legal and Ethical Issues, 334-35
Leukemia, 58, 168, 188, 209, 214,
    325
Lidocaine, 247, 250, 253, 262, 286,
    314, 379
Limb pain, 16, 64, 65, 88, 190, 193,
    206, 371, 372
Limbic system, 11, 23, 51, 66, 268
Listening to children, 9, 25, 37, 75,
    148-49, 334
Lyrica, 257, 261

Massage, xv, 50, 108, 183, 186, 200,
    202, 210-13, 293, 364, 368-70
McCaffery, M., 41, 193, 199, 374
    Medication and imagery, 172
    Safety, 242
Medications *See also* generic
    names
    Administration of, 222, 224,
    230, 233, 242-49
    Antidepressant, 52, 224-25, 237,
    258, 380
    Combinations of, 241
    Dosages, 225-28, 254, 258, 261,
    324
    Methods of taking, 242
    Psychological dependence, 36
Melzack, R., 4, 39, 41, 49, 51, 66-70,
    326, 375
Meperidine, 241
Methadone, 238, 239-41, 246
Migraine *See* Headaches
Mindfulness, 180, 181
Mirror box therapy, 65
Modeling of coping, 311, 313, 338
Modulation, 44 *See also* Gating
    Pain
Morphine, xiv, 13, 35, 48, 53, 54,
    56, 57, 172, 207, 222, 224, 231,
    233, 234, 237-38, 239, 240, 241,
    246, 248, 354, 369, 371, 380
Morris, D., 10, 376
Murdock, M., 163, 376
Music, xiv, 20, 108, 147, 167, 173,
    174-75, 371, 374, 377
Myelination, 25, 26
Myofasdal pain, 61, 186, 373
Myths about pain, 22-37, 85, 88

Naproxen, 230
Needles, coping with *See also*
    Blood;
    Injections, 12, 23, 30-31, 203,
    285, 307